SYMBOLIC PATTERNS OF CHILDBIRTH

ANJA HÄNSCH

SYMBOLIC PATTERNS OF CHILDBIRTH

PETER LANG
Bern · Berlin · Bruxelles · Frankfurt am Main · New York · Oxford · Wien

Bibliographic information published by die Deutsche Nationalbibliothek
Die Deutsche Nationalbibliothek lists this publication in the Deutsche Nationalbibliografie; detailed bibliographic data is available on the Internet at ‹http://dnb.d-nb.de›.

British Library Cataloguing-in-Publication Data: A catalogue record for this book is available from The British Library, Great Britain.

Library of Congress Control Number: 2016930791

This book has been published with a financial subsidy from the European University Institute. This publication is based on the EUI Ph.D. thesis «Symbolic Orders of Childbirth» defended at the European University Institute Florence, Department of Political and Social Sciences, 2000.

ISBN 978-3-03910-432-1 pb. ISBN 978-3-0351-0886-6 eBook

This publication has been peer reviewed.

Hochfeldstrasse 32, CH-3012 Bern, Switzerland
info@peterlang.com, www.peterlang.com

To my mother

To Nina Salzano, mia seconda madre

To Adelheid Hausen, my first teacher and Socratic midwife

Per Maria Carmela De Bellis con grande affetto e gratitudine

To Paola Iop, midwife and "sage-femme"

To Yasmin: it's with you that everything started

Wonder at the mystery is itself a fruitful act of understanding, in that it affords a point of departure for further research. It may even be the very goal of all understanding, since it means penetrating through the greatest possible amount of knowledge to authentic nescience, instead of allowing Being to disappear by absolutising it away into a self-enclosed object of cognition.

Das Staunen vor dem Geheimnis ist selber ein fruchtbarer Erkenntnisakt als Ausgang weiteren Forschens, dann aber vielleicht gerade das Ziel all unseres Erkennens, nämlich durch maximales Wissen zum eigentlichen Nichtwissen vorzudringen, statt das Sein verschwinden zu lassen in der Verabsolutierung zum in sich geschlossenen Erkenntnisgegenstand.

Karl Jaspers

Contents

Preface 13

Acknowledgements 15

I. Childbirth as Symbolic Patterns, Experience and Performance 19

II. A Conception of Childbirth 25
- 1. The Paradigm: Hannah Arendt's Philosophy of Natality 25
  - 1.1 Primary, Political, Theoretical and Spiritual Natality: Four Ways of Accessing a Beginning 26
  - 1.2 Natalities and Immortalities 30
- 2. Childbirth, Sex and Gender 34
- 3. Conceiving of the Birthgiving Woman 37
  - 3.1 From an Existential Definition of Death to an Existential Definition of Giving Birth 37
  - 3.2 Thrownness and Anxiety 41
  - 3.3 Pain as Disclosing Mystery, Standstill and Non-Relationality 43

III. Symbolic Patterns of Childbirth 47

III.1 The Supremacy of the Male 49
- 1.1 Creation as Procreation in Egyptian Cosmogony 50
- 1.2 The Twelfth Tablet of the Gilgamesh-Epic 53
- 1.3 Hesiod: On *Anadyomène* 56
- 1.4 Genesis: Woman of Man Born 57
- 1.5 The Genealogies of the Old Testament and of Prophet Muhammad 58
- 1.6 Mimesis: The Births of Athena and Dionysos 60

1.7 The Semen and the Stars: Aristotle's *De Generatione Animalium* and the Gender of *Pneuma* 64
1.8 Foundations for a "Dubious" Supremacy of the Male: Tertullian and Augustine on the Transmission of Original Sin 73
1.9 On the Heels of Aristotle: The *Summa Theologica* of Thomas Aquinas 79
1.9.1 From "Semen and the Stars" to "Semen and Sin" 79
1.9.2 The Agency of the Holy Ghost 83
1.9.3 Reflections on Male Divinities Intervening into Women's Wombs 85
1.10 The Divine in the Prophet: The Procreation of Muhammad in the *Sirat* of Ibn Hisham 87
1.11 Twentieth Century Examples for the Supremacy of the Male 90

III.2 THEORETICAL, SPIRITUAL AND POLITICAL NATALITY VERSUS CHILDBIRTH 101
1. The Babylonian Myth of Creation and the Creation Myth of the Bible 103
2. Plato's *Symposium* and the Deathless Children of Philosophers 105
2.1 Discussion: Reflections on *Theorein*, Doing and Childbirth 113
3. Creation Abandoned for the Idea of Good: The Justinian Myth of Edem and Elohim 114
4. Abraham and the Binding of Isaac (in the Reading of Kierkegaard) 116
5. From Abraham to Agamemnon: *Iphigeneia at Aulis* of Euripides 120
6. Christian Devotion versus Childbirth 126
6.1 Luke 11: 27–28: The Word's Supremacy over the Womb 127
6.2 The Martyrdom of Perpetua and Felicitas 128

6.3 Birth as Deriving "from the Skins of Brutes": Gregory of Nyssa's Understanding of Marriage and Virginity as Different Conditions of the Soul ... 135
7. On Desks and Cradles: a Letter from Héloise to Abélard ... 138
8. *A World Where Saps Will Have Their Way*: The Opposition of Life and Art in Rainer Maria Rilke's *Requiem for a Friend* ... 141
9. *The Ejaculation is a Promise of Death*: Simone de Beauvoir's Conception of Individuality as Being Opposed to the Human Species ... 147
10. Against the Tyranny of the Fates: Joseph Fletcher's Plea for Rational Procreation as Opposed to Childbirth by Raw Nature ... 155
11. From the Supremacy of *Theorein* over Childbirth to Childbirth in Theory? ... 160
11.1 Günter Grass: Headbirths ... 160
11.2 Edward Albee: Who's Afraid of Virginia Woolf? ... 164

III.3 The Supremacy of the Female ... 169
1. The First Birthgiving: Goddesses as Mothers of the Gods and as the Origin of the World ... 170
2. The Creation of the World by Sophia the "Fallen Wisdom": A Gnostic Myth ... 172
3. Isis and Mary: The Supremacy of the Female and Harmony between Spiritual Birth and Childbirth ... 184
4. Mikhail Epstein: The "Russian-Doll-Principle" ... 184

III.4 Harmony between Spiritual/ Theoretical Natality and Childbirth ... 189
1. Childbirth, Wisdom and Mystery Religion: The Reign of Queen Isis ... 190
1.1 Plutarch's Isis as Idea: The Goddess of Philosophers and the Goddess of Childbirth ... 199

1.2 Lucius Apuleius: Isis as "Blessed Queen of Heaven," "Reliever of the Birth Pangs of Women," and "Sovereign of All Things Spiritual" 204
2. From Isis to Mary 207
3. The Incarnation of the Sacred Through a Woman: Mary as "Spiritual Vessel" 210
3.1 Mary-Theotokos 214
3.2 Mary's Disembodiment and the Painless Virgin Birth 218
3.3 Immaculate Conception 223
3.4 Mediatrix – Corredemptrix – Regina Caeli 227
3.5 Mary-Sophia 240
3.6 Two Examples for Different Conceptions of Mary: Augustine and Friedrich Schleiermacher 241
4. Paula Modersohn-Becker: The Pregnant Mystic 246
4.1 Self-Portrait on the Sixth Wedding Anniversary 247
4.2 Self-Portrait, Two Flowers in the Raised Hand 250
4.3 Self- Portrait with Camellia Branch 250
5. Mikhail Epstein: Towards an Ethics of Childbirth 253

IV. Final Remarks: A Baby Has Been Born – So What? 261

Bibliography 267

In Place of a Preface: Kittens and Kids

One early June morning, I walked down the stairs of my house to learn that one of our cat's five-week-old kittens had died. My three-year-old daughter Yasmin came down and for some time looked silently at the dead kitten on the carpet. *E adesso che facciamo*? ("And what shall we do now?"), she asked me. It was at that moment that I understood the powerful impact of culture on our attitudes and emotions with regard to so-called "natural" phenomena as birth and death. My child wanted to know how to deal with death and only started to cry when I told her that it was a sad thing to lose a kitten, or even people through death, although it belonged to life.

Basically, this work tries to explore some answers to the question of how meaning is given not to death but to childbirth. That is to say, in relation to childbirth it deals with my daughter's question: *E adesso che facciamo*?

Acknowledgements 1

It has been a long way from the defense of my PhD thesis *Symbolic Orders of Childbirth* to the publication of *Symbolic Patterns of Childbirth*. I wish to thank all my dear friends who lovingly helped me to cling to my project. Almut Höfert, Isabella Matauschek, Ivesa Lübben, Karin Schmidt, Letizia Paoli, Mariapaola Ferretti, Matthias Rau, and my sister Edda Lorna were my faithful companions in these years of transition. Karin gave it the final push, "Just let it go now!" and Ivesa kindly offered me her home in Bremen as a refuge to finish the footnotes. Above all it was Gianfranco Poggi who with fatherly admonition insistently kept on saying, "Anja, you are hiding this work for too long," or "accidenti Anja, la tesi!"

Sonja Ammann and Berenike Herrmanns were themselves struggling with turning their PhD thesis into a book and the self-help group character of our conversations often was comforting. Sonja's theological expertise also helped me to revise parts of the book.

I wish to warmly thank Mikhail Epstein for taking the effort to look at the English translations of the quotes from his essay *Fatherhood*. I still feel guilty about fragmenting his wonderful book into symbolic patterns of childbirth. Beth Margulis helped to check the accuracy of the translations. I thank the Peter Lang publisher and Benjamin Fröhlich for taking kind care of this book project and for the endless patience they had with my sheer endless delays.

Yasmin, your blissful birth was the catalyst of this book. In the time span between my thesis defense and the publication you have become a young woman being able to encourage me with the final part of the book, "Mammilein, it will go o.k." Maurits, thank you for embarking on the adventure to have a child with me and for standing lovingly by my side in these years when I was writing about symbolic patterns of childbirth and other things. Isadora, if Plato is right with his conviction that children choose their parents, I infinitely thank you for choosing us.

This book would not be what it is now without the thorough copy-editing by Karen Weeks. Karen, I don't know what to write to thank you for all the effort you put into this: Apparently, we've made it!

Amsterdam, June 28, 2015

Acknowledgements 2

An African proverb says, "It needs a village to make a baby." This could be transposed easily to my thesis about symbolic patterns of childbirth, which was written with the help of two villages, an international academic village and my countryside village Pian di Mugnone. I am very grateful to many people who have given me support in various ways during these last years. Above all, my deepest gratitude goes to my "maestro" Arpad Szakolczai who always encouraged me right from the beginning and had amazing patience with my stubbornness. Barbara MacLennan equally always accompanied me with her warm support. Paola Iop, being the wonderful midwife she is, contributed to the experiental basis of this thesis.

For many important conversations I would like to thank Hanne Petersen, Christa Tobler, Letizia Paoli, Adelheid Hausen (my philosophy teacher, who kindly introduced me to the world of the mind when I was a teenager), Armando Salvatore (whom I also thank for having agreed to a home-birth and for his friendship) and Ivesa Lübben. I would like to especially thank my (former) housemates, Bastiaan van Apeldoorn (we still could not answer the question of whether the lastest developments of capitalism are linked to changing symbolic patterns of childbirth), Amy Verdun (who showed me that one could "do it" as a single mum "with a little help from my friends"), Paul Schure, Roger Hammersland (who cheered up the place so much with his smile and his trumpet), my "big brother" Matthias Rau, Cinzia Ardemagni and Indro Castronuovo. Many "thank yous" also go to Liliana Gilli and Niccolò Bellanca, Isabella Matauschek (for her enthusiasm and her wonderful, breathtaking projects: we may still find "that" book), Emilio Santoro (among many other things, for having crawled under the table with Yasmin when she was six months old), Roberta Sassatelli (for her lucid comments), Luca Guzzetti, Monica Fontanarosa, Karin Westerbeek, Harald Wydra and Anna Pettini (for the great time we had while sharing a working-space), Sari Hanafi, Agnes Horvath, Maarten van den Berg (who ultimately convinced me that the world is a spiral and not a circle), Hans van der Veen (for his fruitful "Apollonian antagonisms"), Sheikh Mohammed Azab, Mirko Sladek, Audrey Verdun, Hage Verdun, Celia Lessa, Ruth and Bernard Gbikpi, Marjet Gunning,

Catarina Botti, Paola Monzini, Dorte Verner, Almut Höfert, Linda and Asef Bayat, Eugene MacNamee and Ioannis Papadopoulos (for encouraging me while I was writing a conception of birthgiving), my sister Edda (who has expressed much better in her art what I tried to express through words), my sister Petra, James Kaye, Nicki Owtram (who did a wonderful job with the English corrections), Wolf and Patricia Sauter, Rita Ricci, Isabella und Frank Heinlein, Jean Pierre Cassarino, Yael Poggi and Mariano Aguas (who gave "Florencio" to Yasmin and me what made life a lot easier), Kerstin Ullrich, Monica Miscari, Anette and Per Mouritsen, Willy Viehöver, Tessa Storey, Olivia Weis, Inda Bevis, Ruth Meyer-Belardini, Jens Steffek, Imco Brouwer, Valeria Russo, Vladimir and Irene Gradev, Anne and Carlo Spagnolo, Gianna and Ferruccio Vannucci, Bruno Cirillo, Pietr Omtzigt, Maria-José de la Torre, Serena Giusti, Simona Mezzera (and the wonderful world of "Il marsupio"), Antonio Zanardi-Landi (after all I wrote that chapter on the birth of Dionysos), Asher Salah, Emidio Diodato, Salvatore Cingari, Giulia Beltrametti, Alessandro Guetta, Per Bauth, Mohammed Arkoun (for comments only he could make), Maria Carmela de Bellis (who with her six daughters and nine grandchildren has always been enthusiastic about anything related to childbirth – even a thesis), Karin Schmidt (for her long lasting friendship and for sharing the birth of Janek with me – after all it's not all theory). There are many people who have been there with a smile, or a good word during these years. These are Françoise Thauvin, Helen Lubertacci, Angela Schenk, Bo Strath, Sylvie Pascucci, Ken Hulley, Beatrijs Hartog, Maren Ipsen (with whom I read quite a pile of "baci-sayings" over time), Marcello Scocci (also the chapter on Ireneus was included), Gisela Deus, Ursula Brose, Eva Breivik, Carlotta Alpigiani, Alessandro Coccoli, Antonio Correto, Luca di Rocco, Gianluca Truppa, Dario Centrone, Clare Tame, Robert Danziger, Bonnie Bonis, Cinzia Ceccatelli, Maria Giolli, Teresa Simoni, Marcella Sassoli, Patrizia Masi and Loriano Baccetti (who always kindly agreed to give it yet another try to cure the reumatisms of my Fiat 128, that is "Florencio"). I would like to thank Elisabetta Raspolli, Teresa, Rolando and Irene Romolini and Andrea Prosperi for long talks on the Pian di Mugnone playground. I would also like to thank the always changing "Via Buffalmacco-Community": Axelle Reiter (for her refreshing anarchism), Schirin Amir-Moazami, Carlo Gualini, Luisa Chiodi, Kira Malamud, Pablo Jauregui, Angelo Cattaneo, Barbara Cimolato and Isabel Sanza. In the end there were some people who supported me when I was running out of breath: Christiane Renger (who has simply always been there), Liz Webb, Peter Wagner, Patrick Masterson, Davide Sparti, Gianfranco Poggi, Sarah Matthews-Griego, David Purdey (who found the crucial word of the conclusions: "perhaps"), Barbara MacLennan and Cristina and Giulio Rossi (without their babysitting there would have been no conclusions!) and Yasmin (who had an amazing patience with her stressed mum).

Burke once wrote that life is a contract between the living and the dead. In this spirit I think of my indebtedness to Knut Mittendorfer (in fact you were right: Isis is tied to *agape*) and Susan Strange, who once asked me whether there was a difference between the birth of children and the birth of animals. In terms of human symbolic construction I would answer "yes" now; in other terms I would say "no": a newborn cat, dog, or elephant testifies as much to the miracle, mystery and gift of life as a newborn baby.

Pian di Mugnone, April 5, 2000

I. Childbirth as Symbolic Patterns, Experience and Performance

Childbirth can acquire manifold meanings in myths, philosophy, literature and religion some of which here will be grouped together and explored as symbolic patterns. By "childbirth" I mean the coming into existence of a child, which is treated differently by the four different symbolic patterns to be analyzed. These symbolic patterns are rather heterogenous, sometimes attributing the coming into existence of a child primarily to male "procreation" ("The Supremacy of the Male"), sometimes more relating childbirth to conception, pregnancy and birthgiving on part of the woman ("The Supremacy of the Female"). Furthermore, the symbolic pattern labeled "Theoretical, Spiritual and Political Natality versus Childbirth" leaves aside the question of which body – male or female – gives the more important contribution to the coming into existence of a child. Here, rather, childbirth is seen as lower in value as the realms of ideas, religion, the political or the arts. In contrast to this the symbolic pattern "Harmony between Spiritual/Theoretical Natality and Childbirth" shows that some kind of a "spiritual" birth and childbirth can also go hand in hand with each other. The symbolic patterns of childbirth to be analyzed may reflect, stabilize, subvert, change and constitute power relations (e.g. with regard to gender).

This work situates itself in the framework of a specific type of sociological study termed "reflexive sociology"[1] which attempts to uncover "the taken for granted structure of the everyday life-world and of the practice of human communication and understanding."[2] In its understanding of childbirth as a symbolic pattern, this study seeks to analyze some codes developed in relation to childbirth which have persisted throughout time and space. In this sense, "Symbolic Patterns of Childbirth" is similar to a

---

1 Arpád Szakolczai, *Max Weber and Michel Foucault: Parallel Life-Works*, (London: Routledge, 1998), 17.

2 Ibid. 16.

study by Mircea Eliades on initiation rites in different times and places.[3] Eliades's discussion of the problems inherent in such an approach also holds for this work: "Although it is risky to compare […] documents belonging to such different ages and cultures, I have taken the risk because all these […] facts fit into a pattern."[4]

"Symbolic Patterns of Childbirth" has a historical dimension in so far as the four different ways of constructing childbirth can be traced in texts of different times, places and cultures. Although many of these texts enjoyed an important status in a particular time and place, I do not want to claim that they represent a dominant symbolic construction of childbirth in a given society, but rather, that they all testify to some kind of a continuing pattern in relation to the intellectual discourse on childbirth. That is to say, I leave aside the question as to whether certain ways of giving meaning to childbirth were or are socially dominant, or deviant. This huge task has to be left to historians.

As the interest of this work lies with identifying symbolic patterns of childbirth in a broad comparative perspective there equally is no room for situating the texts chosen for analysis in the frame of the history of the body. However, it has to be pointed out that the texts unfold on a variety of historical backgrounds determining what is male, what is female and how gender related to childbirth is experienced. Barbara Duden's major contributions to the history of childbirth[5] have shown that there is no such a thing as a timeless relationship between a "natural" female body and the experience of such a body. Even the notion of "having a body" is a relatively recent one going back to the 18th century.[6] The same reflections can of course be applied to the history of the "male" body and "procreation". An illustrative example for the historicity of the body in relation to childbirth is the varying understanding of the uterus according to different times and places. Thus, for example, while in modern medecine the uterus is conceived of as having one location only, in Ancient Egypt a woman could be considered to have fallen ill as a result of her uterus having moved to a

3 See Mircea Eliade, *Rites and Symbols of Initiation: The Mysteries of Birth and Rebirth*, trans. Willard R. Trask (1958; reprint, New York: Harper & Row, 1975).

4 See ibid., 58.

5 See e.g. Barbara Duden, *A Doctor's Patients in Eighteenth-Century Germany*, trans. Thomas Dunlap (Cambridge, MA: Harvard University Press, 1991).

6 See ibid., 2.

"wrong spot."[7] In this case the treatment of the "wandering womb"[8] could consist of luring the uterus into descending again by taking measures such as applying fragrant substances to the lower parts of the woman's body.

Though the historical dimension of the body in relation to childbirth will be occasionally touched upon,[9] in general it stays in the background. What is foregrounded here, however, are some symbolic patterns of childbirth, which in manifold variations, can be traced through time and space. As the specific interest of this book lies with this broad comparative perspective, the single texts here grouped together and analyzed as symbolic patterns of childbirth can thus neither be considered in historical nor in philological depth. Because the sources cover a broad range of languages it was necessary to work with translations. And with this, the risk of shortcomings and altered meaning is taken. However, on the whole, the chosen sources will still testify to different symbolic patterns of childbirth even if occasionally a misinterpretation based on translation may have crept in.

The continuities of the symbolic patterns of childbirth presented here can hardly be explained by specific socio-historical configurations. One might think of psychology as a tool to understand them. For instance, in his study of the social construction of masculinity,[10] David D. Gilmore used psychology to explain the recurrent patterns he encountered from Homer to modern and non-modern societies. In the case of the symbolic constructions of childbirth it will instead be necessary to turn to anthropology and to philosophy to explain the continuities found. Victor Turner's ideas on experience and performance are of crucial importance here as they become intertwined with the question of how cultural codes are perpetuated.[11]

Victor Turner elaborates on experience by drawing upon Dilthey's conception of *Erlebnis*. According to Turner experience should not be regarded as a "self-enclosed unity."[12] Rather, it is deeply relational in two

7 See for this and the following Ilza Veith, *Hysteria: The History of a Disease* (Northvale, NJ: Aronson, 1993), 3–5.

8 Ibid., 2.

9 See e.g. the chapters on Aristotle, Thomas Aquinas and Tertullian in section III.1. "The Supremacy of the Male."

10 See David D. Gilmore, *Manhood in the Making. Cultural Concepts of Masculinity* (New Haven and London: Yale University Press, 1990).

11 See Victor Turner and Edith Turner, *On the Edge of the Bush: Anthropology as Experience* (Tucson, Arizona: The University of Arizona Press, 1985), 205–226.

12 Ibid., 211.

senses: First of all with regard to the life and past of an individual because "the category of *meaning* arises in *memory*,"[13] secondly, with regard to the social environment of the individual. It is to the latter that Turner connects the notion of "performance" which is crucial for the understanding of the perpetuation of cultural codes (in our case regarding childbirth).

Cultural codes are the products of condensed experiences. The moment that they are performed, they render it possible for individuals to access the experiences of people who lived before them. Turner writes:

> For our species meaning is entwined with inter-subjectivity, how we know, feel, and desire one another. Our means of communication (language, cultural codes) are saturated, whether we know this or not, with the experiences of our progenitors and forerunners. But these codes can never be experienced unless they are periodically, or at least occasionally, *performed*. We have to try to re-experience in performance, whether as ritual, festival, theatre, or other active modalities of religion, law, politics, or art, as best we can, the socially bequeathed sparks of lives now biologically extinguished.[14]

The perpetuation of cultural codes may have an important influence on the individual's experiental perception:

> Culture is [...] to be regarded as the crystallized secretion of once living human experience [...] which is still capable of liquefaction back into similar if not identical lived-through experience under favorable conditions, like the reputed miracle of Saint Januarius' dried blood.[15]

Turner's theory about the transmission of cultural codes may contribute to solving some of the problems related to the history of ideas. In his study of gnostic worldview,[16] Ioan P. Couliano sees ideas as forming "systems that can be envisaged as 'ideal' objects." However, "these ideal objects cross the surface of history called time [...] in an apparently unpredictable sequence of temporal events ... At this stage of research we are unable to

---

13 Ibid., 214.

14 Ibid., 207.

15 Ibid., 224. In Napels three times a year feasts are celebrated during which a miracle may occur: the coagulated blood of the Christian martyr Saint Januarius which is preserved in two ampoules may liquefy then.

16 See Ioan Peter Couliano, *The Tree of Gnosis: Gnostic Mythology from Early Christianity to Modern Nihilism*, trans. by H.S. Wiesner (San Francisco: Harper San Francisco, 1992).

go much beyond the mere recognition of systems in their logical dimension."[17]

Couliano's statement about the unpredictability of the (re)manifestation of ideas would mean in Turner's language, to talk about the unpredictability of the (re)activation of a cultural code. As has been shown above, for Turner, culture as condensed experience may always lead to an experience of a feeling or a situation located in history. This would account for the possibility of ideas moving from the background of the stage of history to the foreground and vice versa. However, the question remains why certain ideas are (re)activated in certain times and others not. As has already been pointed out this question can only be answered by historians.

Turner's ideas on experience and performance are helpful to explain the perpetuation of cultural codes (ideas included), and even experiences in relation to childbirth. However, for a better understanding of the internal logic of the four symbolic patterns of childbirth chosen for analysis, a general conception of childbirth from a philosophical point of view seems to be necessary. In the following, the attempt will be made to conceive of birth on the basis of the philosophy of Hannah Arendt and Martin Heidegger. Hannah Arendt's philosophy of natality provides the frame for conceptualizing birth as one way of accessing both a beginning and a "mortal immortality." Furthermore, Heidegger's understanding of the situation of the dying person will be explored as a paradigm for conceiving of the birthgiving woman.

---

17 Ibid., 3, 7.

II. A Conception of Childbirth

1. The Paradigm: Hannah Arendt's Philosophy of Natality

Hannah Arendt is most probably the only philosopher who has introduced birthgiving as a central category of philosophical and political thought.[18] Although scattered in her work, her conception of natality is omnipresent in her thinking. This is why Hannah Arendt's work is an ideal point of departure for any investigation into birthgiving/procreation. An excellent study by Patricia Bowen-Moore on Hannah Arendt's philosophy of natality[19] has allowed Arendt's reflections on the topic to be systematized and thus to be evidenced as an underlying principle of her thought. According to Bowen-Moore, by natality Arendt describes three human experiences: "Factual natality – birth into the world; political natality – birth into the realm of action; and theoretical natality – birth into the timelessness of thought."[20]

Hannah Arendt's importance to the symbolic patterns of childbirth lies in her having placed primary natality among political and theoretical natality, all three being different ways of accessing a beginning. Her reflections can be connected to all four symbolic patterns of childbirth to be presented here but are particularly helpful for understanding "Theoretical, Spiritual and Political Natality versus Childbirth."

---

18 See Parekh Bhikhu, *Hannah Arendt and the Search for a New Political Philosophy* (London: Macmillan, 1981), xi.

19 Patricia Bowen-Moore, *Hannah Arendt's Philosophy of Natality* (London: MacMillan, 1989). I am very grateful to Per Mouritsen for pointing Bowen-Moore's work out to me.

20 Ibid., 1.

1.1 Primary, Political, Theoretical and Spiritual Natality: Four Ways of Accessing a Beginning

1.1.1 Primary and Political Natality

Hannah Arendt translates childbirth into an existential and conceptual category.[21] She dared to break with a long held tradition in Western philosophical thought also represented by her teacher Heidegger, whose philosophy of Being as meaning existentially "Being-towards-death" can be considered as the culminating point of a tradition defining human existence through mortality. Hannah Arendt starts from the exact opposite perspective on life by defining human experience in terms of natality. She states, "natality, not mortality, may be the central category of political as distinguished from metaphysical thought."[22] Arendt argues for this in the following way:

> The life span of man running toward death would inevitably carry everything human to ruin and destruction if it were not for the faculty of interrupting it and beginning something new, a faculty which is inherent in action like an ever-present reminder that men, though they must die, are not born in order to die but in order to begin.[23]

Hannah Arendt links the human faculty of beginning ontologically back to childbirth, which thus becomes a conceptual category. Childbirth means the beginning par excellence, or one could say: "The birth of the human being and the appearance of the principle of beginning are contemporary with each other."[24] Such a conception of natality immediately takes on a political dimension, by way of equating the human faculty for beginning with the human faculty to act: "Action as beginning corresponds to the fact of birth, [...] it is the actualisation of the human condition of natality."[25] (Public) action is to be conceived of as a second birth:

---

21 See for the following ibid., 21–26.

22 Hannah Arendt, *The Human Condition* (Chicago and London: The University of Chicago Press, (1958), 9th Impression 1974), 9. At a later stage the question of whether the category of natality is not only applicable to the realm of the political, but also has importance for the metaphysical will be dealt with in the context of natality in its relationship to spirituality.

23 Ibid., 246.

24 Bowen-Moore, *Hannah Arendt's Philosophy of Natality*, 25.

25 Arendt, *The Human Condition*, 178.

> With word and deed we insert ourselves into the human world, and this insertion is like a second birth, in which we confirm and take upon ourselves the naked fact of our original physical appearance, [...] its [this insertion's] impulse springs from the beginning which came into the world when we were born and to which we respond by beginning something new on our own initiative. To act, in its most general sense, means to take an initiative, to begin[26]

Hannah Arendt insists that political action is possible only because men and women are in possession of a principle of beginning by virtue of their births.

In the context of her understanding of natality as the principle of beginning, Arendt emphasizes her affiliation to the political philosophy of Augustine. *"[Initium] ergo ut esset, creatus est homo, ante quem nullus fuit"* ("that there be a beginning, man was created before whom there was nobody"),[27] Augustine wrote in *De Civitate Dei*, where he uses two words for beginning: *initium* and *principium*. *Principium* is used in the semantic context of the creation of the world and in Arendt's interpretation carries with it a much less radical meaning than *initium*, as it "does not mean that nothing was made before (for the angels were)."[28] With the creation of men referred to by *initium*, Augustine emphasizes instead that nobody [nothing] was made before him. Hannah Arendt is thus with Augustine in writing that "with the creation of men [and not with the creation of the world], the principle of beginning came into the world itself."[29]

How does man's principle for beginning manifest itself? Hannah Arendt's answer is: "The new always happens against the overwhelming odds of statistical laws and their probability, which for all practical everyday purposes amounts to certainty; the new therefore always appears in the guise of a miracle."[30]

To Hannah Arendt the miraculous in political philosophy and her conception of natality are intertwined closely with one another. She goes on to write:

> The fact that man is capable of action means that the unexpected can be expected from him, that he is able to perform what is infinitely improbable. And this again is possible only because each man is unique, so that with each birth something uniquely

26 Ibid., 176–177.
27 Augustine, *De Civitate Dei*, quoted in Arendt, *The Human Condition*, 177.
28 Ibid., 177.
29 Ibid.
30 Ibid., 178.

new comes into the world. With respect to this somebody who is unique it can be truly said that nobody was there before.[31]

Arendt's idea of the uniquely new coming into the world through the miracle of every new man born, may be seen as being confirmed by anthropology. The Norwegian anthropologist Unni Wikan, referring to a study about New Guinea by Fredrik Barth, claimed that: "Not even in the stone-age did children become like their parents."[32] The other way round one could say that through the birth of a child, parents gain privileged access to a beginning that can sometimes be conceived of as a spiritual rebirth of the parent himself/herself. Mikhail Epstein expresses this thought very well when he writes: "When a child is born, it is not merely that we bring it into the world. At the same time it brings us into the world, leading us out of the dark, chaotic depths of our inner being, giving us a new sight and a new language."[33]

Although natality as a miracle and as a principle of the beginning is linked to the political in Arendt's thought, childbirth also has for her a

---

31 Ibid.

32 Unni Wikan, *Culture, Identity and Emotion: Lessons from Research on New Immigrants into Europe* (Lecture given at the European University Institute/Florence, March 11, 1996).

33 Mikhail Epstein, *Tagebuch für Olga: Chronik einer Vaterschaft,* trans. by Otto Markus (München: Roitman Verlag, 1990), 118. Similarly, Epstein, *Fatherhood,* 198–199: "In the child, as it were, you see in advance the whole course of your own resurrection: in it you are willing to live on renewed. … We are the first to introduce them [the children] into this life, and they are the first to introduce us into other life."
I have worked with Mikhail Epstein's essay *Fatherhood* in different sections of "Symbolic Patterns of Childbirth." *Fatherhood* was originally published in Russian as *Ottsovstvo* ("Fatherhood. An Essay"), Tenafly, New Jersey: Hermitage Publishers, 1992. It was translated into German and published in Germany as *Tagebuch für Olga*: *Chronik einer Vaterschaft*, trans. Otto Markus (München: Roitman Verlag, 1990). I have worked with this German translation. The page numbers referring to the quotes are from *Tagebuch für Olga*. The English translations from *Fatherhood* are the outcome of a collaboration for which I am most grateful. I have first translated the quotes from German into English. Mikhail Epstein most generously offered to check parts of them against the Russian originals. Gladson Jathanna read the translations for me and Beth Margulis checked them from the perspective of a mother tongue speaker and embellished them by suggesting to use the verb "to envelop" in the text. I am very grateful to Mikhail, Beth and Gladson for the work they put into these translations. Any shortcomings are of my own responsibility.

non-political, or even anti-political side to it, namely its mysteriousness.[34] Bowen-Moore, elaborating on Hannah Arendt, gives an account of the three-fold mystery inherent in birth:

> Birth's mystery is revealed by three factual situations: the event itself as the mystery of the sheer givenness of human existence; the appearance of the child in the world as a stranger; and the meaning the newcomer will give to his own birth (existence) is yet unknown both to him and to the world. Birth itself is an existential mystery.[35]

Hannah Arendt explains why mystery is opposed to the political by referring to the Eleusinian Mysteries in ancient Greece which most probably had the secret of birth and death at their centre. Although the Eleusinian Mysteries provided for a common and quasi-public experience, because everybody participated in them, they were at the same time kept secret from the public realm. This was because "the mysteries concerned the unspeakable, and experiences beyond speech were non-political and perhaps antipolitical by definition."[36]

Neither Bowen-Moore nor Arendt reflected upon the tension created by characterizing primary natality as both a miraculous principle for beginning in that it is tied to the political and as a mystery beyond speech – and going thus beyond the political. Instead of trying to dissolve this tension, I propose to maintain it, considering it inherent in primary natality.

It seems that here a distinction has to be introduced into the conception of primary natality, namely the one between the mother and the newborn. Indeed, with birthgiving the political and the mysterious seem to be intertwined with one another. The child is tied to the political because s/he is in possession of a principle for beginning and to the mystery inasmuch as the meaning of his/her birth is unknown to him/her and the world. The mother – whom Hannah Arendt in fact never mentions – is connected both to the principle of beginning and to the mystery to whom she is giving birth. Moreover – as will be shown in the section on pain – the non-communicability of labour pain also links the birthgiving woman to the mystery. In addition to this, birthgiving and procreation become mysterious if one links them – either implicitly or explicitly – to a metaphysical instance (god/goddess, spiritualized nature…) identified as the ultimate source for the births of children.

---

34 Hannah Arendt, *The Human Condition*, 62–63.

35 Bowen-Moore, *Hannah Arendt's Philosophy of Natality*, 32.

36 Arendt, *The Human Condition*, 63.

1.1.2 Theoretical and Spiritual Natality

From primary miraculous natality – bestowing the principle of beginning on men, then activated in political natality, Arendt, according to Patricia Bowen-Moore, moves to a third realm. She implicitly connects natality to the realm of thought: "From Heidegger, Arendt learned of thinking's passion for the experience of beginning in thought itself; in other words, she learned that thinking, too, is a kind of birthing."[37] To think, in Arendt's interpretation of Socratic philosophy, means to always begin anew, and it is here that the paradigm of (theoretical) natality shines through. As in the realm of the political, where the actor – by virtue of his/her natality – is enabled to make new beginnings, the thinker's mind always starts all over again. That is to say, in a never-ending chain of beginnings s/he indulges in a quest for meaning: "Thinking must always begin afresh; it is an activity that accompanies living and is concerned with such concepts as justice, happiness, virtue, offered us by language itself as expressing the meaning of whatever happens in life and occurs to us while we are alive."[38]

In the context of this work on symbolic patterns of childbirth, theoretical natality is placed next to still another type of natality that can be termed "spiritual natality." This way of accessing a radical beginning is connected to religious experiences. In his *Rites and Symbols of Initiation,*[39] Mircea Eliade studies initiation rites in tribal societies and the experience of the spiritual rebirth they entail. What Eliade writes here may also be used for a general description of spiritual natality: "Attaining to another mode of being – that of spirit – is equivalent to being born a second time, to becoming a new man."[40]

1.2 Natalities and Immortalities

In the previous section, with the help of Patricia Bowen-Moore's work on Hannah Arendt, primary, political, theoretical and spiritual natality were discussed as four different ways of accessing a beginning. In the following, it will be demonstrated that the birth of children is not only to be placed

37 Bowen-Moore, *Hannah Arendt's Philosophy of Natality*, 7.

38 Ibid., 178.

39 See Mircea Eliade, *Rites and Symbols of Initiation.*

40 Ibid., 60.

among political, theoretical and spiritual natality because it shares with them the possibility of putting the individual in a condition to access a new beginning but, furthermore, all four realms of natality are ways of attaining a "mortal immortality," or, to express it as Kierkegaard does, they are ways of making a "movement of infinity."[41]

The link between theoretical natality and a mortal immortality is dealt with in the third chapter of *The Life of the Mind,* where Arendt examines the different answers to the question "What makes us think?" from a historical perspective. Arendt points out that the Greeks conceived of philosophy as "enabling mortal men to dwell in the neighborhood of immortal things,"[42] as in the *Theaitetos* where it says that through philosophy men can reach "immortality in the fullest measure that human nature admits."[43] Arendt here gives an analysis of the shift concerning the means of attaining "immortality," that is, a way of approaching the divine, as far as possible. It was a "general Greek estimate that all mortals should strive for immortality, and this was possible because of the affinity between gods and men."[44] Compared to other living beings, man, in Greek antiquity, is considered a god, "whose chief task therefore consists in an activity that could remedy his mortality and thus make him more like the gods, his closest relations."[45]

One way of attaining immortality was by performing great deeds, which – through the praise of the poets – would bestow ever-lasting fame on the actor/hero, and lead to an eternal place in men's memory. Philosophy, according to Arendt, allowed for a new way of dwelling in the neighborhood of the gods, namely, in that the thinking activity itself pushes the philosopher into a new dimension: "The way to the new immortality was to take one's abode with things that are forever, and the new faculty making this possible was called nous or mind. .... By using his *nous* and by withdrawing mentally from all perishable things, man assimilates

41 Søren Kierkegaard, *Fear and Trembling: Repetition*, trans. and ed. Howard V. Hong and Edna H. Hong (Princeton, New Jersey: Princeton University Press, 1983), 42.

42 Hannah Arendt, *Thinking*, vol. 1 of *The Life of the Mind* (London: Secker and Warburg, 1978), 129.

43 Plato, *Theaitetos*, quoted in Arendt, ibid.

44 Arendt, *Thinking*, 134.

45 Ibid.

himself to the divine."[46] It can be said that philosophy "set itself the original Greek goal of immortality."[47]

Furthermore, Arendt's reflections on thinking suggest a deep link between the notion of immortality and the experience of thinking, even when immortality is not perceived as the goal. An important characteristic of thinking is that it makes the thinking person unaware of having a body.[48] Thus the element in man that is most directly experienced as being the object of decay is not perceived any more. Instead, what characterizes the experience of the thinking ego is the sensation of timelessness – not to be exchanged with eternity.[49] Springing from the clash between past and future, of a no-more and a not-yet, the thought train moves towards the infinite. Arendt sees the thinking-ego in a "gap between past and future, in [a] present which is timeless."[50] It seems that from the notion of timelessness and infiniteness, together with the unawareness of the body, the step to a sensation of immortality is only a small one. Thinking can be understood as a direct "experience" of immortality, due to the sensation of timelessness and "bodilessness" of the thinking ego.

Additionally, Arendt makes a link between political natality and "mortal immortality." She connects political natality back to the principle of beginning (coming into the world with primary natality) and sees it as a realm where the possibility exists to acquire immortality by great deeds that are remembered by posteriority. As Arendt points out, this kind of immortality is highly dependent on others. In antiquity, lasting fame was dependent on the poet's praise of a person's deeds,[51] and in general, one may say that immortality in the political realm cannot be separated from some kind of collective memory. In the same way one could see the immortality of thought as depending on reception by others. However, reception bestows a rather dynamic immortality on the products of mind.

In a chapter entitled *Poetry and Immortality* of his *European Literature and Latin Middle Ages* Ernst Robert Curtius collected references to the immortality that stems from the thinking activity. The poets and

46 Ibid. In this context Arendt emphasizes that "logos as distinguished from nous is not divine, and the translation of the philosopher's vision into speech – aletheuein, in the philosophers' strict sense – created considerable difficulties." Ibid., 137.

47 Ibid., 138.

48 See ibid., 163.

49 See ibid., 211.

50 Ibid., 212.

51 See ibid., 135.

philosophers enlisted by Curtius (Horatius, Lucian, Cerippus, Reginald of Canterbury, Boudri de Bourgueil, Abélard, Benzo d'Albe, Gauthier de Châtillon, Ariosto) partially refer to the fact that the poet bestows fame on others, and partially point to the immortalizing effect that the writing of poetry and philosophy may have on its author.[52]

Like theoretical and political natality also spiritual natality is connected to "mortal immortality." This link is touched upon by Hannah Arendt when she writes that Christianity replaced thought with faith as the bringer of immortality.[53] In general one may argue that religious belief systems tend to bestow some kind of "mortal immortality" on the believer, most often on the condition that the rules of the belief system are followed. Religious ideas such as paradise, afterlife, or nirvana after death are expressing the immortality stemming from spiritual natality. Furthermore, religious acts such as praying may just like the activity of thinking confer a sensation of timelessness and bodilessness upon a person. Thereby s/he may experience "mortal immortality."

What about primary natality whose connection to immortality has not been mentioned yet? It is Plato to give the answer: procreation and birth-giving can be understood as a way to partake of immortality. By generation "mortal nature [...] can always leave behind it a new creature in place of the old."[54] In Plato's *Symposium*, Diotima says to her interlocutor Socrates: "All men are pregnant, Socrates, both in body and in soul: on reaching a certain age our nature yearns to beget. ... It is a divine affair, this engendering and bringing to birth, an immortal element in the creature that is mortal."[55]

Quite a similar link between a "mortal immortality" and primary natality can be found in the Gilgamesh-Epic. The king Gilgamesh is haunted by the fear of death. On his way to visit Utnapishtim, the only human being on whom the gods have bestowed the gift of immortality, he encounters the divine Siduri, she who gives. Siduri who lives in the sea gives Gilgamesh the following advice:

> Gilgamesh, wherefore do you wander?
> The eternal life you are seeking you shall not find.

---

52 Ernst Robert Curtius, *Europäische Literatur und lateinisches Mittelalter* (1948; reprint, Tübingen and Basel: Francke Verlag, 1993), 471–472.

53 See Arendt, *Thinking*, 138.

54 Plato, *Lysis, Symposium, Gorgias*, trans. W.R.M. Lamb (1925; reprint, Cambridge, Mass.: Harvard University Press, 1975), 195.

55 Ibid., 191.

When the gods created mankind,
They established death for mankind,
And withheld eternal life for themselves.
As for you, Gilgamesh let your stomach be full,
Always be happy, night and day.
Make every day a delight,
Night and day play and dance.
Your clothes should be clean,
Your head should be washed,
You should bathe in water,
Look proudly on the little one holding your hand,
Let your mate be always blissful in your loins,
This, then, is the work of mankind.[56]

Siduri in these verses tries to comfort Gilgamesh by poining out the joys of life to him: clean dressing, eating, dancing, playing, erotic pleasure. Among these joyful aspects of life she counts having children as a means to counterbalance death: "Look proudly on the little one holding your hand,"[57] she tells the hero Gilgamesh who had reached her reign looking for eternal life.

The link between a mortal immortality and childbirth is made quite explicit by Mikhail Epstein, when he writes: "When we give life to a child, we sentence it to death whereby the child gives immortality to us."[58]

2. Childbirth, Sex and Gender

In the previous section with the help of Hannah Arendt's philosophy, primary natality was localized among political, theoretical and spiritual natality as one way to access a beginning and a "mortal immortality." Nevertheless, it seems that a conception of childbirth does not exhaust itself by these characteristics but also has to take into consideration the relation between gender and childbirth. Highlighting the constructions of gender and gender relations along the lines of childbirth is one way of accomplishing this. For example, Judith Butler in a critical reading of

56 *The Epic of Gilgamesh: A New Translation, Analogues, Criticism*, ed. and trans. Benjamin R. Foster (New York and London: Noton & Company, 2001), 75.

57 Ibid.

58 Epstein, *Tagebuch für Olga,* 116.

Julia Kristeva points out that defining the female body primarily by its "reproductive function" constructs the "institution of motherhood as compulsory for women."[59] Similarly, of course also "procreation" or fatherhood can function as a decisive element for defining masculinity. To a certain extent the question of defining gender along the lines of childbirth relates to the symbolic patterns "The Supremacy of the Male" and "The Supremacy of the Female." These may also be read as contributing to configurations of power in society based on gender constructions.

However, though the investigation into the construction of masculinity and femininity on the grounds of childbirth and procreation seems to be a promising field of study, it is not the main focus of this work. The question of cultural images picturing men as having to procreate to be men, or women as having to give birth to be women, here, on the whole is left aside. Though moving on difficult ground here it will be argued that despite the constructedness of the body implied in its historicity there is some *potential* of meaning, which is inherently attached to childbirth. Andrea Maihofer has drawn attention to the fact that there is a tendency in feminist philosophy to ignore the question of whether bodily practices such as giving birth may have a meaning constitutive of society and culture.[60] For her, the avoidance of this topic results from the fact that claiming a natural difference of the sexes would easily lead to a legitimisation of the existing gender system, declaring it immutable. In fact, going in this direction, Judith Butler reveals her epistemological doubts concerning reflections on the body by stating that she would wish to assure her critics that there are "minimally, sexually differentiated parts, activities, capacities, hormonal and chromosomal differences that can be conceded without reference to 'construction.'"[61] However, Butler literally writes about an "anxiety" to do so, as for her, "to 'concede' the undeniability of 'sex' or its 'materiality' is always to concede some version of 'sex', some formation of 'materiality.'"[62] Though Butler's arguments against differentiating between the sexes on the whole are plausible, radically sticking to her

59 Judith Butler, *Gender Trouble: Feminism and the Subversion of Identity* (1990; reprint, New York: Routledge, 2008), 126.

60 See Andrea Maihofer, *Geschlecht als Existenzweise* (Frankfurt: Helmer, 1995), 77.

61 Judith Butler, *Bodies That Matter: On the Discursive Limits of Sex* (1993; reprint, New York: Routledge, 2011), XIX.

62 Ibid.

position would rather limit the investigation into symbolic patterns of childbirth.[63] It is "women" and not "men" who give birth. Thus the *potentials* of meaning and experience related to childbirth to a certain extent are also informed by this "difference."

On a "corporeal" level man's relationship to childbirth is largely marked by exclusion. Apart from the moment of "conception"/"procreation,"[64] childbirth is attached to the woman's body through the period of pregnancy and through birthgiving. Man may or may not be part of childbirth to the degree that he identifies with "procreation," or with the child in general. Thus Mikhail Epstein writes: "In the fatherly body, there is no place of origin for the baby. He is connected to it more through his will than by his flesh."[65]

The symbolic pattern "The Supremacy of the Male" to be presented later can be read as an effort to come to terms with the distance to childbirth that the male "*physis*" imposes/can impose. This may be done either by symbolically attributing more importance to procreation than to conception, pregnancy and birthgiving, or by symbolically excluding the female body all together from the births of children. On the other hand woman's deep corporeal involvement with childbirth has most probably led to the symbolic pattern "The Supremacy of the Female."

Though it will not add to a deeper understanding of the symbolic patterns of childbirth to be presented, conceiving of childbirth from a philosophical point of view without reflecting upon the situation of the woman giving birth seems negligent. Thus the following reflections will be dedicated to a conception of woman and birth.

63 For a more comprehensive analysis of body theory and childbirth see Anja Hänsch, "Barbara Duden, Judith Butler, and Birth: Contentions about Body Theory Revisited," in *Birth and Death in British Culture: Liminality, Power, and Performance*, ed. Anette Pankratz, Claus-Ulrich Viol, and Ariane de Waal (Newcastle upon Tyne, UK: Cambridge Scholars Publishing, 2012), 15–32.

64 To analyse the construction of "conception" and "procreation" would be a study on its own.

65 Epstein, *Tagebuch für Olga,* 220.

3. Conceiving of the Birthgiving Woman

The following attempt to conceive of childbirth with the focus on the birthgiving woman parallels Martin Heidegger's existential conception of death, as illustrated in paragraphs 46 to 62 of *Being and Time*.[66] This is because birthgiving for the woman seems to bear many of the outstanding features that Heidegger assigns exclusively to death.

3.1 From an Existential Definition of Death to an Existential Definition of Giving Birth

Here, Heidegger's understanding of death will serve as a paradigm for a conception of birthgiving. First of all, one has to take a closer look at the Heideggerian definition of death as an existential phenomenon towards which *Dasein* comports itself, in order to deduce a definition of birthgiving. In summary, Heidegger's definition of death runs as follows: "Death is that possibility which is one's ownmost, which is non-relational, and which is not to be outstripped [*unüberholbar*]."[67] What does this mean? To Heidegger death is the possibility of life, which is one's ownmost because in death nobody can represent another person, as is the case in the world of everyday concern: "Dying is something that every *Dasein* itself must take upon itself at the time."[68] The dying person cannot hide behind the "they" of everyday concern. S/he has to say "I die" and cannot say "they die" or "one dies."

Death is furthermore non-relational for "with death, *Dasein* stands before itself in its ownmost potentiality-for-Being." Thus all relations of *Dasein* "to any other *Dasein* have been undone."[69] Moreover, death is that possibility "which is not to be outstripped" *[unüberholbar]* for the reason

66 Martin Heidegger, *Being and Time*, trans. John Macquarrie & Edward Robinson (Oxford: Blackwell, (1962) 1978), 252. In the following the numbers of the pages quoted will always correspond to those of the original German text which have also been reported in the English translation. The German edition of *Being and Time* used is: Martin Heidegger, *Sein und Zeit*, 17th ed. (Tübingen: Max Niemeyer Verlag, 1993).

67 Heidegger, *Being and Time*, 250.

68 Ibid., 240.

69 Ibid., 250.

that "death is the possibility of the absolute impossibility of *Dasein*." Thus "as potentiality-for-Being, *Dasein* cannot outstrip the possibility of death."[70]

The question to be posed here is: Do these characteristics of death equally apply to birthgiving? Although, of course, everybody has to die and not everybody gives birth, it seems that the situation of birth, like death, could also be conceived of as a possibility that is one's ownmost. The same characteristic of unrepresentability applies equally to both. The birthgiving woman cannot be substituted by another person. She has to say: "I give birth" and cannot hide behind a "one gives birth" or a "they give birth."

To conceive of birth as one's ownmost does not mean that childbirth defines what a woman *is* or desires or should desire. In this context I wish to build on Kerreen Reiger and Rhea Dempsey's approach of seeing birth as collectively and individually performed.[71] Dempsey and Reiger apply the idea of birth as performance to the natural birth movement as well as to advocates of medicalised birth.[72] This understanding of birth may also be related to a conception of birth as one's ownmost. Thus there are different performances of birth actualising or not actualising birth as one's ownmost on the level of experience. In this sense technological interventions into both birthgiving and dying could not alter their above mentioned characteristic of irrepresentability but rather did alter the possibilities of actualising birth and death as one's ownmost on the level of experience.

Furthermore, following the Heideggerian matrix, birthgiving, as death, may be conceived of as non-relational. This is because the woman's *Dasein*, while giving birth, as with death, stands before itself in its ownmost potentiality for being. Her *Dasein* is only as far as it is a "Being-towards-birth," or a "Being-towards-a-potential-*Dasein*," which implies that "all its relations to any other *Dasein* have been undone." Here, birth and death can be conceived as the most extreme situations to which the particular loneliness that accompanies all "limit," or "liminal" experiences is

70 Ibid.: „Als Seinkönnen vermag das Dasein die Möglichkeit des Todes nicht zu überholen. Der Tod ist die Möglichkeit der schlechthinnigen Daseinsunmöglichkeit."

71 See Kerreen Reiger and Rhea Dempsey, "Performing Birth in a Culture of Fear: An Embodied Crisis of Late Modernity," *Health Sociology Review* 15, no. 4 (2006): 364–373.

72 See ibid., 366–367.

attached.[73] As with regard to death the birthgiving woman stands before her ownmost potentiality for being. However, characterizing birthgiving as a potentiality, which is the woman's ownmost, contains a dynamic element that does not apply to death. It is true that making a firm distinction between the pregnant woman and the unborn child means to apply the notion of the individual desperately where it is not applicable. As it was once put in a non-chalant way: "Certainly the distinction between me and not-me becomes a little blurry to say the least, when one has been inhabited as a mother."[74]

For the birthgiving woman a situation which is her ownmost and in which she cannot be represented, is produced by an uttmost relationality[75] not to be exchanged with relationality to another *Dasein* in the Heideggerian sense. The birthgiving woman cannot be represented with regard to the isolating "Being-towards-birth." Nevertheless, her non-relationality to other *Dasein*s actualizes itself in a relationality, namely a relationality inside a dyad.[76] To give birth means an accentuation of the state of "being-towards" in pregnancy. It means to give oneself up not with regard to one's *Dasein* but with regard to the potential *Dasein* that is part of one's *Dasein*.

This reasoning already leads closely to the third existential characteristic of death/birthgiving, namely the one of death/birthgiving as a possibility that is not to be outstripped. Heidegger writes with regard to

73 I am grateful to Arpad Szakolczai for pointing this out to me.

74 Nancy F. W. Passmore, "A Consciousness Manifesto," in *The Politics of Women's Spirituality*, ed. Charlene Spretnak (New York: Anchor Press, 1982), 169.

75 I am grateful to Catarina Botti whose insightful critique helped me with the development of this thought.

76 The epistemological problem to describe this dyad aedequately is illustrated very well in a short story by Rafik Schami. (See for the following Rafik Schami, *Die Sehnsucht fährt schwarz. Geschichten aus der Fremde* (München: Deutscher Taschenbuch Verlag, 1988), 98–100. Schami describes his struggle with the writing of a story in which he refers to one of the female characters in the plural because she is pregnant. After he has sent his manuscript to his editor he gets it back full of corrections: all the plural forms have been changed back to the conventional singular. There is no generally accepted language which would pay attention to the special state a pregnant woman is in. Schami suspects language to center around the male body because he is missing the aedequate language to describe the state of the pregnant woman: „Sicher haben die Männer die Sprache unter ihrer Herrschaft nach ihrem Willen gebogen. Sie werden nie schwanger, und deshalb hatten sie aus Neid die Dualform aus allen Sprachen herauszensiert" (Ibid., 100).

death that "Being towards this possibility enables *Dasein* to understand that giving itself up impends for it as the uttermost possibility of its existence."[77] This applies equally to birthgiving. While a woman gives birth, all her Being is directed towards the effort of bringing a human being into life. This means that her Being becomes a "Being-towards-a-potential-Dasein," which–curiously enough–forms a part of her *Dasein*. Therefore, while a woman is giving birth, there can be no "ahead-of-itself" for a certain amount of time, which may well be thought of as a standstill of the woman's Being in favour of a "Being-towards-a-potential-Dasein." Such a standstill reveals an analogy with the moment of death in the sense that for the woman giving birth, with her Being transformed into a "Being-towards-a-potential-*Dasein*" nothing is outstanding anymore. The fact that nothing is outstanding anymore lets the birthgiving woman reach a moment of wholeness, a moment in which the "*ständige Unabgeschlossenheit*" of *Dasein* becomes a "*Abgeschlossenheit*."

On the other hand with regard to the mother-child dyad there is a second reason why birthgving presents itself as a possibility that is not to be outstripped. Given that birthgiving is a time of passage, during which it is not clear whether the woman and the unborn will continue to live or die, two possibilities present themselves as immanent possibilities: death as the "possibility of the absolute impossibility of *Dasein*"[78] and life as the possibility of the absolute possibility of *Dasein*.

Thus birthgiving is by definition a possibility-of-Being in which *Dasein* itself becomes a possibility. In this distinctive possibility-for-Being, the birthgiving woman, as with death, "has been fully assigned to her ownmost potentiality-for-Being."

As has been shown above, an existential definition of birthgiving can be modeled on Heidegger's existential definition of death. In the following section, two important Heideggerian categories, namely those of "thrownness" (*Geworfenheit*) and "anxiety" (*Angst*) will be connected to birthgiving.

77 Heidegger, 1962, 264.

78 Ibid., 250.

3.2 *Thrownness and Anxiety*

Though at a first glance Heidegger seems to ignore birthgiving as a phenomenon of existence, it is not all together absent from his philosophy, as birthgiving is included in the category of "*Geworfenheit*" (thrownness). In the Heideggerian language "to be thrown" is a metaphor for "to be born," e. g. he writes: "As being, *Dasein* is something that has been thrown; it has been brought into its 'there', but *not* of its own accord."[79] In fact, Heidegger has a very particular approach to birthgiving. This becomes obvious if one analyses the German term *Geworfenheit* linguistically. *Geworfenheit* is a substantive, which Heidegger deduces from the passive voice of the verb *werfen* (*geworfen werden*) meaning to be thrown. However, "*werfen*" is also a term that is used as a synonym for birthgiving, in the case of animals giving birth. Hence, *Geworfenheit* refers to the animal-like nature Heidegger attributes to birthgiving. Moreover, Heidegger does not focus on the one who gives birth, the woman, but on the one who is born, the child. Additionally, it should be noted that "to be thrown" is both a rather violent and inappropriate metaphor for "being born." This is because the baby is usually not abandoned in a hostile world after birth, but continues to be fused with the mother e.g. through breastfeeding for quite some time. Young babies cannot distinguish their body from their mother's.[80]

Despite the linguistical and epistemological problems of the category of thrownness mentioned here, I will keep it as a term, because I will continue to use the Heideggerian conception of death as a *matrix* for a conception of birthgiving.

In Heideggerian language, the relationship between thrownness and death consists of the fact that, if *Dasein* exists, it has already been thrown into that distinctive possibility of *Dasein*.[81] The state-of-mind that displays thrownness into death is anxiety. Heidegger specifies that "anxiety in the face of death must not be confused with fear in the face of one's demise,"[82]

79 Ibid., 284.

80 As Arpád Szakolczai pointed out to me, the idea of thrownness is profoundly Gnostic. He argues that, contrary to being "thrown" into the world as a stranger, the child is born into the "world of home."

81 Heidegger, *Being and Time*, 251.

82 Ibid.

but has to be understood as anxiety "in the face of that potentiality-for-Being which is one's ownmost, non-relational, and not to be outstripped."[83] Moreover, anxiety, far from being a mood of "weakness" in some individuals, is "a basic state-of-mind of *Dasein*," which "amounts to the disclosedness of the fact that *Dasein* exists as thrown Being towards its end."[84]

In the following, thrownness and anxiety will be linked to birth(giving). This may imply a completely different understanding of life than the Heideggerian one. Can a "thrownness into birth" be substituted for the Heideggerian "thrownness into death"? This step would indeed come close to Hannah Arendt's philosophy of natality. Her "men, though they must die, are not born in order to die but in order to begin"[85] is ontologically linked back to primary natality: "This beginning is guaranteed by each new birth; it is indeed every man."[86] Arendt's implicit critique of Heidegger consists of substituting "thrownness into death" with what could be called a "thrownness into the beginning," which for her is rooted in primary natality. Nevertheless, women as "agents of primary natality" in Hannah Arendt's writing are left entirely in the dark.

However, on the basis of Arendt's philosophy the notion of "thrownness into beginning" can be adopted. The supreme expression of this category is childbirth, which leads to the appearance of the beginning par excellence: every new human being born. In this sense, the roots of beginning go back to generation: When male and female *Daseins* are thrown into existence, they are not only "thrown into death" but also into the possibility of giving new life and/or nurturing new life. With women most often potentially capable of actually giving birth, a "thrownness into birth" is most tangible.

How does anxiety disclose "thrownness into birth"? Pregnant women's anxiety in the face of birthgiving can be equated with anxiety regarding death. Thus, the anxiety related to birthgiving may be interpreted as an anxiety regarding a potentiality-for-Being, which is one's ownmost, non-relational, and not to be outstripped. In this sense, birthgiving for women may constitute the second possibility-of-Being which bears the

83 Ibid.

84 Ibid.

85 Arendt, *The Human Condition*, 9.

86 Hannah Arendt, *The Origins of Totalitarianism* (New York: Harcourt Brace Jovanovich, (1951) 1978), 478–479.

features of such a distinction. If in the Heideggerian perspective, anxiety discloses the thrownness into death and therefore "the fact that *Dasein* exists as thrown Being towards its end,"[87] in this reasoning anxiety has to be conceived of as also disclosing the fact that *Dasein* may exist as thrown Being towards the beginning of another *Dasein.*

3.3 Pain as Disclosing Mystery, Standstill and Non-Relationality

The twofold character of primary natality as both political (as a principle of beginning) and non-political (for its quality of a mystery) has already been pointed out. Looking at primary natality from the viewpoint of the birthgiving woman, the question of the non-political element inherent in birthgiving comes up again. The potential experience of pain during birthgiving is another characteristic, along with its mystery, that ties primary natality to the non-political. Hannah Arendt elaborated on the experience of pain as the opposite of the public realm, constituting itself through communication. For her "the experience of great pain, is at the same time the most private and least communicable of all."[88] If we assume with Arendt that appearance as "something that is being seen and heard by others as well as by ourselves"[89] is constitutive of reality, then intense pain creates a peculiar relationship between the suffering person and reality: "Pain, in other words, truly a borderline experience between life as being among men *(inter homines esse)* and death, is so subjective and removed from the world of things and men that it cannot assume an appearance at all."[90]

Arendt, at this point, quotes some verses from a poem on pain from Rilke's deathbed:

> Come thou, thou last one, whom I recognize
> Unbearable pain throughout this body's fabric ....
> Is it still I, who there past all recognition burn?
> Memories I do not seize and bring inside.

---

87 Heidegger, *Being and Time*, 251.
88 Arendt, *The Human Condition*, 51.
89 Ibid.
90 Ibid.

O life! Living! O to be outside!
And I in flames. And no one here who knows me.[91]

Applying Arendt's and Rilke's reflections on pain to the pain felt during labour, one can say that it discloses both the non-relational character of birthgiving and the standstill of the woman's being in a "Being towards-another-being." As it was already pointed out, the woman's *Dasein*, while giving birth – as with death – stands before itself, before its own potentiality-for-Being. The non-communicability of labour pain discloses the fact that all her relations to any other *Dasein* have been undone in her (second) distinctive potentiality-for-Being. In a different context, Peter Schwenger writes about body-knowledge in general: If this "knowledge is by definition uncommunicable, that is because it is largely body-knowledge, which [...] is the very opposite of words."[92] Labour pain here can be seen as a special instance of "body-knowledge."

91 Rilke, quoted by Arendt, *The Human Condition*, 51: "Komm du, du letzter, den ich anerkenne,/ heilloser Schmerz im leiblichen Geweb..../ Bin ich es noch, der da unkenntlich brennt?/ Erinnerungen reiß ich nicht herein./ O Leben, Leben: Draußensein./ Und ich in Lohe. Niemand, der mich kennt."

92 Peter Schwenger, *Phallic Critiques: Masculinity and Twentieth-Century Literature* (London: Routledge and Kegan Paul, 1984), 113. An early advocate of "body-knowledge" can indeed be found in Tertullian. In *De Anima* he starts a dispute with Plato's ideas on the soul. Whereas for Plato the soul is ungenerated and enters the human body right after birth with the first breath, Tertullian argues that both soul and body come into existence with conception. To support his argument, he refers to the "body knowledge" of pregnant women. According to Tertullian they feel the soul of the unborn and he harshly tells men and infertile women to keep silent in front of pregnant women's body-knowledge: "Give us your testimony, then, ye mothers, whether yet pregnant, or after delivery (let barren women and men keep silence), – the truth of your own nature is in question, the reality of your own suffering is the point to be be decided. [Tell us, then,] whether you feel in the embryo within you any vital force other than your own, with which your bowels tremble, your sides shake, your entire womb throbs, and the burden which oppresses you constantly changes its position? Are these movements a joy to you, and a positive removal of anxiety, as making you confident that your infant both possesses vitality and enjoys it? Or, should his restlessness cease, your first fear would be for him; and he would be aware of it within you, since he is disturbed at the novel sound; and you would crave for injurious diet, or would even loathe your food – all on his account; and then you and he, [in the closeness of your sympathy,] would share together your common ailments – so far that with your contusions and bruises would he actually become marked, – whilst within you, and even on the selfsame parts of the body, taking to himself thus peremptorily the injuries of his mother!" (Tertullian, *On the Soul*, vol. 2

If intense pain in general confers the sensation of a standstill of one's own being upon the suffering person – Rilke questions himself whether it is still him burning "past all recognition" – in the case of birthgiving this standstill, is of a very peculiar kind: Labour pain discloses a standstill of the woman's being in favour of a "Being-towards-another-Being."

Thus, with regard to birthgiving, we encounter the peculiar phenomenon that pain acquires a gender dimension. Still the divine punishment of Eve in Genesis 3:16, "I will greatly multiply thy sorrow and thy conception; in sorrow thou shalt bring forth children," points out that the pain of birthgiving is a special one a man will never feel (and in Genesis more normatively, should never feel). Thus labour pain – like any other intense pain – belongs to the least communicable of experiences. However, women who have given birth with labour pain "share" such an experience, which cannot assume an appearance at all. It seems that here Hannah Arendt's views on the Eleusinian Mysteries may be equally applied to birthgiving, conceptualized from a gender perspective. As has already been mentioned, the Eleusinian Mysteries provided for a common and quasi-public experience, because everybody could participate in them. At the same time they were kept secret from the public realm. This was because "the mysteries concerned the unspeakable, and experiences beyond speech were non-political and perhaps antipolitical by definition."[93] Analogously birthgiving can be thought of as constituting a common and quasi-public experience because it is shared by a large number of women. On the other hand, as the unspeakable, birthgiving may assume the characteristics of a mystery as opposed to the political.

---

of *The Writings of Quintus Sept. Flor. Tertullianus*, trans. Peter Holmes (Edinburgh: T. & T. Clark, 1870), XXV).

93 Arendt, *The Human Condition*, 63.

III. Symbolic Patterns of Childbirth

Childbirth can acquire manifold meanings in myths, philosophy, literature and religion some of which here will be grouped together and explored as symbolic patterns. Four of these symbolic patterns have been chosen for analysis and can be traced through space and time:

1. The supremacy of the male
2. Theoretical, spiritual and political natality versus childbirth
3. The supremacy of the female
4. Harmony between spiritual/theoretical natality and childbirth

These four ways of accessing giving birth through different registers are not randomly grouped together, but are assumed to be linked by an internal logic based on the conception of childbirth outlined in the previous chapter. On the grounds of Hannah Arendt's philosophy of natality it was possible to place childbirth (primary natality) on one line with the thinking activity of the mind, the performance of great deeds and a spiritual rebirth due to religious experiences. All these realms are ways of accessing a beginning and a mortal immortality.

The link between primary natality and "mortal immortality" may explain one peculiar phenomenon in the history of thought regarding our topic, namely the symbolic exclusion or devaluation either of the role of the male or of the role of the female sex in relation to the birth of children (symbolic patterns 1 and 3). Such a way of symbolically attributing childbirth more to the man, or more to the woman, may be considered an endless symbolic contention over the question of which body has more, or which body has *the* access to a certain way of attaining a beginning and/or a mortal immortality. This "symbolic contention" is particularly visible with regard to the first symbolic pattern of childbirth ("The Supremacy of the Male") probably originating in the comparatively larger distance of the male body to childbirth. A strong symbolic appropriation of the whole process of giving birth/generation to the man, to be discussed in the context of the first symbolic pattern of childbirth, may be read as the male desire to appropriate childbirth to himself.

The second symbolic pattern of giving birth/procreation starts from a settling of the question which body may be responsible for the birth of a child. Independently of whether supremacy, in matters of childbirth, is attached to the woman (symbolic pattern no. 3), or to the man (symbolic pattern no. 1), birthgiving and procreation are devalued in view of other ways of gaining a mortal immortality and/or an access to a beginning. The realms of the political, ideas, religion or the arts are depicted as a more noble way than childbirth to attain a mortal immortality. In this sense, one could speak about an establishment of a hierarchy of mortal immortalities where childbirth (primary natality) figures on a lower level than the other types of natality. However, as will be shown by the symbolic pattern "Harmony between Spiritual/Theoretical Natality and Childbirth" the different forms of attaining a mortal immortality or accessing a beginning, do not have to be played out against each other.

Of course the symbolic patterns of childbirth to be presented are a mere tool to facilitate the investigation into different meanings attributed to childbirth. Thus some of the texts selected to represent one symbolic pattern may also be interwoven with another symbolic pattern. In this context it is significant to note that "The Supremacy of the Female" and "Harmony between Spiritual/Theoretical Natality and Childbirth" are overlapping with regard to two important examples chosen for analysis, namely the Isis and the Mary cult.

III.1 The Supremacy of the Male

Femaleness existed,
but she was not
in the beginning.

Apocryphon of John

Have compassion on thy offspring ....
and let not this seed of Pelops' line be blotted out;
for then, in spite of death, thou art not dead.
For children are voices of salvation to a man, though he be dead.

Electra on the tomb of her father Agamemnon in
The Libation-Bearers of Aeschylus

I came forth from the Father, and am come into the world:
again, I leave the world, and go to the Father

Gospel of John

The first symbolic pattern of childbirth to be analyzed here, presents itself as accentuating the importance of the man for the coming into existence of a child. Woman to different extents is symbolically excluded from the realm of childbirth. Men procreate, sometimes they give birth, and on the whole women are not given much, if any importance with regard to the generation of new life. This can also be done by transferring the spiritual part of childbirth to the man and constructing birthgiving and pregnancy as mere physical acts. "Obviously" women give birth to children after pregnancy. However, both pregnancy and giving birth may be constructed as totally unimportant, or as less important than the short moment of "procreation" on behalf of the man.

Elements of "The Supremacy of the Male" are not completely alien to contemporary culture as illustrated by a short example. On the first page of his manual for family therapy, the psychologist and psychiatrist Michael Wirsching writes: "Every human being was procreated by a father and born by a mother."[94] It is interesting to reflect upon the construction of procreation in this sentence. Here "procreation" on part of the man is equal to birthgiving on the part of the woman. Furthermore, the fact that the woman plays a part during "procreation" is completely ignored.

Maybe, "The Supremacy of the Male" in a peculiar way testifies to the long involvement of the woman with childbirth during pregnancy and giving birth on the one hand and the comparatively greater physical distance of the man to childbirth on the other. In this sense, the symbolic pattern "The Supremacy of the Male" may "balance" such an inequality between the sexes by an emphasis laid on the importance of procreation, male spiritual intervention into childbirth, or a mimetical appropriation of pregnancy and birthgiving on part of the man. To proclaim a supremacy of the male over the female in matters of childbirth can be read as an effort to symbolically bridge or undo the larger distance of the man to childbirth. In this way man gains a privileged access to a beginning and to a mortal immortality. As will be shown in the following chapter, the procreational supremacy of the male over the female is connotated mostly positively. However, a "dubious" supremacy of the male over the female in matters of childbirth comes into play with Christian thinkers such as Ambrose, Augustine, Tertullian and Thomas Aquinas. This is because they state that male semen not only transmits "the soul," but also original sin.

1.1 Creation as Procreation in Egyptian Cosmogony

One of the oldest creation myths, if not *the* oldest, portraying the supremacy of the male over the female in terms of generation, comes from Ancient Egypt. As old as the *Pyramid Texts* is the myth of the sun god Ra who created the world by first willing into being his own physical existence and then creating Shu, the god of air and Tefnut, the goddess of mist. The divine couple thus began the long genealogical line of Egyptian gods. From their union comes Geb, the god of the earth, and Nut, the goddess of the sky. As Robert A. Armour puts it humorously, Nut and Geb "provided

94 Michael Wirsching, *Paar- und Familientherapie: Grundlagen, Methoden, Ziele* (München: Beck, 2005), 7: "Jeder Mensch wurde von einem Vater gezeugt und von einer Mutter zur Welt gebracht."

the universe with a population of gods and goddesses who were to be the dramatis personae of Egyptian mythology."[95]

However, Ra is the creator of the world as a result of both self-creation and the creation of Shu and Tefnut. As will be shown in two sources, male procreation emerges as a dominant theme in the Ancient Egyptian creation myth. There are separate parts of the Ancient Egyptian myth of creation spread over the Pyramid Texts. Secondly, *The Book of Overthrowing Apophis,* which is more recent than the Pyramid Texts, has the advantage that its account of the creation of the world is not fragmented, but rather tells a complete story. Creation myths of antiquity are often characterized by a close relationship to male or female fertility as in the creation myth of Ra. In contrast to this, the creation myths of the Bible and the Qur'an present the creation of the world as a-sexual. Genesis starts with the words: "In the beginning, when God created the heavens and the earth, the earth was a formless void and darkness covered the face of the deep, while a wind from God swept over the face of the waters. Then God said, 'Let there be light'; and there was light."[96] In the Qur'an "Allah need only say 'be, and it is.'"[97] A body-neutral conception of God is by no means a dominant paradigm for creation myths in general, though. As will be shown in the following with the creation myth of Ra, creation can be depicted as the first act of procreation. Robert A. Armour summarizes it elegantly as follows:

> In the beginning were the primeval waters, named Nun [...] which, since they were unconscious and inanimate, were incapable of independent action. Out of the waters Ra raised himself on a hill and created himself. Ra says that at the moment of his creation nothing else existed, neither the heavens, nor the earth, nor the things upon the earth. Until this moment he had lived alone in the primeval waters, where he developed in darkness and contained both male and female principles. For reasons that remain obscure to mortals, he conceived the idea of creation and willed his

95 Robert A. Armour, *Gods and Myths of Ancient Egypt* (1986; reprint, Cairo: The American University in Cairo Press, 1987), 22.

96 Genesis 1:1–3. If not stated otherwise, all biblical quotes are from *The New Oxford Annotated Bible*, ed. Michael D. Coogan, 3rd ed. (Oxford: Oxford University Press, 2007).

97 Faruq Sherif, *A Guide to the Contents of the Qur'an* (Reading: Ithaca Press, 1995), 26. See also Sura II., 111. The Qur'an makes an explicit statement that procreation is something human. In verse 3 of Sura 112 it says that God did neither procreate, nor was he procreated ("*lam yalid wa-lam yulad*"). I am grateful to Mohammed Arkoun for pointing this verse out to me.

> own physical existence. What happened next is open to some controversy, but the most widely accepted version follows the concept as expressed in the Pyramid Texts, which tell us that Ra was the god "who once came into being, who masturbated in On. He took his phallus in his grasp that he might create orgasm by means of it, and so were born the twins Shu and Tefnut." The exact details are hazy and what happened seems to have been anatomically possible only for a chief god, but Ra said that he embraced his own shadow during this remarkable act and "poured seed into my own mouth." His children were formed and he spat them out: Shu was to be the god of the air and Tefnut the goddess of the mist. Ra said that he "became from one god three gods." This act resulted in the immediate existence of light and the dispersal of chaos. ....
>
> After creating himself and his two children Ra wept, and the tears that fell gave birth to mortal men and women.[98]

Before commenting on Armour's summary of the Egyptian myth of creation, the *Book of Overthrowing Apophis* has to be taken into consideration as it allows for accessing the myth more directly. In the version of the creation myth of *The Book of Overthrowing Apophis* Ra himself talks about his creation. Here he appears as Khepri, the scarab beetle god. Ra's procreation of the world is told as follows:

> The Lord of All, after having come into being says: I am he who came into being as Khepri (i.e., the Becoming One). When I came into being, the beings came into being, all the beings came into being after I became. Numerous are those who became, who came out of my mouth, before heaven ever existed, nor earth came into being, nor the worms, nor the snakes were created in this place. I, being in weariness, was bound to them in the Watery Abyss. I found no place to stand. I thought in my heart, I planned in myself, I made all forms being alone, before I ejected Shu, before I spat out Tefnut, before any other who was in me had become. Then I planned in my own heart, and many forms of being came into being as forms of children, as forms of their children. I conceived by my hand, I united myself with my hand, I poured out of my own mouth. I ejected Shu, I spat out Tefnut .... After having become one god, there were (now) three gods in me .... I created all snakes, and all that came into being with them. Shu and Tefnut produced Geb and Nut; Geb and Nut produced out of a single body Osiris, Horus the Eyeless One, Seth, Isis, and Nephtys, one after the other among them. Their children are numerous in this land.[99]

---

98 Ibid., 19–20.

99 Alexandre Piankoff and Natacha Rambova, *The Shrines of Tut-ankh-amon* (New York: Pantheon Books, 1955), 24, quoted in Mircea Eliade, *Gods, Goddesses and Myths of Creation: A Thematic Source Book of the History of Religions* (New York: Harper & Row, 1974), 96–97.

In both the *Pyramid Texts* and the *Book of Overthrowing Apophis* Ra creates by means of his divine body. It is from divine semen that Shu and Tefnut come into being. As the creator is thought of as masculine, the gestation of the god of air and the goddess of mist who are at the origin of the world, takes a peculiar form. Ra pours his semen in his mouth and he gives birth to the first divine couple by spitting them out. With his ironic comment on the whole act that it "seems to have been anatomically possible only for a chief god,"[100] Armour also in a sense points to the core meaning of the story if it is interpreted from the perspective of symbolic patterns of childbirth. On a symbolic level here generation takes place without any female being involved. Woman is not present in the act of the creation of the world, which comes into being by ejaculation and the appropriation of childbirth by the male god.

1.2 The Twelfth Tablet of the Gilgamesh-Epic

The twelfth tablet of the Gilgamesh-Epic may be read as an early example of a text testifying to a supremacy of the male over the female in matters of childbirth. It was added to the rather homogeneous eleven-tablet composition of the Gilgamesh-Epic and mostly consists of an Akkadian translation of the latter part of the Sumerian poem "Bilgames and the Netherworld," dated back to 1800 B.C.[101] Heidel sees a connection to the rest of the epic in the themes of death and afterlife.[102]

In the following, the twelfth tablet of the Gilgamesh-Epic will be commented on from the perspective of symbolic patterns of childbirth. The text assigns more importance to men than to women with regard to the the process of generation. The context is the story of the hero Enkidu going to fetch his friend Gilgamesh's drums after they fell into the underworld. Although Enkidu is kept by the earth goddess among the dead, he is allowed to see Gilgamesh as a spirit again. Gilgamesh asks his friend about the underworld and more precisely about the state of mind of men who had different numbers of sons:

100 See Armour, *Gods and Myths of Ancient Egypt*, 20.

101 *The Babylonian Gilgamesh Epic: Introduction, Critical Edition and Cuneiform Texts*, ed. A. R. George (Oxford: Oxford University Press, 2003), 47–49.

102 See *The Gilgamesh Epic and Old Testament Parallels*, trans. Alexander Heidel, 2nd ed. (Chicago: Chicago University Press, (1949) 1963), 10–12.

(G.) Did you see him who had one son?
(E.) I saw him.
(G.) How does he fare?
(E.) He weeps bitterly at the peg driven into his wall.[103]

(G.) Did you see him who had two sons?
(E.) I saw him.
(G.) How does he fare?
(E.) He sits on two bricks and eats bread.[104]

(G.) Did you see him who had three sons?
(E.) I saw him.
(G.) How does he fare?
(E.) He drinks water from a waterskin kept filled by a youth.

(G.) Did you see him who had four sons?
(E.) I saw him.
(G.) How does he fare?
(E.) He rejoices like a man hitching up a team of four asses.

(G.) Did you see him who had five sons?
(E.) I saw him.
(G.) How does he fare?
(E.) His hand is deft as a master scribe's, he enters the palace directly.

(G.) Did you see him who had six sons?
(E.) I saw him.
(G.) How does he fare?
(E.) He rejoices like a man hitching up his plow.

(G.) Did you see him who had seven sons?
(E.) I saw him.
(G.) How does he fare?
(E.) He sits on a throne with the lesser gods to hear legal proceedings.[105]

In these verses we find that a link is made between a "mortal immortality" and procreation. The text suggests a hierarchy of serenity among the spirits of men who had different numbers of sons. From the weeping man who had procreated only one son, the hierarchy extends to the father of seven sons who is supposed to dwell in the neighbourhood of the gods after his death. He sits on a throne with them. However, the symbolic pattern of

103 Benjamin Foster comments on this verse: "This shows his house has been sold" (see Foster, *The Epic of Gilgamesh*, 138).

104 Benjamin Foster comments on this verse: "His two sons, symbolized by the bricks, maintain his funerary offerings" (see ibid., 139).

105 Ibid., 138–139.

childbirth in the twelfth tablet of the Gilgamesh-Epic is of the kind that bestows a mortal immortality through childbirth exclusively on men. The male body procreating many sons may approach the divine, whereas the female body does not seem to have any access to such an immortality. No verses on the birth-giving woman parallel the verses on procreating men. Thus, what is not said can become as meaningful as what is said. This becomes even more obvious by taking a closer look at the context of the verses quoted above. The verses on men in the underworld who had different numbers of sons are followed by parallelisms drawn between men and women with regard to infertility and people who died young without living their sexuality:

> (G.) Did you see him who has no heir?
> (E.) I saw him.
> (G.) How does he fare?
> (E.) He eats bread hard as a kiln-baked brick....
>
> (G.) Did you see the woman who never gave birth?
> (E.) I saw her.
> (G.) How does she fare?
> (E.) She is discarded like a defective pot, no man takes pleasure in her.
>
> (G.) Did you see the able-bodied young man who did not bare his wife's loins?
> (E.) I saw him.
> (G.) How does he fare?
> (E.) He endlessly knots rope and you see him blubbering over it.[106]
>
> (G.) Did you see the able-bodied young woman who did not bare her husband's loins?
> (E.) I saw her.
> (G.) How does she fare?
> (E.) She endlessly plaits reeds and you see her blubbering over it.[107]

In these verses the absence of generation both in the form of procreation and in the form of giving birth is seen as a disgrace. However, the only mention of giving birth is in the guise of its disgraceful absence on the twelfth tablet of the Gilgamesh-Epic whereby – as illustrated above – the procreation of many sons (symbolically taking place without women) may make men dwell in the neighbourhood of the gods.

---

106 Benjamin Foster comments on this verse: "Because he never untied his wife's clothes, he is doomed to tie knots forever" (Ibid., 140).

107 Ibid., 139–140, verses 296–299 and 304–315.

1.3 Hesiod: On *Anadyomène*

The Greek myth about the birth of the love-goddess Aphrodite resembles the myth of the creation of the world by Ra in that the Greek goddess – just like Shu and Tefnut in the Egyptian myth – exclusively owes her existence to a male divinity. In Hesiod's *Theogony*, dating from the eighth century BC, it is described how the god Kronos overpowers his father Ouranos, the sky. Ouranos refused to allow his children to emerge into the light insisting rather, that they remain in the womb of his wife Gaia, the earth. Kronos dismembers his father using a sickle that Gaia has given him. Aphrodite is then born from the members of Ouranos thrown into the sea:

> But the members themselves, when Kronos
> had lopped them with the flint,
> he threw from the mainland
> into the great wash of the sea water
> and they drifted a great while
> on the open sea, and there spread
> a circle of white foam
> from the immortal flesh, and in it
> grew a girl, whose course first took her
> to holy Kythera,
> and from there she afterward made her way
> to sea-washed Cyprus
> and stepped ashore, a modest lovely Goddess,
> and about her
> light and slender feet the grass grew,
> and the gods call her
> Aphrodite, and men do too,
> and the aphro-foam-born
> goddess, and garlanded Kythereia,
> because from the sea-foam
> she grew, and Kythereia because she had gone
> to Kythera,
> and Kyprogeneia, because she came forth
> from wave-washed Cyprus,
> and Philommedea, because she appeared
> from medea members.[108]

---

108 Hesiod, *The Works and Days, Theogony, The Shield of Herakles*, trans. Richmond Lattimore (1959; reprint, Ann Arbor, MI: The University of Michigan Press, 1991), 134–135.

As in the Ancient Egyptian myth of Ra creating the world, a male divinity procreates from and with his genitals only, without a female force being present. In the case of Aphrodite this becomes particularly meaningful because, according to Hesiod's verses, Aphrodite would be older than all the other Olympian gods who came to power with Zeus, the son of Kronos. Walter Burkert explains the extraordinary status of Aphrodite in Ancient Greece as follows:

> At the very first cosmic differentiation, the separation of heaven and earth, the power of union also emerged. Aphrodite is thereby caught up in a tradition of cosmogonic speculation which continued to be richly exploited through Orpheus down to Parmenides and Empedocles: begetting and the mingling of love is what drives the world onwards.[109]

Seeing Aphrodite as "what drives the world onwards" lets the fact that she is derived from the genitals of Ouranos appear in a special light. The peculiar way in which she is generated exclusively from her father may thus be read as symbolically ensuring male supremacy over the life-perpetuating principle itself.

1.4 Genesis: Woman of Man Born

In *Genesis*, as in the Egyptian myth of creation, man replaces woman with regard to birthgiving. While Ra both procreates and gives birth to the world without the help of a woman, in Gen. 2:21–23, man with the help of divine intervention gives birth to the first woman:

> So the LORD God caused a deep sleep to fall upon the man, and he slept; then he took one of his ribs and closed up its place with flesh.
> And the rib that the LORD God had taken from the man he made into a woman and brought her to the man.
> Then the man said,
> "This at last is bone of my bones
> and flesh of my flesh;
> this one shall be called Woman

109 Walter Burkert: *Greek Religion*, trans. John Raffan (Cambridge, Mass.: Harvard University Press, 1985), 154.

> for out of Man this one was
> taken."

The fact that in *Genesis* Eve is born from Adam's rib, means to Erich Fromm that "even the natural course of events that women give birth to men, is reversed."[110] Actually, such a symbolic reversal of the order of things constitutes a way of appropriating the female generational capacities to the male. Eve, the first woman whose name means "the living"[111] derives from Adam. The very origin of the perpetuation of human life is thus constructed as male and not as female.

1.5 The Genealogies of the Old Testament and of Prophet Muhammad

It is in the genealogies of the patriarchs from Adam to Noah, in Genesis 5, that we encounter still more symbolic exclusions of the woman from childbirth:

> And Adam lived a hundred thirty years, and begot a son in his own likeness, after his image; and called his name Seth ….
> And Seth lived a hundred and five years, and begot Enos ….
> And Enos lived ninety years, and begot Cainan.[112]

The patriarchs are symbolically born of no woman. It is mostly the male body that is attached to the births of children. Men are strongly identified with procreation. By this the father and the first-born son are thereby intimately linked to one another. Furthermore, there is a caesura in a

110 See Erich Fromm, *The Forgotten Language: An Introduction to the Understanding of Dreams, Fairy Tales and Myths* (1951; reprint, New York: Grove Press, 1957), 234.

111 See Othmar Keel and Silvia Schroer, *Eva – Mutter alles Lebendigen: Frauen- und Göttinnenidole aus dem Alten Orient,* 2nd ed. (Fribourg, Switzerland: Academic Press Fribourg Schweiz, 2006), 10.

112 This is not the only construction of childbirth in Genesis. "In between" the birth of Eve from Adam and the procreation of patriarchs in Gen. 5:3, Eve gives birth to Cain and to Abel (Gen. 4:1–2). This quote and the following quotes are from the King James Bible because the translations of these passages in the King James Bible are more literal than the ones of the "New Oxford Annotated Bible." I am grateful to Sonja Ammann for her advice on this matter.

patriarch's lifetime brought about by the birth of the first son because the lifetime of every patriarch is counted by tallying up the years before and the years after he has procreated his male successor. This caesura in a patriarch's lifetime may be read as a symbolic expression of the patriarch's access to a new beginning by procreation:

> And Adam lived a hundred thirty years, and begot a son in his own likeness, after his image; and called his name Seth ….
>
> And the days of Adam after he had begotten Seth were eight hundred years: and he begot sons and daughters.
>
> And all the days that Adam lived were nine hundred and thirty years: and he died.
> And Seth lived after he begot Enos eight hundred and seven years, and begot sons and daughters.
>
> And all the days of Seth were nine hundred twelve years; and he died.
> And Enos lived ninety years, and begot Cainan.
>
> Enos lived after he begot Cainan eight hundred and fifteen years, and begot sons and daughters.
>
> And all the days of Enos were ninehundred and five years: and he died.

A similar pattern of attributing sons to men only, without mentioning women, appears in the list of names of sons, e.g. of Ishmael (Gen. 25:13), of Jacob (Gen. 46:8), of Reuben (Gen. 46:9), of Levi (Gen. 46:11) and of Juda (Gen. 46:12). Also in the king lists in Gen. 36:31–39 there is mention of the fathers of kings but not of the mothers.

Though "the supremacy of the male" establishing strong links between fathers and sons is by far the dominant symbolic pattern of childbirth in Genesis, birthgiving women are not all together absent from the genealogical lines. Thus for example in Genesis 36:4 it says: "Adah bore Eliphaz to Esau; Bashemath bore Reuel." Genesis 25:1–2 reads: "Abraham took another wife, whose name was Keturah. She bore him Zimran, Jokshan, Medan, Midian, Ishbak, and Shuah." However, thereafter the text immediately switches back to the dominant symbolic pattern of childbirth found in other parts of Genesis. Thus "Jokshan was the father of Sheba, and Dedan. The sons of Dedan were Asshurim, Letushim, and Leummim" (Gen. 25:3).

In Islam, the genealogies of Prophet Muhammad follow the same principle as the dominant scheme of the genealogies of the Old Testament. Syed Ahmed Khan Bahador identifies five authors who attempted to write a genealogy for Muhammad: Baihakee, Ibn Hisham[113], Ibn Arabee, Barookhh and Jerah.[114]

The first three genealogists traced the genealogy of Mohammed down from Abraham to Moid, son of Adnan. They all adopted the same system of giving the names of sons originating from their fathers, e.g.: "Adnan, son of Adad, son of Sam, son of Yashab" and so forth.

Barookh and Jerah operated with a different system resembling the genealogies found in the Old Testament – by making reference to procreation. Starting with Abraham, they set up long chains of fathers who procreate their sons: "Abraham begat Ishmael, and Ishmael begat Kedar, and Kedar begat Awam, and Awam begat Aws" and so on.

However, independently of the way in which fathers and sons are linked to one another, the genealogical lines of Baihakee, Ibni Hisham, Ibn Arabee, Barookhh and Jerah function through the exclusion of women: men procreate, or are procreated, but they are not born.

1.6 Mimesis: The Births of Athena and Dionysos

Up to now the texts that have been chosen to illustrate the first symbolic pattern of childbirth have all followed a similar logic. The supremacy of the male over the female in relation to childbirth was expressed in terms of the male body. Male generational power was considered to be at the origin of the world (Ra), at the origin of a cosmic principle (Ouranos), at the origin of (important) men (the genealogies of the Old Testament and of prophet Muhammad, the Gilgamesh Epic) and at the origin of humanity (Eve born from Adam's rib). The Greek myth of the births of Athena and Dionysos represents a different mode of symbolically manifesting the generational supremacy of the male over the female. As will

113 I will treat Ibn Hisham in depth in section 10 of "The Supremacy of the Male."

114 See Syed Ahmed Khan Bahador, *Essays on the Life of Mohammed and Subjects Subsidiary Thereto* (1870; reprint, Delhi, India: Idarah-i Adabiyat-i Delli, 1991), 4–8.

be shown in the following, in case of the births of Athena and Dionysos, Zeus by an act of mimesis, appropriates female generational potency to himself.[115]

1.6.1 Dionysos

There are many references to the myth of the birth of Dionysos. However, here two of the most complete versions, namely that of Apollodorus in his *Library*, most probably written in the middle of the first century B.C., and that of the *Metamorphoses* of Ovid, written between the years 1–8 C.E. will be presented. The account of Apollodorus runs as follows:

> But Zeus loved Semele and bedded with her unknown to Hera. Now Zeus had agreed to do for her whatever she asked, and deceived by Hera she asked that he would come to her as he came when he was wooing Hera. Unable to refuse, Zeus came to her bridal chamber in a chariot, with lightnings and thunderings, and launched a thunderbolt. But Semele expired of fright, and Zeus, snatching the sixth-month abortive child from the fire, sewed it in his thigh. On the death of Semele the other daughters of Cadmus spread a report that Semele had bedded with a mortal man, and had falsely accused Zeus, and that therefore she had been blasted by thunder. But at the proper time Zeus undid the stitches and gave birth to Dionysos.[116]

Ovid's version of the birth of Dionysos is essentially the same as that of Apollodorus. The verses relating to the death of Semele and the birth of her son run as follows:

> Then her mortal frame
> Could not endure the tumult of the heavens;
> That gift of love consumed her. From her womb
> Her baby, still not fully formed, was snatched,
> And sewn (could one believe the tale) inside
> His father's thigh, and so completed there
> His mother's time.[117]

115 See Adriana Cavarero, *Nonostante Platone: Figure femminili nella filosofia antica* (Roma: Editori Riuniti, 1990), 110.

116 Apollodorus, *The Library*, trans. Sir James George Frazer (1921; reprint, Cambridge, Mass.: Harvard University Press, 1939), III. IV. 3.

117 Ovid, *Metamorphoses*, trans. A. D. Melville, with an introduction and notes by E. J. Kenney (Oxford and New York: Oxford University Press, 1986), III. 311–317.

In the myth of the birth of Dionysos we encounter a "mimesis of maternity,"[118] as Adriana Cavarero puts it. In fact, after Zeus has procreated Dionysos in Semele, all the subsequent stages of female generational activity are reproduced in mimetic acts. The conception of Dionysos takes place through the snatching of the child from Semele's womb; the pregnancy in the thigh follows. Afterwards, the undoing of the stitches can be considered as the period of labour followed by birthgiving. In fact, Ovid writes about Dionysos as of a "babe twice born." In her interpretation of the myth, Adriana Cavarero insists on the fact that in order to appropriate female generational power for himself Zeus has to kill. It is only after Semele's death that he can take over the maternal role. In the myth of the birth of Athene a similar pattern will be encountered.

1.6.2 Athena

There are several sources for the story of the birth of Athena. The oldest version comes from the *Theogony* of Hesiod. Here the myth runs as follows: Zeus swallows his first wife Metis out of fear that she could give birth to a son capable of overpowering his father:

> Zeus, as King of the gods,
> took as his first wife Metis,
> and she knew more than all the gods
> or mortal people.
> But when she was about to be delivered
> of the goddess, gray-eyed
> Athene, then Zeus, deceiving her perception
> by treachery
> and by slippery speeches,
> put her away inside his own belly.
> This was by the advices of Gaia,
> and stormy Ouranos,
> for so they counseled,
> in order that no other everlasting
> god, beside Zeus, should ever be given
> the kingly position.
> for it had been arranged that, from her,
> children surpassing in wisdom
> should be born, first the gray-eyed girl,

118 Cavarero, *Nonostante Platone*, 110.

> the Tritogeneai
> Athene; and she is the equal of her father
> in wise counsel
> and strength; but then a son to be King
> over gods and mortals
> was to be born of her, and his heart
> would be overmastering:
> but before this, Zeus put her away
> inside his own belly.[119]

Several verses on from this account, Hesiod writes about the birth of Athena: "Then from his head, by himself, / he [Zeus] produced Athene of the gray eyes."[120] Apollodorus and Pindar both add some details to the story of the birth of Athene. They introduce the figure of Hephaistos[121] who fulfils the function of a midwife. Apollodorus writes: "And when the time came for the birth to take place, Prometheus or, as others say, Hephaestus, smote the head of Zeus with an axe, and Athene, fully armed, leaped up from the top of his head at the river Triton."[122] The description of the birth of Athene by Pindar is very similar to that of Apollodorus. In the *Olympian Odes* we find the following lines: "By the cunning craft of Hephaestus, at the stroke of the brazen hatchet, Athene leapt forth upon the crest of her father's head, and cried aloud with a mighty shout, while Heaven and Mother Earth trembled befor her."[123]

The myth of the birth of Athene structurally resembles the myth of the birth of Dionysos. This is because of the fact that here again, step by step, the different aspects of female fertility are imitated and coupled with a matricide. In case of the Dionysos myth, Zeus fulminates Semele, and in the case of the Athene myth, the chief god swallows up Metis, before her maternal powers can unfold. In both cases the pregnancy of Zeus follows the killing of the mother, which in case of Metis is planned and in case of Semele is depicted as an accident due to a complicated interplay of love and jealousy. With regard to the birth of Athene the mimesis of female

---

119 Hesiod, *Theogony*, trans. Richmond Lattimore, 886–899.

120 Ibid., 924.

121 Apollodorus does not make up his mind between Hephaistos and Prometheus for the midwife like function during the birth of Athene. See Apollodorus, *The Library*, I., 3, 6.

122 Ibid.

123 Pindar, *The Odes of Pindar*, trans. Sir John Sandys, 2nd ed. (1915; reprint, Cambridge, Mass.: Harvard University Press, 1968), VII, 34–45.

generational activity is even more evident, because pregnancy takes place in Zeus' belly-a more explicit allusion to the female uterus than Zeus' thigh in the Dionysos myth. Athene's birth is woven even deeper into a symbolic pattern of childbirth that enhances the supremacy of the male over the female, as Zeus is given a male midwife to be helped while he gives birth. The violence in the imagery of Hephaistos, the god of craftsmen, splitting Zeus' head, recalls the general violence of the story, which is necessary for the transfer of female generational potency to the male.

1.7 The Semen and the Stars: Aristotle's *De Generatione Animalium* and the Gender of *Pneuma*

The previous examples that were used to illustrate the first symbolic pattern of childbirth, "The Supremacy of the Male," demonstrate a superiority defined in terms of physiology, or of a mimesis of physiology. The man's procreational activity was considered to be more important than pregnancy and birthgiving on the side of the woman, or pregnancy and giving birth were mimetically performed by the male. With Aristotle's *De Generatione Animalium* we move towards a "spiritual" supremacy of the male over the female with regard to childbirth. As early as the Gilgamesh-Epic, proximity of the male fertile body to the gods is alluded to (should a man have many sons). Aristotle philosophically elaborates upon such a *rapprochement* of the divine and the human male through procreation. In *De Generatione Animalium*, he gives precise reasons as to why male procreational activity is more spiritual than that of the female. His version of the symbolic pattern of childbirth, which is characterized by a supremacy of the male over the female, may be read as being informed by what Karl Jaspers called the culture of the axial age (*Achsenzeit*).

In 1949, Karl Jaspers published his book *The Origin and Goal of History*[124] (*Vom Ursprung und Ziel der Geschichte*[125]) where he introduced the term "axial age." Jaspers assumes that in different parts of the world

124 Karl Jaspers, *The Origin and Goal of History*, trans. Michael Bullock (London: Routledge, 1953).

125 Karl Jaspers, *Vom Ursprung und Ziel der Geschichte* (München: Piper, 1949).

(India, China, Iran, Palestine, Greece), between 800 and 200 BC, cultural processes took place which had a long-lasting influence.[126] According to Jaspers, the ideas of a need for salvation and a transcendence of one's bodily existence, go back to the axial age.[127]

Shmuel Eisenstadt, who elaborates on Jaspers' work, defines the axial age civilizations as civilizations "in which there is an emphasis on the chasm between the transcendental and the mundane order and a conception of a higher moral or metaphysical order."[128] In contrast to axial age civilizations, pre-axial societies can be understood as "societies in which the mundane and transmundane worlds are defined in relatively homologous terms." In the pre-axial age, the "search for immortality is on the whole envisaged in terms of some physical continuity. It is usually seen as conditional to the fulfillment of one's concrete obligation to one's group."[129]

With these ideas on the axial age in mind, one could argue that Aristotle relates the axial age chasm between the transcendental and the mundane to gender. The mundane aspect of generation is attached to the female body while the spiritual element in procreation comes from the male. Additionally, Aristotelian thinking splits male semen itself in material and spiritual parts. How this exactly works will be shown in the following analysis of *De Generatione Animalium.*

De Generatione Animalium was written with other zoological works, namely, the *Historia Animalium* and *De Partibus Animalium* between the years 347 and 335 BC.[130] In Aristotle's writing there is a pattern, frequently found in philosophy, that Hilde Hein highlighted: "Where male and female are opposed, spirituality is derivatively affirmed of the one and denied of the other."[131] With regard to Aristotle, as will be shown in the following, it is the female generational activity that is to be de-spiritualized.

On the first pages of *De Generatione Animalium* Aristotle clearly places the male and the female in opposition to each other. He states that

---

126 See ibid., 19–20.

127 See ibid., 22, 33.

128 S. N. Eisenstadt, ed., *The Origins and Diversity of Axial Age Civilisations* (New York: SUNY Press, 1986), 3.

129 Ibid.

130 Arthur Leslie Peck, introduction to *Generation of Animals*, by Aristotle (1942; reprint, Cambridge, Mass.: Harvard University Press, 1979), viii.

131 Hilde Hein, "Liberating Philosophy: An End to the Dichotomy of Spirit and Matter," in *Beyond Domination: New Perspectives on Women and Philosophy*, ed. Carol Gould (Totowa, NJ: Rowman & Allanheld, 1984), 124.

“they differ in their *logos*, because the male is that which has the power to generate in another […], while the female is that which can generate in itself, i.e., it is that out of which the generated offspring, which is present in the generator, comes into being.”[132] The male possesses the principle of movement and of generation while the female possesses the principle of matter.[133] That this dualism, like all dualisms, implies a hierarchy is evident right from the outset of *De Generatione Animalium*. In as much as the male is in possession of a principle of movement, the male body is already associated with the divine, because the principle of movement (*kinesis*) refers linguistically to the “unmoved mover,” who is the divine origin of all life in Aristotelian thought. Meanwhile the female’s principle of matter has no relation to the divine whatsoever. As Hilde Hein points out,[134] matter must, in fact, not necessarily stand in opposition to spirituality. This has already been shown by the examples of the Gilgamesh-Epic, the creation of the world by Ra and the genealogies of the Old Testament, where the male body was attached to the divine through its physical activity of procreation, thereby securing man access to mortal immortality. However, in Aristotle’s writings such a mortal immortality is only possible by rendering the male body as non-physical as possible and the female body as physical as possible. This is done by his theory on the nature of semen.

Aristotle defines semen as “residue” which means that it is left over as surplus from useful nourishment.[135] Furthermore, in Aristotle’s reasoning, in blooded animals, blood must be considered as the final form of nourishment, and semen as concocted blood. Now, according to Aristotle, males and females both produce “residues” for generation; in the case of the female this is menstrual fluid and in the case of the male it is semen. However, the difference between these two types of residues is one of quality. The female, “weaker creature […] produces a residue, greater in amount and less thoroughly concocted.”[136] The result is that menstrual fluid can be considered only as a kind of “semen, not indeed semen in a pure condition, but needing still to be acted upon.”[137] Aristotele thus defines the female

132 Aristotle, *Generation of Animals*, trans. Arthur Leslie Peck (1942; reprint, Cambridge, Mass.: Harvard University Press, 1979) I., II., 716a, 20–25.

133 See ibid., 716a, 1–7.

134 See Hein, *Liberating Philosophy*, 128–129, 135–137.

135 See Aristotle, *Generation of Animals*, 725a.

136 Ibid., 726b 30–34.

137 Ibid., 728a 26–28.

by a deficiency: "Woman is as it were an infertile male; the female, in fact, is female on account of inability of a sort, viz., it lacks the power to concoct semen out of the final state of the nourishment."[138] The ultimate reason for the inability of the female to produce semen lies with the heart. "All concoction works by means of heat"[139] and the part of the body possessing the principle of natural heat is the heart.[140] Aristotle's statement that "male animals are hotter than female ones"[141] points to a difference between the sexes in relation to the heart.

However, what is interesting in the context of the first symbolic pattern of childbirth, are the details of this opposition between menstrual fluid and male semen. Apart from assigning an inferior state of concoction to menstrual fluid, Aristotle specifies, "the male provides the 'form' and the 'principle of movement', the female provides the body, in other words, the material."[142] Furthermore, Aristotle makes the association between male and active, and female and passive. The male is the "active partner, the one which originates the movement" while the "female [is] the passive one."[143] To fully understand the meaning of these most famous statements of *De Generatione Animalium* one has to take a closer look at the Aristotelian conception of movement (*kinesis*) which, together with the ideas of soul (*psyche*), *dynamis* and *pneuma* forms a complex system. In the end it is these four categories and their interplay that bring the male closer to the divine than the female. How does each part of that system work?

First of all, the term *kinesis* (movement) is used exclusively in relation to the male. *Kinesis* is one of the Aristotelian categories of change (*metabole*).[144] While genesis is the change from non-existence to existence and death is the change from existence to non-existence, *kinesis* circumscribes change in existing things. There are three types of *kinesis*, namely quantitative, qualitative and locomotive *kinesis*. As has been pointed out already, linguistically this term evokes the divine in its description of the "unmoved mover," the ungenerated source of all being, the ultimate source of all movement. "The first principle and primary reality is immovable,

138 Ibid., 728a 17–20.
139 Ibid., 765b 15–17.
140 See ibid., 766a 34–37.
141 Ibid., 765b 18–19.
142 Ibid., 729a 10–13.
143 Ibid., 729a 27–30.
144 See for the following Arthur Leslie Peck, *Introduction*, lix–lx.

both essentially and accidentally, but it excites the primary form of motion [*kinesis*], which is one and eternal."[145] In *De Generatione Animalium* it is said that the male semen contains *kinesis* and that this movement stands in close relationship to Soul: "Now semen, and the movement and principle which it contains, are such that, as the movement ceases each one of the parts gets formed and acquires Soul."[146] Here it is important to specify that in Aristotelian thinking there are different types of Soul – nutritive, sentient, appetitive, locomotive and rational Soul.[147] Female matter is considered to possess nutritive Soul[148] whereas the male is related to sentient soul and rational soul. Aristotle writes: "Thus, if the male is the factor which produces the sentient Soul, in cases where male and female are separate, it is impossible for the female all by itself and from itself to generate an animal; because the faculty just mentioned is the essence of what is meant by 'male.'"[149]

The male is not only linked to sentient Soul but is also closely associated with rational Soul. This again places him in the proximity of the divine, because rational soul is the part of Soul which continues to exist after the death of the body. Aristotle states that rational soul comes "to be formed within the male from some outside source."[150] How does this process take place exactly? To explain the link between rational/sentient Soul and semen, Aristotle introduces the category of *pneuma* which is the vehicle allowing Soul to function through the body. *Pneuma* can be defined as "the corporeal substance with which the sort of Form known as Soul is specially and regularly connected."[151] *Pneuma* also stands in a close relationship to *kinesis*. Peck puts it like this: "It is this *pneuma* and the substance in the *pneuma*, which is the vehicle of Soul, and it is *pneuma* which Soul uses as its 'instrument,' through which it brings about kinesis both in moving the full-grown body and in 'moving' i.e., developing the embryo."[152]

---

145 Aristotle, *The Metaphysics*, trans. Hugh Tredennick (Cambridge, Mass.: Harvard University Press, 1962), XII, 1073a 23–26.

146 Ibid., 734b 23–25.

147 See Aristotle, *On the Soul*, trans. W. S. Hett (1936; reprint, Cambridge, Mass.: Harvard University Press, 1975).

148 See Aristotle, *Generation of Animals*, 736a 32–37, 737a 23–33.

149 Ibid., 741a 14–20.

150 Ibid., 736b 20–23.

151 Peck, xiii.

152 Ibid., lix.

Aristotle accentuates the divine nature of the *pneuma* contained in semen by making an analogy between *aither*, the fifth element, and *pneuma*. In *De Caelo* (On the Heavens), Aristotle writes on *aither*: "From all these premises therefore it clearly follows that there exists some physical substance besides the four in our sublunary world, and moreover that it is more divine than, and prior to, all these."[153] *Aither* is considered to be "ungenerated and indestructible, and susceptible neither to growth nor alteration,"[154] and it contains the heavenly bodies, the sun, the moon and the stars. Finally, Aristotle describes the analogy between *aither* and the *pneuma* contained in semen as follows:

> The faculty of Soul of every kind has to do with some physical substance which is different from the so-called "elements" and more divine than they are; and as the varieties of Soul differ from one another in the scale of value, so do the various substances concerned with them differ in their nature. In all cases the semen contains within itself that which causes it to be fertile – what is known as 'hot' substance, which is not fire nor any similar substance, but the pneuma which is enclosed within the semen or foam-like stuff, and the natural substance which is in the pneuma; and this substance is analogous to the element which belongs to the stars.[155]

Apart from the fact that the female lacks *kinesis* and *pneuma* – which is the reason why only the male can transmit sentient/rational soul to the embryo – she also lacks *dynamis*. *Dynamis* means the capacity to do, the potency, and it is linked exclusively to male semen: "The male does not emit any part such as will remain situated within the fetus, but begets the young animal simply by means of the dynamis residing in the semen."[156] Peck points to the fact that the *dynamis* is regularly associated with the male while the female is defined by a lack of *dynamis*.[157]

The "spiritualization" of the male body by means of the concepts of *kinesis,* rational soul, *pneuma* and *dynamis* is carried further by a "decorporealisation" of the semen. Aristotle insists on the fact that the contribution of the male to the fetation is of a purely spiritual nature: "The secretion from the male provides no material at all for the creatures which

153 Aristotle, *On the Heavens*, trans. W. K. C. Guthrie (1939; reprint, Cambridge, Mass.: Harvard University Press, 1971), 269a, 31–33.

154 Ibid., 270a 13–15.

155 Aristotle, *Generation of Animals*, 736b 30–737a.

156 Ibid., 730a 1–3.

157 See Peck, *Introduction*, lii.

get formed."[158] He argues that "there is no necessity for any substance to pass from the male; and if any does pass, this does not mean that the offspring is formed from it as from something situated within itself during the process, but as from that which has imparted movement to it, or that which is its 'form.'"[159]

Aristotle continues to elaborate his ideas on the non-physicality of the male body by stating that the physical part of the semen evaporates after fetation is set. In this sense, it is useless to try to detect it.[160] Aristotle's division of the semen into physical and non-physical parts can be seen as a transposition of the axial age gap between the spiritual and the mundane into the realm of male procreation. The gap cuts right through the male body.[161] In other words, as the body is generally associated with the mundane ("physical activity has nothing whatever to do with the activity of reason"[162]), male semen has to be at least partially disembodied in order to become a transmitter of rational soul, by which it is connected to the divine. Reason as such is considered to be divine in its opposition to matter.[163]

Up to this point, my main concern has been to show how Aristotle associates the male procreating body with spirituality and the female procreating body with matter, and that in this way he proclaims the supremacy of the male over the female in relation to childbirth. Perhaps one of his most explicit statements in the setting up of such hierarchies combined with normative judgements, is the following:

> And as the proximate motive cause, to which belong the *logos* and the Form, is better and more divine in its nature than the Matter, it is better also that the superior one should be separate from the inferior one. That is why wherever possible and so far as possible the male is separate from the female, since it is something better and more

158 Aristotle, *Generation of Animals,* 764b 10–13.

159 Ibid., 729b 19–24.

160 Ibid., 737a 11–17: "This physical part of the semen, being fluid and watery, dissolves and evaporates; and on that account we should not always be trying to detect it leaving the female externally, or to find it as an ingredient of the fetation when that has set and taken shape, any more than we should expect to trace the fig-juice which sets and curdles milk. The fig-juice undergoes a change; it does not remain as a part of the bulk which is set and curdled; and the same applies to the semen."

161 Further on, the symbolic pattern of childbirth attached to Mary will show that the axial age gap may also cut through the female body (see section III.4.3.).

162 Ibid., 736 26–29.

163 See ibid.

> divine in that it is the principle of movement for generated things, while the female serves as their matter. The male, however, comes together with the female and mingles with it for the business of generation, because this is something that concerns both of them.[164]

Although the sentences quoted above could very well be considered the quintessence of the Aristotelian position on childbirth, it should not go unmentioned that Aristotle himself did try to bridge his gendered spirit-matter dichotomy. While maintaining the hierarchies he admits that, after all, male and female, viz., form and matter, cannot be strictly separated from each other:

> After all, the carpenter is close by his timber, and the potter close by his clay; and to put it in general terms, the working or treatment of any material, and the ultimate movement which acts upon it, is in all cases close by the material, e. g., the location of the activity of house-building is in the houses which are being built.[165]

Peck links this passage from *De Generatione Animalium* to the last section of Aristotle's *Metaphysica* where Aristotle writes that Matter in its ultimate stage is identical with Form.[166] However, this type of thought does not dominante *De Generatione Animalium* and even where there is a bridge between the two, the chasm continues to separate male and female, divine and matter, *pneuma* and the physical part of the semen, the transcendental and the mundane. Through the conception of a chasm of this type, on an ideological level, the woman plays a minor part in generation and thus gains less access to the mortal immortality attached to it. Here it is important to specify that Aristotle identifies generation as a means of approaching the divine very explicitly. In *De Anima* (On the Soul), he writes on nutritive soul that "its functions are reproduction and the assimilation of food," and he continues his thoughts by stating that reproduction is a way of partaking of mortal immortality:

> For this is the most natural of all functions among living creatures, provided that they are perfect and not maimed, and do not have spontaneous generation: viz., to reproduce one's kind, an animal producing an animal, and a plant a plant, in order that they may have a share in the immortal and divine in the only way they can; for every creature strives for this, and for the sake of this performs all natural functions. "That for

164 Ibid., 732a 3–12.
165 Ibid., 730b 3–9.
166 See Peck, *Introduction*, xii.

the sake of which" has two meanings: (1) that for the purpose of which, and (2) that for the benefit of which. Since, then, they cannot share in the immortal and divine by continuity of existence, because no perishable thing can remain numerically one and the same, they share in these in the only way they can, some to a greater and some to a lesser extent; what persistes is not the individual itself, but something in its image, identical not numerically but specifically.[167]

In *De Generatione Animalium* Aristotle again associates generation with mortal immortality: "There are the causes on account of which generation of animals takes place, because since the nature of a class of this sort is unable to be eternal, that which comes into being is eternal in the manner that is open to it."[168]

Thus, as has been shown, generation, in Aristotelian thinking, is a means to approach the divine. However, right from the start, some bodies are closer to the divine than others. More precisely, the male generational residue contains the *pneuma* (upon which the divine can act in order to transmit rational soul), while the female is associated with matter which remains unconnected to the divine. In this sense, the male has a greater share of the mortal immortality that comes with the generation of children. By way of the *pneuma* contained in his semen he contributes the more important part to the formation of the fetus. *Pneuma* is linked to the divine because it is analogous to aither, the fifth element, the element of the stars.

Far into late antiquity, *De Generatione Animalium* exercised a lot of influence over the understanding of generation. Traces of *De Generatione Animalium* can also be found in gnostic thought[169] and in the Middle Ages it became the leading text on generation.[170] Until the discovery of the ovum by William Harvey in the 17th century, the Aristotelian theory of generation was widely accepted. The reception and the dominance of Aristotle's theory of generation is a prominent example of how issues of power and gender relations may be linked to symbolic patterns of

167 Aristotle, *On the Soul*, II, 415a, 25–34.

168 Aristotle, *Generation of Animals,* 731b 30–34.

169 See e.g. Hippolytus' summary of the ideas of the gnostic thinker Simon Magus on the different contributions of men and women to generation. Hippolytus, *Philosophumena or the Refutation of All Heresies*, trans. F. Legge (New York: The Macmillan Company, 1921), VI.17.

170 This was due to a chain of translations. The Arabic translation by the physician Ibn al-Batriq dates from the 9th century. Michael Scot then translated the text from Arabic into Latin around 1217 and thereby made it accessible to the Europe of the Middle Ages (See Peck, *Introduction*, xi and xx).

childbirth, considering that already in the second century C.E. the scholar Galen maintained that the female also contained seed.[171] Aristotle did not only prevail over Galen in antiquity, but also when Galen's theory was conveyed to Europe via the Arabs in the 14th century, it was not received with enthusiasm. Indeed, a Spanish physician of the 16th century wrote about Galen's theory that, if it was true, it should be kept secret from women lest they become "all the more arrogant by knowing that they [...] not only suffer the pain of having to nourish the child within their bodies [...] but also that they too put something of their own into it."[172]

One of the most prominent followers of Aristotle in the Middle Ages was Thomas Aquinas. As will be shown in chapter nine of this section, in his *Summa Theologica* he re-elaborated the Aristotelian theory of the supremacy of the male over the female in matters of childbirth. However, to better understand Thomas Aquinas it is necessary to first take a closer look at the conception of childbirth in the writings of Tertullian and Augustine.

1.8 Foundations for a "Dubious" Supremacy of the Male: Tertullian and Augustine on the Transmission of Original Sin

The previous examples chosen to illustrate the supremacy of the male in matters of childbirth had rather positive connotations. That man could symbolically appropriate the female generational forces to himself, or simply, could be seen as more important with regard to the generation of new life, did not constitute a problematic fact.

However, in some strands of Christian thought, the Aristotelian idea of male semen transmitting soul was fused with the idea of original sin because original sin was conceived of as being transmitted by the soul. As will be shown in the following chapter, Thomas Aquinas discussed this topic in depth. However, it was the early Christian thinkers such as Tertullian and

171 See Frances Gies and Joseph Gies, *Women in the Middle Ages* (New York: Crowell, 1978), 50–52.

172 I. de Valverde, *Historia de la composicion del cuerpo humano*, Rome 1556, quoted in Julia O'Faolain and Lauro Martines, *Not in God's Image: Women in History from Greeks to Victorians* (Lonon: Virago, 1973), 121–122.

Augustine who laid the foundations for the transformation of the Aristotelian supremacy of the male in matters of childbirth into what can be described as a "dubious" supremacy. In the following, the main focus will be on Tertullian's *De Anima* and on Augustine's *Anti-Pelagian Writings*.

De Anima was composed around 210 C. E.[173] and is mainly intended as a response to Platonic and gnostic theories about the soul. Tertullian does not agree with gnostic thinkers such as Marcion, Valentine, Simon Magus and Carpocrates, who rely on the strict, hierarchical Platonic division of body and soul that informed the gnostic conception of sin. As Martino Menghi states with regard to Valentinian gnosis, the central idea here is that human beings sin because of the body and not because of the soul. Thus, if one succeeds in freeing oneself from one's material part with the help of *gnosis*, one does not sin.[174]

In *De Anima* Tertullian takes an altogether different standpoint. To him it is not the body but the soul which is capable of sinning, given that he understands the body as an instrument of the soul.[175] In addition to inverting gnostic theory, by claiming that it is the soul and not the body which sins, Tertullian differs from Platonic and gnostic thought on the coming into existence of both body and soul. This then necessarily leads to the question of his attitude towards childbirth. Plato and the gnostics see souls as ungenerated. That is to say, in their view the souls reside in the Hyperuranium from whence they descend to earth and are incorporated into the newborn with the first breath after birth. Tertullian's ideas contrast

173 See Mario Vegetti, introduction to *L'anima*, by Tertullian, ed. Martino Menghi (Venezia: Marsilio Editori, 1988), 22.

174 See Tertullian, *L'anima*, ed. Martino Menghi (Venezia: Marsilio Editori, 1988), 244.

175 Tertullian, *On the Soul*, 40.2–3: "Now although the flesh is sinful … yet the flesh has not such ignominy on its own account. For it is not of itself that it thinks anything or feels anything for the purpose of advising or commanding sin. How should it, indeed? It is only a ministering thing, and its ministration is not like that of a servant or familiar friend – animated and human beings; but rather that of a vessel, or something of that kind: it is body, not soul. Now a cup may minister to a thirsty man; and yet, if the thirsty man will not apply the cup to his mouth, the cup will yield no ministering service. Therefore the differentia, or distinguishing property, of man by no means lies in his earthly element; nor is the flesh the human person, as being some faculty of his soul, and a personal quality; but it is a thing of quite a different substance and different condition, although annexed to the soul as a chattel or as an instrument for the offices of life." The here exposed idea of the innocence of the flesh will be developed by Thomas Aquinas with regard to Mary and the question of why Jesus was conceived without sin.

this sharply. According to *De Anima* the soul is not only generated, but moreover both soul and body are seen right from the beginning as being in close union. The soul derives from the breath of God, which was bestowed upon Adam ("From the breath of God first came the soul"[176]). Both the soul substance and the body substance are at work with the creation of the first man: "Forasmuch, therefore, as these two different and separate substances, the clay and the breath, combined at the first creation in forming the individual man, they then both amalgamated and mixed their proper seminal rudiments in one."[177]

Tertullian does not limit himself to theorizing about the coming into existence of the first man, but also develops precise ideas regarding generation in general. This is where we encounter the idea of the supremacy of the male over the female in matters of childbirth in *De Anima*. Tertullian imagines that what God transmitted to Adam is then transmitted by Adam to the human species. To put it more concretely, the male semen is the carrier of both the body and the soul substance. In this logic, Tertullian writes:

> Even now the two substances, although diverse from each other, flow forth simultaneously in a united channel; and finding their way together into their appointed seed-plot, they fertilize with their combined vigour the human fruit out of their respective natures. And inherent in this human product is his own seed, according to the process which has been ordained for every creature endowed with the functions of generation. Accordingly from the one [primeval] man comes the entire outflow and redundance of men's souls.[178]

In terms of generation Adam is the "matrix" of humanity. Men (in the literal sense of the word) are connected back to that origin and therefore become the transmitter of life, whereas woman in *De Anima* is seen as the vessel for making new life grow:

> [The] soul [of the human being] (which may be compared with the nascent sprout of a tree) has been derived from Adam as its root, and has been propagated amongst his posterity by means of woman's generative organs, to which it has been entrusted for transmission, and thus has sprouted into life with all its natural apparatus, both of intellect and of sense![179]

176 Tertullian, *De Anima*, ed. J. H. Waszink (Amsterdam: North-Holland Publishing Company, 1947), 27.7.: "Ex afflatu dei anima."

177 Ibid., 27.8.: "Cum igitur in primordio duo diversa atque divisa, limus et flatus, unum hominem coegissent, confusae substantiae ambae iam in uno semina quoque sua miscuerunt."

178 Tertullian, *On the Soul*, 27.8.-9.

179 Ibid., 19.6.

It is easy to recognize traces of Aristotelian thought in Tertullian. Just as in Aristotle's *De Generatione Animalium* it is man who transmits the soul. However, Tertullian goes one step further in the logic of the supremacy of the male than Aristotle. This is because in his thinking male semen does not only contain the soul but also the bodily substance which Aristotle, after all, had still left to the female. Additionally, Aristotle and Tertullian differ with regard to what could be called the "ethical status of the soul." The Aristotelian soul transmitted via male semen, containing the star-like *pneuma*, becomes infected by original sin in Tertullian's reasoning. This is because Tertullian links original sin back to Adam: "The evil of sin was developed in him [Adam]."[180] As Adam's soul has sinned and all souls derive from him[181] it follows that male semen as the transmitter of soul also transmits original sin. In relation to Tertullian, Ernst von Aster writes of a somehow physiological explanation of sin in *De Anima*.[182]

With the introduction of the notion of original sin, the supreme role of man with regard to the transmission of soul becomes dubious. Procreation linked to the divine in Aristotle's writings now suffers from the blot of sin that can be undone only by a spiritual re-birth in Christ. At this point Tertullian develops an idea that will be at the core of the second symbolic pattern of childbirth to be examined in section III.2. of this work. The second symbolic pattern of childbirth is based on an opposition of spiritual birth and giving birth/procreation. Tertullian places the spiritual birth in Christ above procreation, which becomes inseparable from sin:

> Every soul, then, by reason of its birth, has its nature in Adam until it is born again in Christ; moreover, it is unclean all the while that it remains without this regeneration; and because unclean, it is actively sinful, and suffuses even the flesh (by reason of their conjunction) with its own shame.[183]

Tertullian's ideas about the transmission of original sin correspond closely to Augustine's reflections on the same matter. Partially, Augustine's ideas arose as a response to the theologian Pelagius and his disciple Caelestius, who fled to Sicily and then to Catharge after the sack of Rome

---

180 Ibid., 21.3.

181 See ibid. 20.5.

182 See Ernst von Aster, *Geschichte der Philosophie* (1932; reprint, Stuttgart: Kröner, 1980), 123–124.

183 Tertullian, *On the Soul*, 40.1.

on August 24, 410 by the Goths under Alaric.[184] Pelagius went on to Palestine, whereas Caelestius remained in Catharge where he was accused of heresy by Paulinus of Milan, the biographer of St. Ambrose, at a synod in 411. Among the accusations were the following, of great interest for an investigation into different constructions of childbirth/procreation. Caelestius was considered as a heretic because he taught "that the sin of Adam injured only himself" and "that infants at the time of birth are in the same condition in which Adam was before his transgression."[185]

In the following, a closer look will be taken at Augustine's notion of original sin and its meaning for a special construction of procreation. However, it should be kept in mind that the theology of original sin was most probably not Augustine's "personal brainchild."[186] Tertullian is an important forethinker of the idea of original sin which gains more weight in Augustine's writings. Moreover, although Augustine was not present at the above-mentioned synode, "a basically 'Augustinian' view of original sin was put forward on behalf of the North African Church by Aurelius, Bishop of Carthage, and also espoused by Paulinus, from the Church of Milan."[187]

Augustine mentions his ideas about original sin in all of his anti-Pelagian writings. First of all, Augustine sees human nature as initially created without sin: "In the beginning man's nature was created without any sin."[188] However, this beatified state of mankind ended with Adam's sin which was transmitted to humanity: "For they are not without sin, either that which they contracted originally or that which they added through their own misconduct. 'For all have sinned,' either in Adam or in themselves, 'and are deprived of the glory of God.'"[189] Augustine, very much

184 For this and the following see William J. Collinge, introduction to *On Nature and Grace*, by Augustine, in Augustine, *Four Anti-Pelagian Writings: On Nature and Grace, On the Proceedings of Pelagius, On the Predestination of the Saints, On the Gift of Perseverance*, trans. John A. Mourant and William J. Collinge (Washington, D. C.: The Catholic University of America Press, 1992), 12.

185 Ibid., 12–13.

186 Ibid.

187 Ibid., 13.

188 Augustine, *On Nature and Grace*, in St. Augustine, *Four Anti-Pelagian Writings: On Nature and Grace, On the Proceedings of Pelagius, On the Predestination of the Saints, On the Gift of Perseverance*, trans. John A. Mourant and William J. Collinge (Washington, D. C.: The Catholic University of America Press, 1992), 3.

189 Ibid., 4.

like Tertullian, sees the remedy for original sin contracted by every man in a spiritual rebirth in Christ: "A man is born answerable for the sin of the first man and held by the bend of condemnation, unless the guilt contracted through generation is absolved through regeneration."[190] From this logic it derives that infants who do not undergo baptism as a means of spiritual salvation in Christ die in sin: "It remains, therefore, that they [those infants who perish because they die without baptism] are held in bondage by original sin alone, and because of this alone go into damnation."[191]

Like Tertullian, Augustine places spiritual birth in Christ morally above procreation which becomes inseparable from sin. That the transmission of original sin is envisaged as physical becomes clear in *De Gratia Christi* and *De peccato originali libri II.* Here Augustine states that Adam has passed the sin on to the children ("*peccatum ex Adam in paruulos transeat*"[192]). In the same vein, a statement by Augustine makes sexual intercourse equivalent with the transmission of guilt. Christ can be described as truly righteous because "as one who was born of a virgin, he was not bound in any way by the ordinances against a guilty mode of having been begotten."[193]

In summary, the Aristotelian supremacy of the male over the female due to the faculty of the man to transmit the soul via the *pneuma* becomes highly dubious in the writings of Tertullian and Augustine. Man still transmits the soul; however, this soul is now viewed as being infected with original sin.[194]

---

190 Augustine, *On the Gift of Perseverance*, in St. Augustine, *Four Anti-Pelagian Writings: On Nature and Grace, On the Proceedings of Pelagius, On the Predestination of the Saints, On the Gift of Perseverance*, trans. John A. Mourant and William J. Collinge (Washington, D. C.: The Catholic University of America Press, 1992), 4.

191 Ibid., 23.

192 St. Augustin, *De Gratia*, in St. Augustin, *Oeuvres*, Vol. 22, *La crise Pélagienne II: De Gratia Christi et de peccato originali libri II, De natura et origine animae libri IV,* introduction, traduction et notes par J. Plagnieux et F.-J. Thonnard (Paris: Desclée, de Brouwer, 1975), XII. 13.

193 Augustine, *Against Two Epistles of the Pelagians*, IV. Xi 29, quoted in Jaroslav Pelikan, *Mary Through the Centuries: Her Place in the History of Culture* (New Haven and London: Yale University Press, 1996), 190.

194 The supreme role of man with regard to the "transmission" of body and soul is not the only way in which early Christian thinkers express a supremacy of the male over the female in matters of childbirth. On a theological level Tertullian dethrones the Ancient Roman birthgoddesses and sides them with the devil. The goddesses who formerly presided over birth in all its various aspects, are now replaced by the "new,"

1.9 On the Heels of Aristotle: The *Summa Theologica* of Thomas Aquinas

In the years between 1265 and 1272 the Domenican Thomas Aquinas (1225–1274) wrote his *Opus magnum* the *Summa* or *Summa Theologiae*, known as *Summa Theologica* by tradition.[195] The *Summa Theologica* fused Aristotelian thought with Christian doctrine and was to become one of the most influential theological works of the Middle Ages. In 1323, Thomas Aquinas, was declared a saint on the basis of his life and writings, and in 1879 his philosophy was made the official teaching on matters theological and philosophical in the seminaries of the Catholic Church.[196]

1.9.1 From "Semen and the Stars" to "Semen and Sin"

One of the basic ideas that Thomas Aquinas took from Aristotle with regard to generation was the sharp distinction between male and female, which was reproduced with its clear notion of hierarchy:

"male" god. Tertullian (*De Anima*, 39.1–2) inveighs against the birth goddesses: "All these endowments of the soul, which are bestowed on it at birth are still obscured and depraved by the malignant being who, in the beginning, regarded them with envious eye, so that they are never seen in their spontaneous action, nor are they administered as they ought to be. For to what individual of the human race will not the evil spirit cleave, ready to entrap their souls from the very portal of their birth, at which he is invited to be present in all those superstitious processes which accompany childbearing? Thus it comes to pass that all men are brought to the birth with idolatry for the midwife, whilst the very wombs that bear them, still bound with the fillets that have been wreathed before the idols, declare their offspring to be consecrated to demons: for in parturition they invoke the aid of Lucina and Diana; for a whole week a table is spread in honour of Juno; on the last day the fates of the horoscope [Fata scribunda] are invoked; and then the infant's first step on the ground is sacred to the goddess Statina."

195 See Anton C. Pegis, introduction to Thomas Aquinas, *Summa Contra Gentiles*, by Thomas Aquinas, vol. 1, *God*, trans. Anton C. Pegis (1955; reprint, Notre Dame, Ind.: University of Notre Dame Press, 1975), 17.

196 See William P. Baumgarth and Richard J. Regan, S. J., *On Law, Morality and Politics: Saint Thomas Aquinas* (Indianapolis/Cambridge: Hackett Publishing Company, 1988), xiii.

> Woman is defective and misbegotten, for the active force in the male seed tends to the production of a perfect likeness in the maculine sex; while the production of woman comes from a defect in the active force or from some material indisposition, or even from some external influence; such as that of a south wind, which is moist, as the Philosopher observes.[197]

Aquinas also follows Aristotle with regard to his ideas about the different contributions of men and women in the process of generation: "The active force is in the semen of the male, as the Philosopher says; but the foetal matter is provided by the female."[198]

Like Aristotle, Thomas Aquinas associates the active force of the semen, which acts upon the passive female matter, with rational soul. Here Thomas Aquinas is actually less precise than Aristotle about the connection between male semen and the rational Soul because he does not give a precise definition of *pneuma*, which in Aristotelian thought serves as the transmitter of rational soul in the semen. However, Thomas Aquinas writes about the "power in the semen": "Although the soul is not transmitted because the power in the semen is not able to cause the rational soul, nevertheless the motion of the semen is a disposition to the transmission of the rational soul: so that the semen by its own power transmits the human nature from parent to child."[199]

As in Aristotle's writings there is an outside source for the intellectual soul in the *Summa Theologica.* The "unmoved mover" of Aristotelian vocabulary becomes God with Aquinas.[200] Thus in the *Summa Theologica* we find a descending hierarchy where God acts upon male semen which in turn acts upon female matter. Such reasoning is developed in analogy to Aristotle's philosophy and installs supremacy of the male over the female in terms of generation. Moreover, like Aristotle, Thomas Aquinas also has the tendency to conceive of the male semen as, at least partially, a non-physical substance. This idea is elaborated upon in the Aquinean reasoning about heritage, which is attributed to those parts of the semen derived directly from the soul:

---

197 Thomas Aquinas, Summa Theologica, trans. Fathers of the English Dominican Province (1948; reprint, Westminster, MD.: Christian Classics, 1981), I Q 92, 1. In the *Summa Theologica*, Thomas Aquinas writes about "*the* Philosopher" when he refers to Aristotle.

198 Ibid., II Q 118, 1.

199 Ibid. I–II, Q 81, 1.

200 See ibid., II Q 118, 2.

> Wherefore in order for a man to be like his grandfather, there is no need that the corporeal seminal matter should have been in the grandfather; but that there be in the semen a virtue derived from the soul of the grandfather. .... For kinship is not in relation to matter, but rather to the derivation of forms.[201]

As in Aristotelian philosophy, the "de-corporealization" of male semen enables the male body to come closer to the divine than can the female body. It is through intellectual Soul and Reason that man partakes of God's wisdom.[202] Thus the transmission of intellectual Soul by exclusively the male body leads to a proximity of God and man that the woman will never be able to obtain.

Furthermore, Thomas Aquinas supplements Aristotelian thought with a Christian argument that accentuates the disparity between men and women in relation to generation. He thus reflects upon the statement in Genesis that Eve was created from Adam's rib, and he deduces from that fact that "even the corporeal matter, which is supplied by the mother [...] is originally derived from Adam."[203] As shown in the last section, Tertullian had already maintained that male semen contained both body substance and soul substance. Thus with the Aquinean idea that "the rib was in Adam as the principle of the human race, as the semen in man, who is a principle through generation,"[204] the supremacy of the male over the female in matters of generation becomes a twofold supremacy.

However, the supremacy of the male over the female in matters of generation also has its problematic sides in the *Summa Theologica*. This has to do with the fact that the attitude towards generation itself has changed, if compared to Aristotle's *De Generatione Animalium*. In Aristotelian thinking, generation has exclusively positive connotations. By contrast, Thomas Aquinas fuses the notion of original sin with Aristotelian ideas about generation. The soul is thus not only a means to approach the divine but is also related to guilt. Thomas Aquinas, like Tertullian, explicitly states that guilt is located in the soul and not in the body.[205] Thus, according to Thomas Aquinas, "the motion of the semen is a disposition to the transmission of the rational soul,"[206] but the semen is also the transmitter of guilt:

201 Ibid., II Q 119, 2.
202 See ibid., I–II Q 91, 2 ad 3.
203 Ibid., II Q 119, 2.
204 Ibid., I Q 97, 2.
205 See ibid., I–II Q 83, 1.
206 Ibid., I–II Q 81, 1.

> The semen by its own power transmits the human nature from parent to child, and with that nature the stain which infects it: for he that is born is associated with his first parent in his guilt, through the fact that he inherits his nature from him by a kind of movement which is that of generation. Although the guilt is not actually in the semen, yet human nature is there virtually, accompanied by that guilt.[207]

Guilt is thus associated with male generational activity and not with female matter, which in itself cannot sin: "Hence the soul is more infected by the semen, than by the flesh which is already perfect, and already affixed to a certain person."[208] The link between male semen and sin, on the one hand, and between female matter and the absence of sin, on the other, becomes even clearer as Thomas Aquinas discusses the conception of Christ. Relying on Augustine, he departs from the idea that Christ "took the visible substance of His flesh from the Virgin's flesh."[209] He argues that "the virtue of His conception did not spring from the seed of man but far otherwise – from on high."[210] It is not the female matter deriving from Adam, but the male semen deriving from Adam, that is linked to sin. Thus Christ is free from original sin, because he received his matter from the Virgin Mother, and it was the Holy Ghost that acted upon that matter:

> But Christ is said to have been in Adam according to the corporeal substance, not according to the seminal virtue. Because the matter from which His Body was formed, and which was supplied by the Virgin Mother, was derived from Adam; whereas the active virtue was not derived from Adam, because His Body was not formed by the seminal virtue of a man, but by the operation of the Holy Ghost.[211]

So far, the reasoning of Thomas Aquinas in relation to generation comes as a twofold supremacy of the male over the female – the principle of the human race comes from Adam and the male semen is the active, generational power which acts upon the passive, female matter. However, the semen does not only transmit rational soul but also human nature, which is associated with original sin. What has changed in the line of thought from Aristotle to Thomas Aquinas passing by Tertullian and Augustine is not the supremacy of the male over the female in matters of childbirth, but the fact that generation itself becomes a rather dubious activity. As has

207 Ibid.
208 Ibid., I–II, Q 81, Art. 1.
209 Ibid., III, Q 15, 1.
210 Ibid.
211 Ibid., Pt III, Q 32, Art. 4.

already been pointed out, in the thoughts of Thomas Aquinas, reason is the means by which to approach the divine. This stands together with the idea that "good operation in God and the angels is altogether without passion, as it is without a body."[212] Now generation comes under trial precisely because it is associated with sexual pleasure, which lies beyond the control of reason: "That veneral concupiscence and pleasure are not subject to the command and moderation of reason, is due to the punishment of the first sin, inasmuch as the reason, for rebelling against God, deserved that its body should rebel against it, as Augustine says."[213] The absence of reason during the act of procreation means that man can be compared to animals: "Beasts are without reason. In this way man becomes, as it were, like them in coition, because he cannot moderate concupiscence. In the state of innocence nothing of this kind would have happened."[214]

Thus, although there is a supremacy of the male over the female in relation to generational power, generation itself becomes highly problematic. In fact, in the ultimate analysis Thomas Aquinas devaluates generation: "But man is yet further ordered to a still nobler vital action, and that is intellectual operation."[215] However, in the *Summa Theologica* the generation of Christ is the one exception to the rule. As will be shown in the following Aquinas' description of the agency of the Holy Ghost upon the Virgin Mary is a most subtle form of both theorizing the supremacy of the male over the female with regard to generation and of exempting Christ from original sin.

1.9.2 The Agency of the Holy Ghost

In the *Summa Theologica* the conception of Jesus Christ is described as the intervention of the Holy Ghost into female matter. The Virgin Mary is

212 Ibid., Pt I-II, Q 59, Art. 5 ad 3.

213 Ibid., Pt II-II, Q 153, Art. 2. This idea is also developed by the notion that generation in the state of innocence would have been carried out in an altogether different mode. See ibid., Pt I, Q 98, Art. 2.

214 Ibid., Pt I, Q 98, Art. 2. For the negative influence of coitus on reason and spirit see also Pt I-II Q 34, Art. 1 ad 1; Pt II-II, Q 186 Art. 4 and Spl. 41, Art. 3 ad 2.

215 Ibid., I Q 92,1. With this statement Thomas Aquinas places himself in a tradition to be examined further on in section III.2. of this work. It is a tradition of thought that devalues childbirth in comparison to other ways of attaining mortal immortalities, namely, those of political, spiritual or theoretical natality.

said to have brought "Him [Christ] forth, not actively, but passively, just as other mothers achieve this through the action of the male seed."[216] As has already been hinted at above, considering the Virgin Mary as a being of passive matter has the theological function of keeping Christ free from original sin.[217]

As original sin is transmitted only by male semen, Mary's material contribution to the birth of Christ remains a spiritually pure contribution. In this sense, this is an association of the female womb with the absence of sin. Therefore it is not at all problematic that the Son of God should be born of a female womb. On the bodily appearance of the angel of annunciation to Mary, Thomas Aquinas states: "The angel of the annunciation appeared in a bodily vision to the Blessed Virgin [...] it was fitting as regards the dignity of the Mother of God, who was to receive the Son of God not only in her mind, but in her bodily womb."[218]

In the *Summa Theologica*, the supernatural element of Christ's conception also displays the supremacy of the male over the female with regard to generation. The Virgin Mary supplies the matter that is free of sin and is acted upon by the Holy Ghost. The supernatural power intervening in the conception of Christ is not pictured as a gender-neutral one. It merely replaces the male generational power and thus maintains an affinity with the male rather than the female sex: "But the formation of the body is caused by the generative power, not of that which is generated, but of the father generating from seed, in which the formative power derived from the father's soul has its operation. But Christ's body was not formed by the seed of man [...] but by the operation of the Holy Ghost."[219]

The Holy Ghost is a powerful agent, intervening in Mary's womb instead of mortal man. It is pictured as disposing matter like semen, and with that, regarding Christ's conception, divine intervention is portrayed as male. The difference between ordinary man and the Holy Ghost appears to be one of potency. This becomes evident in a passage on the formation of Christ's body:

---

216 Ibid., Pt III, Q 32, Art. 4 ad 1.

217 This reasoning works despite the fact that Mary is seen as bearing the stain of original sin because she was created from human, male semen: "Because the Blessed Virgin was conceived in original sin, she was in Abraham as needing to be healed. Therefore she paid tithes in him, as descending from him according to seminal virtue. But this is not true of Christ's body, as stated above" (Ibid., Pt III, Q 31, Art. 8).

218 Ibid., Pt III, Q 30, Art. 3.

219 Ibid., Pt III, Q 33, Art. 1.

> But the body's very formation, in which conception primarily consists, was instantaneous, for two reasons. First, because of the infinite power of the agent, viz. the Holy Ghost, by whom Christ's body was formed, as stated above. For the greater the power of an agent, the more quickly can it dispose of matter; and consequently, an agent of infinite power can dispose matter instantaneously to its due form.[220]

As has been shown above, the power of the Holy Ghost is essentially presented as a male power, which intervenes in the Virgin Mary's womb. This is yet another expression of the symbolic supremacy of male generational activity over female generational activity. A divine entity appears in the shape of a male numinous figure who basically "procreates" his son. In this sense, it is a male divinity that is in control of a mortal woman's womb.[221]

1.9.3 Reflections on Male Divinities Intervening into Women's Wombs

The pattern underlying the idea of the Holy Ghost intervening in the womb of a woman bears some resemblance to certain aspects of Ancient Hebrew and Ancient Egyptian conceptions of childbirth which shall be briefly sketched out in the following. In her study *God and the Rhetoric of Sexuality*, Phyllis Trible examines how God (Yahweh) relates to women's wombs (*rehem*) in the Old Testament.[222] In her careful philological analysis she comes to the conclusion that "in the Hebrew scriptures the wombs of women belong to God."[223] Among the many examples that Phyllis Trible gives for her thesis, three will be used here to illustrate her argument.

Genesis 20, 1–18 tells the story of the divine punishment of infertility coming upon the house of Abimelech, because the latter had taken Sarah into his harem without knowing that she had already been married to Abraham. It is said: "For Yahweh had closed every womb [kol-rehem] of

---

220 Ibid.

221 Of course, one could also tell the story from a different perspective. A woman, not a man, is chosen to be acted upon by a divine entity. However, Thomas Aquinas does not emphasize this point, which is the matrix for a different tradition in Christianity. On the basis of an elaboration of the figure of Mary, such a tradition belongs to a symbolic pattern of childbirth in which a supremacy of the female over the male is proclaimed. This will be shown in section III.4.3 of this work.

222 See for the following Phyllis Trible, *God and the Rhetoric of Sexuality* (Philadelphia: Fortress Press, 1978), 34–38. The following translations from the Bible are by Phyllis Trible.

223 Ibid., 37.

the house of Abimelech because of Sarah, Abraham's wife." Here Yahweh has the power over fertility by acting upon the female womb. This is also an important idea in the story of Jacob and his two wives Rachel and Leah (Genesis 29–30). Having been used by her father, Laban, to trick Jacob, Leah is now hated by Jacob, her husband. Therefore, "when Yahweh saw that Leah was hated, he opened her womb *[rahmah]*." Later on in the story, God also bestows fertility upon Rachel. It is said that he remembers her and "opens her womb *[rahmah]*." Finally, in the last example taken from the book of Jeremiah, Yahweh is himself given a voice, telling the prophet:

> Before I formed you in the womb [beten] I knew
> you,
> and before you came forth from the womb [rehem]
> I set you apart.

The womb (*rehem*), according to the Hebrew Scriptures, "is a physical object upon which the deity acts."[224] Moreover, in the Old Testament the imagery connected to God is dominantly male.[225]

The ideas of Thomas Aquinas on the conception of Christ, the book of Genesis, and the book of Jeremiah all share the idea that a male God controls the womb of women. The difference, however, is that in one case the divine intervention concerns one special woman, whereas in the other case God acts regularly upon every female womb. Phyllis Trible puts it beautifully like this: "Only God closes and opens wombs in judgement, in blessing, and in mystery."[226]

As far as the idea of the intervention of a male god into the female womb is concerned, this pattern can also be found in the myth of Khnum, one of the Ancient Egyptian gods of creation. Khnum was generally imagined as taking the shape of a ram, forming mankind on a potter's wheel.[227] Apart from being one of the gods of creation, he is also closely associated with birth, in the sense that it is believed that he still fashions every child to be born. As Jaroslav Cerný puts it: "This is only a refinement of the original ascription to Khnum of the creation of all living

224 Ibid., 35.

225 See Paul D. Hanson, "Masculine Metaphors for God and Sex-Discrimination in the Old Testament," *The Ecumenical Review* 27 (1975): 316–324.

226 Phyllis Trible, *God and the Rhetoric of Sexuality*, 38.

227 See Robert Thomas Rundle Clark, *Myth and Symbol in Ancient Egypt* (London: Thames and Hudson, 1959), 265.

things, on account of the extraordinary engendering power of his sacred animal, the ram."[228] Khnum, like Yahweh, is believed to intervene directly into the female womb. On the temple walls of the Egyptian temple of Esna it says: "Respect Khnum, you pregnant women, for he is the builder of the mansion of birth."[229]

1.10 The Divine in the Prophet: The Procreation of Muhammad in the *Sirat* of Ibn Hisham

The last chapter on Thomas Aquinas dealt with the special procreation of Christ. However, Jesus does not stand alone as a founder of a religion who is procreated in a way that testifies to the male's spiritualization through the process of generation. Equally Prophet Muhammad, in the *Sirat* of Ibn Hisham, is described as being selected as the messenger of God by divine intervention into procreation.

The *Sirat* by Ibn Hisham is one of the most important sources regarding Muhammad's life. *Sirat* in Arabic means way of acting, conduct, and biography. In the ninth century C.E. Ibn Hisham systematized the biography of Muhammad written by Ibn Ishaq. As the original scriptures of Ibn Ishaq were almost entirely lost, it was actually impossible to compare the works of Ibn Ishaq and Ibn Hisham. Thus the editor Ibn Hisham became as famous as Ibn Ishaq.[230]

The *Sirat* very quickly became a work of great authority. This can be deduced from the kind of editing it underwent by Ibn el-Magribí. To make the *Sirat* resemble the Qur'an Ibn el-Magribi divided it into 30 sections

228 Jaroslav Cerný, *Ancient Egyptian Religion* (London: Hutchinson's University Library, 1952), 49.

229 I am very grateful to the Egyptologist Jana A. Loose for translating this text for me and for giving me the reference.

230 If one dates the *Sirat* back to Ibn Ishaq's lifetime, it was most probably written in the first half of the second century of the Higra. Thus, it is the oldest book of Arabic literature except the Qur'an and old Arabic poetry. See Ferdinand Wüstenfeld, introduction to *Das Leben Muhammeds*, by Ibn Ishaq, trans. and ed. Ferdinand Wüstenfeld (Göttingen: Dieterichsche Universitäts-Buchhandlung, 1860), 2:xxxvii).

and vocalized it fully, just like the Holy Book.[231] The section entitled *Of the Woman who Offered Herself in Marriage to 'Abdullah* describes the miraculous procreation of Muhammad, which will here be interpreted from the perspective of the supremacy of the male over the female in matters of childbirth. This section of the *Sirat* starts with the father of Prophet Muhammad, Abdullah, setting out to marry his future wife Aminat. 'Abdullah's father 'Abdu Muttalib accompanies him to the tribe of Aminat. On their way, the two men meet a woman who makes a peculiar offer to Abdullah:[232] "When she looked at him she asked, 'Where are you going Abdullah?' He replied, 'With my father.' She said, 'If you will take me you can have as many camels as were sacrificed in your stead.' 'I am with my father and I cannot act against his wishes and leave him', he replied."[233]

Thus Abdullah follows his father and marries Amina, the future mother of the Prophet. When he comes back from his marriage, Abdullah meets the same woman again, and he asks her "why she did not make the proposal that she had made to him the day before." She replied, "that the light that was with him the day before had left him, and she no longer had need of him."[234] Straight after this episode, Ibn Ishaq tells another similar one:

> 'Abdullah went in to a woman that he had beside Amina d. Wahb when he had been working in clay and the marks of the clay were on him. She put him off when he made a suggestion to her because of the dirt that was on him. He then left her and washed and bathed himself, and as he made his way to Amina he passed her and she invited him to come to her. He refused and went to Amina who conceived Muhammad. When he passed the woman again he asked her if she wanted anything and she said 'No! When you passed me there was a white blaze between your eyes and when I invited you you refused me and went in to Amina, and she has taken it away.'

---

231 See ibid., 2:xxxix. Arabic is written in consonants. The diacritical signs for the vowels are usually left out. This cannot be done with a holy text like the Qur'an which has to be fully vocalized to avoid any type of misunderstanding.

232 For the Arabic original see Ibn Ishaq, *Das Leben Muhammeds*, trans. and ed. Ferdinand Wüstenfeld (Göttingen: Dieterichsche Universitäts-Buchhandlung, 1860), 100–101. For the English translation see Ibn Ishaq, *The Life of Muhammad*, trans. and ed. A. Guillaume (1955; reprint, Lahore: Oxford University Press, Pakistan Branch 1970), 68.

233 This passage from the *Sirat* is elegantly translated by Guillaume. In the Arabic original the lady who meets Abdullah is direct. In exchange for the camels that she offers, she asks him: "*waqa' 'alayi 'al-an,*" which means literally "if you fall on me now," that is, "if you make love to me now."

234 Ibn Ishaq, *The Life of Muhammad*, 68–69.

It is alleged that that woman of his used to say that when he passed by her between his eyes there was a blaze like the blaze of a horse. She said: 'I invited him, hoping that he would be in me, but he refused me and went to Amina and she conceived the apostle of God.'[235]

In both episodes from the *Sirat* quoted above, it is emphasized that a divine element was at work in the procreation of Muhammad. Abdullah is filled with a divine light just before uniting himself with the Prophet's future mother Aminat. What is important here to the logic of a symbolic pattern of childbirth is the fact that the divine descends into a masculine, not a feminine body. In other words, the divine blessing is bestowed upon the future prophet by an intervention into his father's, not his mother's, body. The women who want Abdullah to make love to them recognize the divine light in its physical expression. It is the divine element that attracts them to him, not ordinary male beauty. This becomes evident by the chain of events. With the procreation of the Prophet, the divine intervention has fulfilled its function. Thus, after he has united himself with Amina, the illuminated body of Abdullah is again transformed into an ordinary body, and the women concerned lose all interest in him.

Another more recent text than the *Sirat* of Ibn Ishaq also uses the idea of the divine intervention into the male body in order to procreate the Prophet. Abul-Hasan Ahmed ben Abdallah ben Muhammed el Bekri wrote *The Procreation of Lights by the Birth of the Chosen One: His Miracles and his Battles*.[236] The underlying thought of the first part of this book is that the ancestors of Prophet Muhammad, from Adam onwards, transmitted an aureole from father to son. Here we find a special version of the genealogies of the Old Testament and of Prophet Muhammad. Not only do men seemingly procreate their sons without women, but in the special case of the genealogy of Prophet Muhammad, the patriarchs transmit a divine election with procreation. In both the *Sirat* and *The Procreation of Lights by the Birth of the Chosen One*, the supremacy of the male over the female in terms of childbirth manifests itself by the descendance of the divine spirit into male bodies for the sake of the special procreation of the prophet.

235 Ibid., 69.

236 See Wüstenfeld, *Introduction*, 2: LI. The Arabic title of the book is *Intiqal al-anwar fi maulad al-mustafi al-muhtar wa-ma'gizatihi wa-magazihi*. The manuscript is registered as *Hamburg Codex No. 138 and 139*.

1.11 Twentieth Century Examples for the Supremacy of the Male

Constructing childbirth in terms of a supremacy of the male over the female does not belong to a remote past. As has been shown in the introduction to this section, even contemporary manuals on family therapy may espouse the notion that male "procreation" can correspond to birthgiving on part of the woman. In the following I wish to present two examples from 20th century literature for "The Supremacy of the Male," namely Mikhail Epstein's *Fatherhood* and Ernest Hemingway's *Indian Camp*.

1.11.1 Mikhail Epstein: Fatherhood

In 1990 the Russian writer and literary critique Mikhail Epstein published his essay *Ottsovstvo* ("Fatherhood")[237] which he wrote from his experience of fatherhood, from his wife's pregnancy to the moment when his daughter Olga starts to walk and talk. *Fatherhood* illustrates the already mentioned fact that it is an artificial construction to separate the symbolic patterns of childbirth from each other. In general, the practice of this work is to assign a text to one symbolic pattern without, however, omitting its eventual interwovenness with any others in the course of the analysis.

Nevertheless, with regard to Mikhail Epstein's essay three out of the four symbolic patterns of childbirth, here presented, can be identified. Therefore *Fatherhood* will accompany us to the final section of this work showing its manifold facets. "The Supremacy of the Male," however, seems to be the dominant symbolic register of the novel because Epstein places the idea of the father as the giver of new life at the heart of his thinking. The father is the creator of the child: "But the father is giving life to his children with all its gifts: air, light […] and this is also why he ideally wants to be loved more than anything else in life and to be venerated as the source of all being."[238]

In Epstein's *Fatherhood* the *motif* of the father as the creator of life is intrinsically linked to the idea of the father as the origin, and there are

237 See Epstein, *Tagebuch für Olga*.

238 Epstein, *Tagebuch für Olga*, 74–75.

numerous references to this throughout the whole essay. He writes: "You should not completely bare your origin. Already the parable of Noah's sons relates this."[239] Epstein depicts the fatherly origin as both physical and spiritual. The flesh of the daughter is seen as deriving from the flesh of the father,[240] whereas at the same time the child's way of appropriating life to himself/herself is led back to the fatherly origin:

> In general, any unconscious expression of the joie de vivre of the child – her appetite, her strength, her growing, her interest in her environment – is to a high degree a justification which can be felt inside, a 'patriodicee', because she is confirming and multiplying the value of the original paternal gift.[241]

To be at the origin of his child's life grants a mortal immortality not only to the father but also to his wider family. Thus describing a stay at his parents' house, Epstein expresses the feeling of a justification of his whole existence deriving from the fact that he has given life to a daughter:

> Nowhere Olja is loved as much as she is loved here. Nowhere am I by my sheer existence justified as much as I am here because she would not be there without me. In this house where I leisurely stroll around I feel more blissful than at any other time, or anywhere else and nobody else like the grandparents makes you feel this with such an intensity. Everybody else is expecting something from me. It is possible that I will not have success, that I will not make it, that I will end up in fiasco and that I will not achieve anything with my life. However, here I have already achieved as much as I could – a new and perfect life which will not let us die.[242]

The strong physical link that Epstein establishes between father and child is reminiscent of Tertullian and Aquinas, in that all share the idea that the father transmits the decisive life giving substances to the child. It is the semen that appears to be the carrier of life, whereas the womb is pictured as the chaotic primary substance where the semen may either die or live:

> How painful is the road from non-being to being – it leads through myriads of dying sperm cells which are not needed for fecundation. .... How many of them are perishing there in the dark, oceanic womb of life, in the chaos of the original substance, in the whims and inhumanities of evolution.[243]

239 Ibid., 176.
240 Ibid., 200: "The flesh of the daughter has derived from the flesh of the father."
241 Ibid.
242 Ibid., 164.
243 Ibid.

In the logic of establishing an intense physical link between father and child, Epstein writes about the child having been "inside the father," an expression which could also be interpreted as a metaphorical mimesis of pregnancy: "It is impossible to completely conceive of the father as of the other because the child has been in the father just like the father is in the child."[244]

The importance Epstein gives to procreation may be read as a modern "follow up" of creation as procreation in Egyptian cosmogony, the birth of woman in Genesis, Hesiod's Anadyomène, genealogical lines (in the Old Testament and of Prophet Muhammad) and the Gilgamesh Epic. However, this is not the only way of how *Fatherhood* expresses a symbolic supremacy of the male over the female in matters of childbirth.

With the experience of procreation the father comes closer to the mystery of creation, which is the mystery of a male god. Throughout *Fatherhood* the divine appears in the shape of the Judeo-Christian God Father. Making father-procreation and God-creation analogous, human procreation then becomes a means by which to approach the divine.[245] The human father feels a spark from the divine father in himself. The mystery of creation and the mystery of procreation are fused into one:

> I am writing the diary of a father and I do not feel the limits of this word any longer. It becomes bigger and more comprehensive. It is taking on a meaning which goes beyond me and demands to write it with a capital letter. Whose father's? That one and only Father's? Is it not that this whole diary is an involuntary parable on the creation of the world, on the mystery of the paternal?[246]

The human father resembles God who created mankind in his image:

> Parenthood is a mysteriously illuminated condition: Here I enter the true profundity of religious experience because I begin to resemble the father. I grasp what it means to create something out of oneself and to love what one has created. It is not by chance this commandment which is the most original of all (in the first book of Genesis): "Be fruitful and multiply." Man who has been created in the liking of the creator

244 Ibid., 244.

245 Beforehand, we have also seen in Aristotle's writings that the procreating man and the divine can be linked. Aristotle established this link by the idea of *kinesis*, which he attributed to both the "unmoved mover" and male semen.

246 Epstein, *Tagebuch für Olga*, 208. See also 222: "That the father is the first earthly close at hand image of the heavenly father also brings with it an immense danger."

> takes in his image most completely by his own parental materialisation because here he himself creates in his own liking.[247]

The analogy that Epstein draws between God, the father of humanity and the human father also has a dark side. This is the power of the creator over what he has created.[248] The giver of new life also feels the power of being able to take what he has given:

> At first the father transcends himself and gives life to somebody else. And then driven by the desire to transcend even these limits he re-appropriates it to himself as the right to take it away and to annihilate. The well-known "I have procreated you, I will also kill you" wholly finds its place in the nature of the father containing, as it were, two forms of the absolute with an unfathomable thin line becoming blurred between them. [...] However, if the others are one's own children it is sufficient to feel the father within oneself and thereby, as it were, also God: my own flesh and blood – I have given it and I can also take it.[249]

The rapprochement of the procreating father and the creating god is not the only way *Fatherhood* establishes the supremacy of the male over the female in matters of childbirth and generation. Epstein continues in this vein by constructing a spiritual supremacy of the male over the female when it comes to generation. In keeping with a gendered spirit-matter dichotomy he attributes a spiritual role to men and a physical role to women in the process of generation. To a certain extent this feels reminiscent of the Aristotelian idea of man providing the soul and woman providing matter for the formation of new life. Epstein describes the future father's feeling of emptiness during the pregnancy of the woman: "There everything is becoming plain and is swelling and is filling up with strength but inside me there is a damned emptiness painfully sucking at me. I have never experienced such a state of melancholy and futility as the one in this long winter."[250]

---

247 Ibid., 208.

248 Ibid., e. g. 211: "And I understand the compassion and the tenderness which penetrated the heart of the Lord when He saw his beloved creation tremble. And so also my tiny child has already grown up into sinning and there is no place where it could hide from me. My voice must resound over it, seeing everything with unrelenting harshness without leaving it even for a moment to its little but already illicit secrets."

249 Ibid., 219.

250 Ibid., 12.

This impression of "being emptied" during pregnancy is explained by the idea that the father, as if he extended coition, is continuously giving something to the woman, and what he gives are the *saps of the psyche.* Thus, symbolically, the short length of "procreation" is extended to nine months whereby metaphorically the man, both on a physical and on a psychic level, becomes deeply involved with the unborn:

> Our melancholy and our feeling of being disadvantaged this is our share of participating in the destiny of the baby. This is nourishment for it through the saps of our psyche and this is why we feel like being squeezed dry. It is our way of participating in the work of nature both at conception and while the baby is carried to term. We have to give and to empty ourselves. They have to absorb and to conceive in order to give birth to abundance. And when will power and working capacity are leaving us during this time it would be as bizarre and ridiculous to complain about it as about the loss of semen during conception. Pregnancy is but the continuation of the coitus, the gift of the male to the female in the formation of a third–a sexual intercourse which is extending over nine months and is followed by a state of melancholy previously unknown.[251]

The gendered spirit-matter dichotomy in relation to procreation, conception and pregnancy is expressed by Epstein when he writes: "The women, calm and triumphant, could inasmuch not share our psychic burden as we could not share their fleshly burden."[252] Again Aristotle does not seem to be that far away when it comes to Epstein's depiction of semen as intervening into the mother during conception. Here the male appears as the active, forming principle, whereas the female is passive matter: "There the semen parted from him into the mother and reshaped her."[253] As in Aristotle's *De Generatione Animalium*, the father is identified with form and spirit. Thus Epstein conceives of the grandfather in the following way: "He [the grandfather] has still formed my father in his liking […]. He enveloped me from all sides like a spiritual womb."[254]

The symbolic pattern "The Supremacy of the Male" also persists in Epstein's description of birthgiving. Here again he brings the male closer to the spiritual than the female who is sided with matter. The woman in labour is seen as being occupied with a mere physical act. It is the "flesh which opens up" whereas the father indulges in a spiritual birth act. While

251 Ibid., 14.
252 Ibid., 13.
253 Ibid., 69.
254 Ibid., 170.

the mother is in labour, the father starts to pray. His intense praying is depicted as his way of creating the child. The table on which his bible lies is called the "birth table."[255] In a mimetical act of the creation of the world in Genesis, the father gives birth to the child by his prayer, i.e. by his word: "This table where the bible lay was my birth table so that the word, the first in my life, the only word of my countless words could really and truly become flesh."[256] It is interesting to note that Epstein pictures a perfect synchronicity between the mere physical birthgiving of the woman and the spiritual birthgiving of the father. It is this joint effort, which leads to the birth of the child:

> My prayer and her giving birth were basically one trembling, one terrible contraction just as it had been during pregnancy: the fullness of her body and the emptiness of my soul had been one. My whole life I had been speechless before God. Every word had stuck in my throat but as soon as her flesh started to open "immediately his mouth was opened and his tongue freed, and he began to speak praising God."[257]
>
> The same day and according to one will the seal of our lives-up to then closed with no way out-was broken. My words were forcing their way outside on the same paths as the fruit of her womb and her pain was my master. .... "Lord, have mercy upon us, release my little baby from the impenetrable darkness and give it your light." .... These words [...] finding their way out of me under cramps and thus re-enacting the path of the baby under cramps penetrated the deathly obstacle again and again to clear the baby's path to light. Prayer is like giving birth.[258]

1.11.2 Ernest Hemingway's Indian Camp: *The White Male Doctor and Modern Mimesis of Giving Birth*

As has been shown above by the essay *Fatherhood*, in the 1990's it was still possible to write about birthgiving and procreation in terms of a spiritual-physical supremacy of the male over the female. Though in a rather different form than Epstein's *Fatherhood*, Ernest Hemingway's short story *Indian Camp* also testifies to the symbolic pattern labeled "The Supremacy of the Male." In Hemingway's short story the main figure is

255 Ibid., 27.
256 Ibid.
257 Luke 1:64.
258 Ibid., 26–27.

not a future father but a white male doctor whose supremacy of the male over the female in matters of childbirth is based on modern medecine.

Indian Camp was first published in 1925 as part of the book *In Our Time*. It belongs to that circle of Hemingway's short stories commonly called the Nick Adams stories. The figure of Nick Adams is a transfiguration of the young Hemingway. A central theme explored in these stories is the relationship between father and son, the latter observing a model of manhood that his parent represents.[259] In *Indian Camp* the fact that Nick Adams' father is a doctor is of utmost importance. As will be shown in the following, the figure of the doctor in *Indian Camp* belongs to a symbolic network in which the ideas of male self-control and a mimetic control over childbirth are closely intertwined with one another.

In *Indian Camp* the boy Nick Adams accompanies his father and his Uncle George to an emergency case. An Indian woman is suffering from complications during birthgiving, and Nick's father manages to save her and the baby by performing a Caesarian. However, after it is established that the operation has been successful, it is discovered that the woman's husband has committed suicide because of emotional stress. He has cut, his throat during the operation.

In Hemingway's short story a far away echo of the births of Athene and Dionysos[260] can be heard. In the Greek myth as also here, we encounter a male's mimetic appropriation of female potency. On his arrival at the Indian camp, Nick's father replaces the women who have dominated the scene unsuccessfully up to this point. It says that "all the old women in the camp had been helping her [the young woman in labour],"[261] and that "an old woman stood in the doorway holding a lamp,"[262] when the doctor arrived. Traditional ways of giving birth have failed along with the female body.[263] Nick's father comments on the woman in labour: "All her muscles are trying to get the baby born. That is what is happening when she screams."[264] Despite her efforts, the young woman does not succeed in giving birth to her baby on her own. With his medical skills the doctor

259 See Schwenger, *Phallic Critiques*, 42.

260 See chapter III.1.6.

261 Ernest Hemingway, *In Our Time* (1925; reprint, New York: Charles Scribner's Sons, 1958), 16.

262 Ibid.

263 With this analysis and the following I rely on Peter Schwenger's interpretation of *Indian Camp*. See Schwenger, *Phallic Critiques*, 42–44.

264 Ibid.

replaces both the old women's knowledge and the young woman's body; he takes control over both. Peter Schwenger writes about *Indian Camp*: "The Caesarian incision replaces the natural opening of a woman's body to make delivery possible by the male doctor where the woman has failed."[265] The doctor's control over the situation of childbirth goes hand in hand with his own self-control,[266] which does not allow space for his own emotions or the feelings and suffering of the woman in labour: "'I haven't any anæsthetic', his father said. 'But her screams are not important. I don't hear them because they are not important.'"[267]

Instead, what becomes important are the actions of the doctor, because it is through them that the baby is finally born. Through the Caesarian, the doctor opens the female body – which was not capable of opening of its own power, and afterwards he closes the female body – which cannot close naturally as after a natural childbirth. It is the doctor who performs the birth of the child, and it is he who has power over life. He animates the baby and gives it to the old waiting woman who represents the traditional woman's authority over childbirth now relgated to a passive role: "His father picked the baby up and slapped it to make it breathe and handed it to the old woman."[268] During the operation, the woman in labour is forced to become a passive object, subject to the actions of the doctor: "Later when he started to operate, Uncle George and three Indian men held the woman still."[269] The doctor does what the woman was supposed to have done, namely birthgiving. The actual mother is unconscious of the process to which she has become the object: "She was quiet now and her eyes were closed. She looked very pale. She did not know what had become of the baby or anything."[270]

The passivity of the mother contrasts with the doctor's "post-operative exhilaration"[271] regarding his successful execution of the techniques that have replaced the natural birthgiving process: "'That's one for the medical journal, George;' he said. 'Doing a Cæsarian with a jack-knife and sewing

265 Ibid., 42.
266 Peter Schwenger elaborates in depth on the function of self-control and control over emotions for the construction of masculinity in Hemingway. See ibid., 42–43.
267 Hemingway, 16.
268 Ibid., *In Our Time*, 17.
269 Ibid.
270 Ibid., 18.
271 Ibid.

it up with nine-foot, tapered gut leaders.'"[272] The doctor affirms his power over childbirth by picturing it as a process over which he (and only he as a doctor) exercises complete control. To him childbirth means an easy job. In relation to the men waiting for their babies to be born, he says: "They're usually the worst sufferers in these little affairs."[273] The doctor's control over the situation leaves a deep impression on his son Nick, who, under the influence of the events he has witnessed, reflects on life and death. He asks his father: "Is dying hard, Daddy?" The doctor's reply is one of self-assurance: "No, I think it's pretty easy, Nick. It all depends."[274] The way in which his father has dealt both with birth (by performing a Cæsarian) and death (by his composure at the Indian's suicide) have a deep impact on Nick. His father's manly control over birth and his composure when being confronted with death make Nick feel save to such an extent that he experiences a feeling of immortality. At the end of the story he thinks: "In the early morning on the lake sitting on the stern of the boat with his father rowing, he felt quite sure that he would never die."[275]

In *Indian Camp*, the male supremacy over childbirth the doctor stands for, is in contrast with the figure of the Indian husband who kills himself. This is where the construction of masculinity becomes intertwined with questions of race. Although the actions of both figures are based on the mimesis of the woman in labour, they choose different aspects of the situation for mimetic actions. As has been shown above, the doctor appropriates the female generational power to himself by reproducing the act of childbirth. In contrast, as Schwenger remarks,[276] the Indian husband reproduces the transformation of his wife into an object. He mimetically repeats the incision of the Cæsarian by cutting his throat. His wife has become an object in the hands of the doctor while he has become an "object of himself."[277] Thus the doctor attains supremacy in terms of childbirth because he, as the white male on the grounds of Western medicine, remains the subject in control of the situation. At the same time, the Indian husband submits himself to this type of male supremacy by emotionally identifing with his wife, who is transformed into an object. Peter Schwenger asserts

272 Ibid., 19.
273 Ibid., 18.
274 Ibid., 19.
275 Ibid.
276 See Schwenger, *Phallic Critiques*, 45.
277 Ibid.

that by cutting his throat, the Indian husband is symbolically "womanized."[278] This means that the male doctor is the only one of the three to exercise power over the process of childbirth, since the figures of the Indian woman and her empathetic Indian husband are transformed into objects. The white doctor's mimetic enactment of childbirth turns him into the true subject of the story.

278 Ibid., 42.

III.2 Theoretical, Spiritual and Political Natality versus Childbirth

The symbolic pattern of childbirth labeled "The Supremacy of the Male," presented itself as accentuating the importance of the man for the coming into existence of a child. In the symbolic pattern of childbirth entitled "Theoretical, Spiritual and Political Natality versus Childbirth," the question of whether the male or the female plays a greater part in the generation of children is left aside. This question that informed "The Supremacy of the Male" becomes subordinate to the search for different kinds of "mortal immortalities" and new beginnings. What does this mean?

In his *Rites and Symbols of Initiation,* Mircea Eliade studied the religious rituals that may accompany and bring about a spiritual rebirth.[279] Referring to tribal societies Eliade writes that "attaining to another mode of being – that of spirit – is equivalent to being born a second time, to becoming a new man. The most striking expression of newness is birth. The discovery of spirit is homologized to the appearance of life."[280] In the symbolic pattern "Theoretical, Spiritual and Political Natality versus Childbirth" such a homologization of the "discovery of spirit" and "the appearance of life" has fallen apart. Furthermore, the important feature of the symbolic pattern to be dealt with in this section is not only that the desire for a "mortal immortality" and a new beginning is fulfilled by a spiritual rebirth and detached from childbirth, but that "conception," "procreation," giving birth, and sometimes even the children themselves are devalued. In this respect, the second symbolic register of childbirth to be analyzed here relies heavily on the hierarchization of different mortal immortalities and natalities. This can be done in several ways. Sometimes the sphere of the political gains supremacy over childbirth. In other cases, the immortality that springs from philosophy, art and religion, is played out against childbirth.

That the symbolic pattern "Theoretical, Spiritual and Political Natality versus Childbirth" does not belong to a remote past but is still part of

279 See Eliade, *Rites and Symbols of Initiation.*
280 Ibid., 60.

contemporary everyday culture can be illustrated by two short examples. In his autobiography *Killing Time,* Paul Feyerabend mentions a letter by his friend Walter Hollitscher who, after a life of political activism writes the following: "I did not think we could be politically active and have children. … Now I am sure we were mistaken and we regret it."[281] Another short example is a bit non-chalant and comes from my own environment. When one of my friends got pregnant with her first child a relative's comment to her mother was: "I have always thought that she would be too intelligent for such a thing."

The reasons for a hierarchization of childbirth and other types of natalities may have to do with the perpetuation of the culture of axial age civilizations, which has previously been shown at work in the Aristotelian conception of procreation. As Eisenstadt puts it, pre-axial societies can be conceived of as "societies in which the mundane and transmundane worlds are defined in relatively homologous terms." In the pre-axial age, the "search for immortality is on the whole envisaged in terms of some physical continuity. It is usually seen as conditional to the fulfillment of one's concrete obligation to one's group."[282] The following chapters will investigate into the hierarchization and opposition of different mortal immortalities and natalities. In the light of Eisenstadt's reflections on the axial age, the hierarchization and opposition of the immortality coming with the birth of children and the immortality coming with philosophy, religion, the arts or political natality may be read as an expression of the chasm between the transcendental and the mundane, characteristic of axial age civilizations. Childbirth is identified with the mundane and, with such logic, becomes inferior to whatever instance is identified with transcendence, be it of a religious, philosophical, political or artistic nature.

Finally, this section will include some reflections on the peculiar twist the symbolic pattern "Theoretical, Spiritual and Political Natality versus Childbirth" may have taken under the influence of modern rationalization processes. Two literary works to be presented, *Headbirths* by Günter Grass and *Who's Afraid of Virginia Woolf?* by Edward Albee deal with the peculiar phenomenon of childbirth moving into the realm of thought by children remaining fictional or potential children.

281 Paul Feyerabend, *Killing Time* (Chicago and London: The University of Chicago Press, 1995), 74.

282 Eisenstadt, *The Origins and Diversity of Axial Age Civilisations,* 3.

1. The Babylonian Myth of Creation and the Creation Myth of the Bible

Whereas at the beginning of the previous section, Ra, the Ancient Egyptian god, stood for the coming into existence of the world by procreation, the creation myth to illustrate the second symbolic pattern of childbirth comes from the Babylonian epic *Enûma Elish*. Parts of *Enûma Elish* can be dated back to the seventh century B.C. and others to approximately 1000 B.C.,[283] although Alexander Heidel maintains that it already existed during the fifteenth century B.C.[284] The *Enûma Elish* takes its name from the opening words of the poem which literally mean "When above."[285] According to Heidel, the epic mainly represents "a literary monument in honor of Marduk as the champion of the gods and the creator of heaven and earth. Its prime object is to offer cosmological reasons for Marduk's advancement from the position as chief god of Babylon to that of the entire Babylonian pantheon."[286]

In the context of symbolic patterns of childbirth, the interest in the *Enûma Elish* lies with the creation scene as described on tablet IV of the epic. Marduk's supreme position among Babylonian gods is based on the creation and maintenance of the universe.[287] However, in order to have been able to create, Marduk first had to defeat Ti'âmat, the mother of the gods. Tablet I introduces her as "she who gave birth to them all,"[288] together with her husband Apsu, who is called the begetter of the gods.[289]

The conflict between the sun-god Marduk and Ti'âmat can be read as a contention about whether it is male or female creational forces that are supreme. Given the fact that it is Marduk who, in the end, is proclaimed the winner, the Babylonian myth of creation becomes part of the logic of the supremacy of the male over the female in matters of the coming into

283 See Alexander Heidel, introduction to *The Babylonian Genesis*, trans. Alexander Heidel (1942; reprint, Chicago: The Chicago University Press, 1963), 13.
284 See ibid.
285 See ibid., 1.
286 Ibid., 11.
287 See ibid.
288 Alexander Heidel, trans., *The Babylonian Genesis* (1942; reprint, Chicago: The Chicago University Press, 1963), 18.
289 Ibid.

existence of the world. Additionally, the second symbolic pattern of childbirth emerges from the *nature* of the fight between Ti'âmat and Marduk. In his interpretation of the *Enûma Elish* Erich Fromm attributes special importance to the following passage, which describes a test Marduk has to pass before he can become the leader of the male heroic gods and set out to kill Ti'âmat:

> They set up among them a certain constellation,
> To Marduk their first-born said they (these words),
> "Your destiny, O Lord, shall be foremost of the gods",
> "Command destruction or creation, they shall take place."
> "At your word the constellation shall be destroyed",
> "Command again, the constellation shall be intact."
> He commanded and at his word the constellation was destroyed,
> He commanded again and the constellation was created anew.
> When the gods, his fathers, saw what he had commanded,
> Joyfully they hailed, "Marduk is king!"
> They bestowed in full measure scepter, throne, and staff,
> They gave him unopposable
> Weaponry that vanquishes enemies.
> "Go, cut off the life of Ti'âmat."[290]

In Fromm's reading, the test Marduk must pass has greater significance than the mere proof of having magical forces. Before the fight with Ti'âmat, Marduk has to prove that he is not inferior to the great mother, whose main characteristic is the ability to bring forth new life and to create. Fromm writes:

> Since he [Marduk] cannot produce with a womb, he must produce in another fashion; he produces with his mouth, his word, his thought. This, then, is the meaning of the test: Marduk can defeat Tiamat only if he can prove that he can also create even though in a different fashion. The test shows us the deep male-female antagonism, which is the basis of the fight between Tiamat and Marduk and the essential point of contention in this fight between the two sexes. With Marduk's victory male supremacy is established, the natural productiveness of the women is devaluated, and the male begins his domination based on his ability to produce by the power of thought.[291]

---

290 Benjamin R. Foster, trans., *Enuma Elish*, in *Before the Muses: An Anthology of Akkadian Literature*, trans. and ed. Benjamin R. Foster, 3rd. ed. (Bethesda, Maryland: CDL Press, 2005), 457–458.

291 Fromm, *The Forgotten Language*, 233–234.

If one follows the logic of Erich Fromm, *Enûma Elish* thus affirms the superiority of creation by the word over creation by giving birth. Therefore, it can be read as an illustrative myth for a symbolic pattern of childbirth in which theoretical natality is played against the birth of children. Interestingly, however, in the *Enûma Elish,* the female generational forces are not completely annihilated but are subordinated to the male power of the word. Even though Ti'âmat is slain, heaven and earth can only be created from her body. In this process, however, the agency of creation is removed from the female and transferred to the male:

> The Lord calmed down, he began inspecting her carcass,
> That he might divide (?) the monstruous lump and fashion artful things.
> He split her in two, like a fish for drying,
> Half of her he set up and made a cover, heaven.
> He stretched out the hide and assigned watchmen,
> And ordered them not to let her waters escape.[292]

According to Fromm, the biblical myth of creation goes a step further than the *Enûma Elish* in eliminating women from creation. In the bible, the word of the male god provides the means by which everything comes into existence. The recurring formula "God said" precedes God's acts of creation in Genesis. As Fromm puts it: "God creates the world by his word; the woman and her creative powers are no longer necessary."[293] One could add that likewise creation by procreation in the sense of the myth of Ra is equally "no longer necessary" and no longer possible: creation by the word makes both procreation and giving birth superfluous.

2. Plato's *Symposium* and the Deathless Children of Philosophers

Personal love is the main theme of Plato's *Symposium* which centers on the idea of beauty in its connection to love and public virtue. In the history of the reception of the *Symposium*, these themes have been the dominant

---

292 *Enûma Elish*, IV, 135–140, transl. by Foster, Before the Muses, 461–462.
293 Fromm, *The Forgotten Language*, 34.

ones.[294] What has been less widely discussed, however, is that in the *Symposium* the discourse on love is intertwined with the constitution of male spiritual identity that is based not only on a particular perception of male and female bodies, but also on a special view of childbirth. Here, Adriana Cavarero, with her work *Nonostante Platone*, managed to fill an important gap.[295] In the following, Plato's path towards postulating a sharp contrast between childbirth and philosophy will be delineated.

The *Symposium* consists of various speeches held at a dinner party. Socrates, Pausanias, Eryximachus and Aristophanes, among others, are invited to Agathon's house. The guests agree upon honouring the god Eros by holding speeches. It is the speeches of Pausanias, Aristophanes and Socrates/Diotima which prove to be particularly important for the context of symbolic patterns of childbirth.

In the speech by Pausanias, the construction of ideal male love operates through his distinction between two love goddesses; one is called Heavenly, the other Popular. They reveal the twofold nature of Aphrodite. Because Pausanias values one aspect of the goddess over the other the dualism implies a hierarchy. Love proceeding from Popular is a love to be found in the "meaner sort of men; who, in the first place, love women as well as boys; secondly, where they love, they are set on the body more than the soul; and thirdly, they choose the most witless people they can find, since they look merely for the accomplishment and care not if the manner be noble or not."[296]

In contrast to Popular stands the Heavenly Goddess, symbolizing love in its more noble form. The speech of Pausanias links these two aspects of love to the different origins of the two goddesses.The Heavenly Goddess is

294 Here Foucault's analysis of the *Symposium* is an interesting exception. In *L'usage des plaisirs*, he contrasts Christian sexual ethics and Ancient Greek sexual ethics. The *Symposium* is one of the examples Foucault gives for the fact that in Ancient Greece sexual pleasure was not considered to be good or bad in itself – as in Christian ethics – but that the use of these pleasures determined their moral value. See Michel Foucault, *L'usage des plaisirs*, vol. 2 of *Histoire de la sexualité* (1984; reprint, Paris: Éditions Gallimard, 1997), 270, 295–316.

295 As will be shown below Adriana Cavarero (See Adriana Cavarero, *Nonostante Platone*) discusses the devaluation of childbirth in the *Symposium*. However, she does not investigate the meaning of the devaluation of procreation.

296 Plato, *Lysis, Symposium, Gorgias*, trans. W.R.M. Lamb (1925; reprint, Cambridge, Mass.: Harvard University Press, 1975), 181b.

said not to have been born of a mother but to be a daughter of Heaven,[297] whereas Popular is the child of Zeus and Dione. Thus, in Pausanias' reasoning, the nobler sort of love proceeds from the goddess who, from her origins "partakes not of the female but only of the male."[298] Consequently those inspired by this love "betake them to the male, in fondness for what has the robuster nature and a larger share of mind."[299] Noble love, in contrast to mean love, has not only a private but also a public dimension, as it "compels lover and beloved alike to feel a zealous concern for their own virtue."[300] If one was to summarize the semantic fields evolving around the two goddesses, the picture would be the following:

> Popular = daughter of Zeus and Dione, mean (merely physical) love for women and boys, private, non virtuous, wantonness;
> Heavenly Goddess = born from Heaven, love between men, private and public, virtuous, untinged with wantonness.

What seems to lie at the heart of this distinction between the two goddesses is the question of their origins, intertwined with attitudes toward childbirth. The fact that Popular is born from a mother connects her to the realm of the female, which, for Pausanias, has negative connotations, e.g. mere bodily love, wantonness, etc. Childbirth, like all the other references to the realm of women, is characterized by the absence of any spiritual or intellectual element. It thus constitutes a point of non-identification.[301] In contrast to this, what clearly functions as a reference point to which male identity should ideally adhere, is the Heavenly Goddess. Of male origin,

---

297 See section III.1.3. of this work for the birth of Aphrodite from the members of Ouranos.

298 Plato, *Symposium*, 181c.

299 Ibid.

300 Ibid., 185c.

301 This type of identity construction may be linked to the sexual ethics in Greek Antiquity. Michel Foucault underlines the fact that in Greek Antiquity any type of sexual relations – heterosexual or homosexual – was understood as a relation between a dominating person and a dominated person. The dominating person exercised the act of penetration and was considered to be superior. As a result, the person who consented to being penetrated was considered to be inferior. (See Foucault, *L'usage des plaisirs*, 285). These roles can obviously change with men, whereas women, according to such logic are structurally inferior to men. This may be the reason why women and the act of birthgiving as an act performed by women, may have become such a strong point of non-identification in the *Symposium*.

she stands for the exclusion of the maternal womb and of female corporeality. The Heavenly Goddess, in this sense, is a "pure" Goddess, a symbolic carrier of virtuous love, precisely because she is free of the bodily universe, which is connected to childbirth.

The logic at work behind the speech of Pausanias resembles very closely the Ancient Greek construction of male civic identity, which Nicole Loraux examines in her *Les enfants d'Athéna*.[302] She argues that on a symbolic level the Athenian foundation myth of Erichthonios allows for the exclusion of the maternal womb from the discourse of the origin of the *polis*. Erichthonios is born from Hephaistos' desire for Athena. The goddess escapes and as some of the semen of the god falls on her leg she dries it with wool which she then throws on the soil. Gaia is fertilized by this semen and produces the child Erichthonios whom she subsequently hands over to Athena. On several vase paintings Loraux analyses, this scene is depicted with Gaia always figuring on a lower level than Athena herself. The virginal goddess Athena thus becomes a mother without giving birth and Erichthonios becomes the son of Athena[303] without being born from a mother: *proles sine matre creata*, Ovid writes about Erichthonios in the *Metamorphoses*.[304] Moreover, Athena herself, born from the head of Zeus, did not have a mother. Thus in the myth of Erichthonios we encounter the double/triple exclusion of the maternal womb: Athena, of no woman born, has a child to whom she does not give birth. Her child is instead from the soil. Male civic identity is thus constructed upon the first Athenian's affiliation to Athena, according to Loraux; an affiliation without the act of birthgiving usually constitutive of the mother-child relationship.

What about the *Symposium* then? Just like in the foundation myth of Athens here again the point of identification for men is a goddess who is of male origin only. The Heavenly Goddess derives from the members of her father Ouranos. Do we additionally find the same kind of identity construction in the myth of Athenian authochtony and Plato's *Symposium*? It is not easy to decide whether it is a spiritual or a civic identity that is constructed in the speech of Pausanias. In a sense, male spiritual and civic identities become intertwined within the notion that noble love, by being concerned with virtue, opens itself up to the male public dimension.[305]

302 Nicole Loraux, *Les enfants d'Athéna* (Paris: La Découverte, 1984).

303 See ibid., 64.

304 Ovid, *Metamorphoses*, II. 553, quoted by Loraux, *Les enfants d'Athéna*, 59.

305 See Cavarero, *Nonostante Platone*, 97–99.

Socrates, who will give the last speech, continues this line of thought. We are prepared for his speech by the intervention of Aristophanes in which – as Cavarero poignantly demonstrates[306] – a devaluation of the maternal origin is enacted.

Aristophanes tells a myth which honours the god Eros. In this the original features of human beings are described as follows:

> The form of each person was round all over, with back and sides encompassing it every way; each had four arms, and legs to match these, and two faces perfectly alike on a cylindrical neck. There was one head to the two faces which looked opposite ways; there were four ears, two privy members, and all the other parts, as may be imagined, in proportion.[307]

Moreover, according to the speech of Aristophanes, human beings were originally characterized by the existence of three sexes: male, female and hermaphrodites, showing both male and female characteristics. The first human beings were very strong and even conspired against the gods. Thus Zeus decided to punish them by slicing every person into two halves. By this act, love came into the world. This was, because after the divine punishment, each creature would look for its former entirety, the former male creatures looking for the lost male half, the former female creatures looking for the lost female half and the former hermaphrodites looking for their opposite sexual counterpart.

In her analysis of Aristophanes' speech, Cavarero, draws attention to the fact that the divine punishment changes the mode of generation among human beings. That is to say, in the "golden age," they "did their begetting and bringing forth not on each other but on the earth, like the crickets,"[308] instead, in the period following the divine punishment generation depends upon the union of male and female, and above all, upon birthgiving. Cavarero emphasizes that in the myth of Aristophanes, to have to rely on the maternal womb in order to "come to the world," is a direct result of Zeus' punishment inflicted upon humanity. She also argues that female potency, as expressed through childbirth, is generally devalued in the myth.[309] And indeed, Aristophanes exalts love between men as true love, keeps silent on love between women, and despises love between

306 See ibid.

307 Plato: Symposium, 189E–190A.

308 Plato, Symposium, 191b.

309 See Cavarero, *Nonostante Platone*, 95–99.

women and men, which is the means by which children are begot.[310] Men indulging in noble love between men have "no natural interest in wiving and getting children, but only do these things under stress of custom,"[311] and it is these men alone who, "prove in a public career to be men."[312]

Undoubtedly, Aristophanes anticipates the speech of Socrates by understanding childbirth as mere material reproduction. Despite her insightful critique of the *Symposium* Cavarero does not comment on the fact that not only are women devalued in the speech of Aristophanes, but so too are men who indulge in love for women and have children. However, this is a point which has to be emphasized, because also the speech of Socrates, which is the most authoritative speech in the *Symposium*, takes a critical attitude toward both "procreation" and childbirth.

At the beginning of his speech, Socrates reveals that his knowledge about love matters stems from a conversation with a Mantinean woman named Diotima,[313] and he recalls her words. Some critics such as Luce Irigaray and M. E. Waithe have claimed that there did indeed exist a historical Diotima whose words have been reproduced in the *Symposium* and whose ideas might well have been distorted by Socratic-Platonic thought.[314] Cavarero is of the opinion that the discourse of Diotima was modified by the platonic Socrates.[315] In any case, with Diotima a female voice enters the *Symposium*.

---

310 Plato, *Symposium*, 191d–192a: "All the men who are sections of that composite sex that at first was called man-woman are woman-courters; our adulterers are mostly descended from that sex, whence likewise are derived our man-courting women and adulteresses. All the women who are sections of the woman have no great fancy for men. …. Men who are sections of the male pursue the masculine, and as long as their boyhood lasts they show themselves to be slices of the male by making friends with men and delighting to lie with them and to be clasped in men's embraces; these are the finest boys and striplings, for they have the most manly nature. Some say they are shameless creatures, but falsely: for their behaviour is due not to shamelessness but to daring manliness, and virility, since they are quick to welcome their like."

311 Ibid., 192b.

312 Ibid., 192a.

313 Footnote p.173 of Lamb's translation of the *Symposium*: "These names suggest a connexion respectively with prophecy and with the favour of heaven."

314 See Luce Irigaray, *L'éthique de la différence sexuelle* (Paris: Les Éditions de Minuit, 1985), 27; Mary Ellen Waithe, "Diotima of Mantinea," in *A History of Women Philosophers*, ed. Mary Ellen Waithe (Dordrecht: Martinus Nijhoff Publishers, 1987), 1:22.

315 See Cavarero, *Nonostante Platone*, 131.

Initially, Diotima's voice seems to be directed against dualisms. The Pausanian and Aristophanian way of contrasting noble love between men, associated with spirituality, and mean love between men and women, connotated with the body, seems to dissolve. She instead proclaims that love signifies the "begetting on a beautiful thing by means of both the body and the soul."[316] Furthermore, both the male body and the female body indulging in generation, are connected to the divine, which also implies beauty. Generation is considered a way to partake in immortality because "mortal nature [...] can always leave behind it a new creature in place of the old."[317] Thus Diotima says,

> All men are pregnant, Socrates, both in body and in soul: on reaching a certain age our nature yearns to beget. This it cannot do upon an ugly person, but only on the beautiful: the conjunction of man and woman is a begetting for both. It is a divine affair, this engendering and bringing to birth, an immortal element in the creature that is mortal; and it cannot occur in the discordant. The ugly is discordant with whatever is divine, whereas the beautiful is accordant. Thus Beauty presides over birth as Fate and Lady of Travail.[318]

What is remarkable in Diotima's speech is not only that by procreation and childbirth the human body may serve as a means to approach the divine and the beautiful, but also that no distinction is made between the sexes with regard to their partaking of the divine through procreation and childbirth. This is expressed in the words: "It is a divine affair this engendering and bringing to birth,"[319] which means that procreation on the part of the man and pregnancy/birthgiving on the part of the woman are placed on the same level and given the same importance in their connection with the divine and with beauty.

However, in Diotima's speech something occurs which could be labelled the "Diotimean turn." This "Diotimean turn" is brought about by a distinction which she/Socrates makes between two ways of participating in immortality. Thereby s/he reintroduces a gendered body-soul dichotomy. One way to partake of immortality is to have children, as discussed above, the other is to have a "pregnancy of soul" bringing forth prudence and virtue. What is here called the "Diotimean turn" consists of the fact

316 Plato, *Symposium*, 206b.

317 Ibid., 207d.

318 Ibid., 206c.

319 Ibid.

that birthgiving, conception and procreation – previously linked to the divine – now become metaphors for the generation and preservation of spiritual products (poetry, virtues, and laws) of which the origin is love between men:

> For I hold that by contact with the fair one and by consorting with him he bears and brings forth his long-felt conception, because in presence or absence he remembers his fair. Equally too with him he shares the nurturing of what is begotten, so that men in this condition enjoy a far fuller community with each other than that which comes with children, and a far surer friendship, since the children of their union are fairer and more deathless. Every one would choose to have got children such as these rather than the human sort.[320]

In the "Diotimean turn" of the *Symposium*, the "children" of spiritual, male communities are not only contrasted with children of flesh and blood, but are also valued more highly. This also implies a specific attitude towards birthgiving: the children women give birth to are sharply contrasted with the "spiritual children" of men. However, it is metaphors taken from the semantic field of birthgiving which are used to designate a superior way of generating, namely that of intellectual procreation. In this context, Cavarero speaks of a mimesis of childbirth which pervades Diotima's speech in the *Symposium*. By mimesis Plato appropriates to himself the symbolic potency of childbirth: all the technical terms related to childbirth are also used in relation to intellectual birthgiving. In addition, childbirth itself is devalued by the fact that it becomes subordinated to intellectual procreation.[321] However, it is not only birthgiving that is devalued in this context, because "intellectual procreation" among men is also placed above the procreation of children on part of the man.[322]

Cavarero proposes to retrieve the maternal potency through a constructive feminist critique of the *Symposium*. In her view, the *Symposium* is projected towards the future and the certain death it will bring. She criticizes Plato for measuring life from the point of view of death and for using "intellectual birthgiving" as a way to approach the divine and achieve immortality. Instead, Cavarero suggests that a retrieval of maternal

---

320 Ibid., 209c-d.

321 See Cavarero, *Nonostante Platone*, 106.

322 In this context men and women are depicted differently. While men are presented as being able to choose the way in which they "procreate," women figure as being tied to birthgiving (referred to in different ways before and after the Diotimean turn).

potency would attract our attention to the past. To understand life as the result of an endless chain of mothers who give birth to children would be the most important element of a philosophy of natality, which stands in opposition to a philosophy of death.[323] Although Cavarero's ideas are very interesting, they overlook the fact that in the *Symposium* the hierarchization of different "immortalities" places the procreation of spiritual products above both birthgiving *and* "procreation."[324]

Conspicuously, in the *Symposium,* love appears to be a choice between two different realms. Love among men practised in accordance with the Heavenly Goddess is a deliberate choice made not only against the realm of Popular, ie. against the realm of the female and female fertility, but also against the realm of paternity, because fatherhood is formed through contact with the female. If one was to sum up the understanding of childbirth proposed by the *Symposium* after the "Diotimean turn", and anticipated by the speeches of Pausanias and Aristophanes, one would derive a conception of male spiritual life standing in sharp contrast to procreation, birthgiving and children: Poetry, virtues and laws, the ideal children of philosophers, are deathless.

2.1 Discussion: Reflections on Theorein, Doing and Childbirth

In her investigation of thinking in the *Life of the Mind*, Hannah Arendt reflects upon the Greek evaluation of thinking and doing. The Pythagorean notion of spectatorship had, according to her, far-reaching significance for the rise of philosophy.[325] The Greek understanding of the divine led to the idea of the supremacy of *theorein* ("contemplation") over doing. Being free from the necessities of mortal life, the Greek gods were envisaged as looking down on human affairs from the Olympus. For them, human life was nothing other than a "spectacle for their entertainment."[326] Such a conception of the divine brought with it the idea that in order to approach

323 See Cavarero, *Nonostante Platone*, 114–121.

324 Cavarero, infact, reacts only to the devaluation of the female generational forces by suggesting a retrieval of maternal potency, which she conceptualizes as a parthenogenetic potency, leaving no space for men's contribution to generation. Her philosophy is a female version of the Bible's exaltation of male potency, where we can read about the long genealogical lines of fathers generating their sons, seemingly without women (See section III.1.5.).

325 See Arendt, *Thinking*, 130–139.

326 Ibid., 132.

the world of the immortals, one had to privilege god-like contemplation of life over action in life.

What does this characteristic of Greek philosophy have to do with a symbolic pattern of childbirth in which theoretical natality and primary natality are mutually exclusive? It seems that the supremacy of *theorein* over doing may easily lead to the depreciation of birthgiving/procreation, given that generation is a means to be involved in the spectacle. In this sense, Plato's attitude of preferring the deathless children of philosophers over children of flesh and blood in the *Symposium* may be read as just another way of favouring *theorein* over doing.

3. Creation Abandoned for the Idea of Good: The Justinian Myth of Edem and Elohim

The symbolic pattern of childbirth that creates an antagonism between spiritual/theoretical natality and childbirth is also present in the Gnostic myth of Edem and Elohim, which shows remarkable morphological similarities with Plato's *Symposium*. The myth of Edem and Elohim from the Book of Baruch by Justin the Gnostic, as has been summarized by Hippolytus' *Refutation of all Heresies,* fuses Platonism with Judaism. As reported by Hippolytus, Justin departs from the idea that before the creation of the world there were three ungenerated principles, namely, two male and one female.[327]

One male principle is called "the good" and is omniscient. The second ungenerated principle is Elohim. He does not have any knowledge and is called the father of everything generated. Like Elohim, the female principle, called Edem or Israel, lacks knowledge. She is depicted as half-serpent and half-maiden. From the love between Edem and Elohim, twenty-four angels are born, twelve belonging to Edem and twelve to Elohim. All the angels together form paradise. Elohim's angels take some of Edem's 'human' substance to transform it into Adam and Eve, the first human beings. They become the symbol of love between Elohim and Edem. The

327 See Hippolytus, *Philosophumena*, V. 26.

animals are generated from the serpent-part of Edem, who is identified with the earth:

> When Paradise was produced from the mutual pleasure of Elohim and Edem, the angels of Elohim taking (dust) from the fairest earth, that is, not from the beast-like parts of Edem, but from the man-like and cultivated regions of the earth above the groin, create man. But from the beast-like parts … the wild beasts and other animals are produced. Now they made man as a symbol of their unity and good-will and placed in him the powers of each, Edem (supplying) the soul and Elohim the spirit.[328] And there thus came into being a certain seal, as it were and actual memorial of love and an everlasting sign of the marriage of Elohim and Edem, (to wit) a man who is Adam. And in like manner also, Eve came into being as Moses has written, an image and a sign and a seal to be forever preserved of Edem. And there was likewise placed in Eve the image, a soul from Edem but a spirit from Elohim.[329]

This idyllic state of affairs very much resembles the situation in Plato's *Symposium* before the "Diotimean turn," that is, before the split between philosophy and the birth of children is introduced. However, also Justin's myth of the creation of the world has its "turn" because the spiritual is separated from the created world and becomes more important than it. Here, Justin links up with Plato who gives ideas, especially the idea of good, supremacy over the physical world. As will be shown in the following, there is a morphological resemblance between Justin's myth of Edem and Elohim, and the *Symposium*. Just as the spiritual products of men in the *Symposium* become more important than the birth of children, likewise in the Justinian myth, the idea of good becomes more important than the created world. Furthermore, this hierarchy in Justin is clearly gendered, in that the earth is left to Edem whereas Elohim dissolves into pure spirituality. This comes about in the following way.[330]

Elohim wants to verify whether something is lacking in his creation. He therefore ascends to the higher strata of heaven, taking his angels with him. He leaves Edem down in the world and it is further specified that she did not want to follow her husband, as she was the earth. Elohim reaches the third ungenerated principle, that of the hypostasis Good, whose light shines brighter than the light created by Elohim. The Good lets Elohim sit on his right side; subsequently, while there, Elohim turns against his creation: "Suffer me, O Lord, to overturn the world which I have made; for

328 Legge here renders the Greek psyche with soul and *pneuma* with spirit.

329 Ibid.

330 See ibid. for the following.

my spirit is bound in men and I wish to recover it."[331] However, the Good prevents Elohim from destroying his creation and tells him to leave it to Edem: "Let therefore Edem hold creation while she will; but do thou abide with me."[332]

Thus in the myth of Edem and Elohim creation and therefore generation is separated from spirituality. This division has a gender dimension to it. Edem, the earth, is identified with creation whereas the male creator abandons his creation to dwell in the realm of the (idea of the) good.

4. Abraham and the Binding of Isaac (in the Reading of Kierkegaard)

> *After these things God tested Abraham. He said to him, "Abraham!" And he said, "Here I am." He said, "Take your son, your only son Isaac, whom you love, and go to the land of Moriah, and offer him there as a burnt offering on one of the mountains that I shall show you."....*
>
> *When they came to the place that God had shown him, Abraham built an altar there and laid the wood in order. He bound his son Isaac, and laid him on the altar, on top of the wood. Then Abraham reached out his hand and took the knife to kill his son. But the angel of the LORD called to him from heaven, and said, "Abraham, Abraham!" And he said, "Here I am."*
>
> *He said, "Do not lay your hand on the boy or do anything to him; for now I know that you fear God, since you have not withheld your son, your only son from me."...*

---

331 Ibid.

332 Ibid. The Justinian myth of creation also confronts the theodicy problem. Abandoned by Elohim, Edem first seeks to regain her husband by making herself beautiful. Given that she is unsuccessful, she sends her angels out into the world to inflict suffering and pain on mankind, to make the *pneuma* of Elohim suffer, as it is enclosed in all human beings. Elohim, for his part, intervenes with his angels to assist humanity. Justin the Gnostic is ultimately empathic towards Elohim's retreat from creation. Although it is said that Elohim broke the marriage contract with Edem by his behaviour, the blame for suffering having come into the world can be placed more on Edem who appears as quite a dubious entity both with regard to her physical appearance and with regard to her character already in the introductory part of the myth. Her half-serpent like body is ambivalent and it is said that she is ill-tempered.

The angel of the LORD called to Abraham a second time from heaven, and said, "By myself I have sworn, says the LORD: Because you have done this, and have not withheld your son, your only son, I will indeed bless you, and I will make your offspring as numerous as the stars of heaven and as the sand that is on the seashore.
Genesis 22

The biblical and Qur'anic story of Abraham's willingness to obey God, even if it means to sacrifice his only son, is important to Judaism, Christianity and Islam.[333] Indeed, out of all the other features of Abraham's life, it is given special prominence in the Qur'an. The commemoration of God's providence and Abraham's obedience is celebrated annually in the course of the Muslim pilgrimage to the House of Ka'ba.[334] With regard to the Bible, Van Seters identifies three themes that are woven together in the story. These are:

> 1) the testing of God which moves from command (vv. 1–2) to obedience (v.3, 9–12), 2) the testing that calls forth the faith of Abraham in the providence of God (v.1, 6–8), which in turn is answered by the act of God's providence (vv.13–14), and his promise of blessing (vv. 15–18), and 3) the sacred place that is the place of Abraham's obedience and of God's provision (vv.2–5, 9, 14).[335]

In the following reading of the story of Abraham and Isaac as an example for the second symbolic pattern of childbirth, the emphasis will be laid on the first two themes – what does the divine test exactly consist of and who is subjected to it?

The hero of Genesis 22 is nobody other than Abraham who is inserted in the long genealogical lines of the Old Testament where fathers are procreating their sons, most often symbolically without women. In Judaism, Christianity and Islam, Abraham is also the original father in a spiritual sense.

In *Fear and Trembling*,[336] Kierkegaard develops the notion that Abraham becomes the father of faith because he is able to place faith

---

333 According to Susan Ackerman, the story of Abraham and the binding of Isaac may be a mythical testimony to the fact that child sacrifice was part of Yahwe worship at an earlier stage of Jewish religion and that this cultic practice was abolished at a later stage. See Susan Ackerman, *Under Every Green Tree: Popular Religion in Sixth-Century Juda* (Atlanta, Georgia: Scholars Press, 1992), 118–119.

334 Sherif, *A Guide to the Contents of the Qur'an*, 75–76.

335 John Van Seters, *Abraham in History and Tradition* (New Haven and London: Yale University Press, 1975), 237.

336 See Kierkegaard, *Fear and Trembling*.

above the ethical. What is the ethical in the story of the binding of Isaac? "In ethical terms, Abraham's relation to Isaac is quite simply this: the father shall love the son more than himself."[337] Seen from the perspective of social morality, Abraham's drawing of the knife has to be judged as murder.[338] Kierkegaard illustrates this point when, in *Exordium,* the preliminary literary reflections to *Fear and Trembling*, he imagines the following scene: "It was a quiet evening when Abraham rode out alone, and he rode to Mount Moriah; he threw himself down on his face, he prayed God to forgive him his sin, that he had been willing to sacrifice Isaac that the father had forgotten his duty to his son."[339]

What is it then that saves Abraham from the accusation of being a murderer and sinner? In Kierkegaard's terms, what we encounter in the Abraham story is a "teleological suspension of the ethical,"[340] in which the ethical and the universal are congruent with one another:

> The ethical as such is the universal, and as the universal it applies to everyone, which from another angle means that it applies at all times. It rests immanent in itself, has nothing outside itself that is its telos but is itself the telos for everything outside itself, and when the ethical has absorbed this into itself, it goes not further. The single individual, sensately and psychically qualified in immediacy, is the individual who has his telos in the universal, and it is his ethical task continually to express himself in this, to annul his singularity in order to become the universal. As soon as the single individual asserts himself in his singularity before the universal, he sins, and only by acknowledging this can he be reconciled again with the universal.[341]

Kierkegaard attempts to show how the teleological suspension of the ethical in the Abraham story establishes an altogether different pattern than that of the tragic hero. The ordeal, the spiritual trial of Abraham, consists of the fact that the ethical, in this case fatherly duty to the son, becomes a temptation: "As a rule, what tempts a person is something that will hold him back from doing his duty, but here the temptation is the ethical itself, which would hold him back from doing God's will. But what is duty? Duty is simply the expression for God's will."[342] To obey God means to place faith above the universal, whereas, according to Kiekegaard, the tragic

337 Ibid., 57.
338 See ibid., 53, 55, 66, 74.
339 Ibid., 13.
340 Ibid., 54
341 Ibid.
342 Ibid., 60.

hero is in an altogether different position because he is asked to place the universal above his own life:

> The tragic hero is still within the ethical. He allows an expression of the ethical to have its telos in a higher expression of the ethical; he scales down the ethical relation between father and son or daughter and father to a feeling that has its dialectic in its relation to the idea of moral conduct. Here there can be no question of a teleological suspension of the ethical itself.
>
> Abraham's situation is different. By his act he transgressed the ethical altogether and had a higher telos outside it, in relation to which he suspended it. [...] It is not to save a nation, not to uphold the idea of the state that Abraham does it; it is not to appease the angry gods. [...] Therefore, while the tragic hero is great because of his moral virtue, Abraham is great because of a purely personal virtue.[343]

The tragic hero, e.g. Agamemnon sacrificing Iphigeneia, may, in Kierkegaard's reading, find rest and security in the universal on behalf of which he is acting. By contrast, Abraham, a "knight of faith," remains lonely and detached from the universal[344] because he is tried by an ordeal in which the universal becomes a temptation. This particular situation explains why Abraham does not tell either Sarah or Eliezer or Isaac about the ordeal, according to Kierkegaard. By obeying God he steps out of the universal and thus cannot be understood by anybody. He "bypassed these three ethical authorities, since for Abraham the ethical had no higher expression than family life."[345] Here again Kierkegaard contrasts Abraham and the tragic hero, above all Agamemnon, who is allowed to reveal his conflict to his environment because he remains in the realm of the ethical/universal, and his conflict can thus be understood by everybody.[346]

343 Ibid., 59.

344 Ibid., 79.

345 Ibid., 112.

346 Ibid., 114–115. Kierkgaard's reflections on Abraham rely heavily on the comparison between Abraham and the tragic hero Agamemnon. He only marginally touches upon the female figures in the two stories, Abraham's wife Sarah and Agamemnon's wife Clytemnestra. These two characters are nevertheless worth looking at, if one wants to gain a more complete picture of the ethical questions at stake. After all, what makes Sarah and Clytemnestra similar is that they do not have unconditional faith. Sarah laughs when she is told that she will still become pregnant in her old age (Gen. 18:12), and Clytemnestra, as will be shown in the following chapter, doubts the legitimacy of both divine authorities and the moral authority of the *polis* when she is faced with her daughter's upcoming sacrifice.

However, from the perspective of symbolic patterns of childbirth the distance between Abraham and Agamemnon narrows considerably. This is because in both cases hierarchies between childbirth and political/spiritual natality are established. What is at the top of such a hierarchy may change, be it the state, as in the example of the following chapter on *Iphigeneia at Aulis*, or God, in the case of Abraham.

Abraham, with his intention of sacrificing his own son, is willing to renounce the mortal immortality that comes with a male successor. In other words, he is ready to sacrifice his access to a new beginning, which is so strikingly illustrated by the symbolic censura that the begetting of a son constitutes for a patriarch's life-time in the Hebrew Scriptures.[347] The original father renounces his fatherhood and with this act becomes the spiritual father of all three world religions. In Hannah Arendt's *Life of the Mind* we have already encountered the idea that Christianity replaced thought with faith as the bringer of immortality.[348] In the story of Abraham and the binding of Isaac, faith, as a means to attain immortality, replaces the immortality that comes with children. Furthermore, Abraham's obedience to God establishes a hierarchy between the procreation of children and faith. It is only through the willingness to sacrifice his son's life to the creator of *all* life, that Abraham, by God's mercy, is also granted the privilege of becoming an original father. Abraham's descendants are made as numerous as the stars precisely because, put to the test, he views obedience to God, that is to say his spiritual birth, to be a higher good than the births of descendants.

5. From Abraham to Agamemnon: *Iphigeneia at Aulis* of Euripides

Kierkegaard's comparison between Abraham and Agamemnon leads to the question of how Greek drama deals with the theme of moral conflict between ethical obligations towards one's child and other ethical obligations. In Euripides' play *Iphigeneia at Aulis,* which will come into focus

347 See section III.1.5. of this work.

348 See Arendt, *Thinking*, 138.

in the following, the main moral question centers on the question of the legitimacy to sacrifice a child for the sake of the state. Thus, in terms of symbolic patterns of childbirth, the interest in *Iphigeneia at Aulis* lies with the play thematizing contentions between political natality and the birth of children.

Together with Aeschylus and Sophocles, Euripides forms the triad of dramatists who epitomise the culturally and politically flourishing Athens of the fifth century B.C.[349] The setting of Euripides' play *Iphigeneia at Aulis* is the onset of the Trojan War. The Greek want to avenge the rape of Helena but their galleries are stuck in Aulis. There is no wind to bring them to the shores of Troja. The seer Calchas reveals that the goddess Artemis is holding back the winds because King Agamemnon has insulted her; she is demanding that Agamemnon's daughter Iphigeneia be sacrificed to her. Agamemnon is convinced that the sacrifice should be performed and sends for his daughter and wife Clytemnestra, to come to Aulis. He uses his desire for Iphigeneia to marry Achilles as a pretext. Once in Aulis, Clytemnestra meets Achilles and they discover that his name has been used to cover up Agamemnon's intention of slaying Iphigeneia. They then decide to rescue her. However, she refuses their help and decides to offer herself as a sacrifice to Artemis. As she is about to be slain the goddess miraculously substitutes a hind for her and takes Iphigeneia to the island of Tauris.

The moral conflicts presented by the drama of Euripides are two. On the one hand, Agamemnon has to decide whether he should sacrifice his child for the fatherland. On the other, Iphigeneia must make up her mind whether to sacrifice herself for Greece or to attempt to save herself with the help of Achilles.

For our context of a symbolic pattern of childbirth that subordinates the births of children to a mortal immortality attained by political action, it is the attitudes of the father, Agamemnon, of Agamemnon's brother Menelaus and of Iphigeneia that become especially important. At the beginning of the first scene of the drama, Euripides depicts Agamemnon mortified by the decisions he has made. His intense feelings for his daughter are stressed through the mention that he procreated her: "The seer Calchas

349 See G. P. Goold, introduction to *Iphigeneia at Aulis*, by Euripides, in *Euripides. In Four Volumes*, G. P. Goold ed., Arthur S. Way trans. (1912; reprint, Cambridge, Mass.: Harvard University Press, 1978), 1:x–xi.

bade […] /Slay Iphigeneia, her whom I begat."[350] Agamemnon regrets to have been in favour of the sacrifice and in a dispute with his brother Menelaus, even wants to undo his decision. By contrast, Menelaus uses two arguments in favour of the sacrifice. If Agamemnon should refuse to slay his child for the sake of Greece, it would endanger his position as king and, furthermore, the honour of Hellas would suffer:

> Many and many a man is like thee, toileth with unflagging will
> Up the heights of power; thereafter from its summit falls with shame,
> Some through blindness of the people, some be all themselves to blame,
> They whose nerveless hands can ward the city not that they have won.
> But, for me, 'tis hapless Hellas most of all that I bemoan:
> Fain she is of high achievement, yet shall caitiff aliens make
> Her a mock, who 'scape her hands for thine and for thy daughter's sake.[351]

Both the arguments made by Menelaus subordinate childbirth to the political sphere. The life of a child is less important than the royal position of its father and the honour of Greece. This is the final solution to the moral conflict of Euripides' play although it is by no means a simple one to achieve. Menelaus changes his mind only after his brother has cried. Agamemnon, in his turn, is convinced by the initial reasoning of Menelaus, which he uses in the dispute he later has with Clytemnestra and Iphigeneia (after they have learnt the will of the goddess Artemis, revealed through the seer). Here, Agamemnon, talking to Iphigeneia, presents the idea that it is the freedom of Hellas, above all, that has to be defended:

> 'Tis Hellas for whom – will I, will I not –
> I must slay thee: this cannot we withstand.
> Free must she be, so far as in thee lies,
> And me, child; nor by aliens' violence
> Must sons of Hellas of their wives be spoiled.[352]

At the moment in which Iphigeneia sides with her father by making the decision of self-sacrifice, she becomes the heroine of the play. Like Agamemnon, she prefers the mortal immortality that comes with political action to the mortal immortality she could attain if she should decide to

350 Euripides, *Iphigeneia at Aulis*, in *Euripides. In Four Volumes*, ed. G. P. Goold, trans. Arthur S. Way (1912; reprint, Cambridge, Mass.: Harvard University Press, 1978), verses 89–90.

351 Ibid., verses 366–372.

352 Ibid., verses 1271–1275.

have children: “Sacrifice me, raze ye Troy; for this through all the ages is / My memorial: children, marriage, glory – all are mine in this!”[353]

Following the logic of Agamemnon and Menelaus, Iphigeneia also tries to convince her mother of the righteousness of her behaviour. She tells Clytemnestra that the glory deriving from her self-sacrifice will pass on to her mother: “Thy glory shall I be.”[354] That is to say, Iphigeneia argues that through her political action, Clytemnestra will attain a mortal immortality that she would otherwise attain by her daughter surviving her.

Nevertheless, Clytemnestra remains an opponent to subordinating her daughter’s life to the *polis*. She continues to blame her husband’s decision to sacrifice Iphigeneia for the sake of Greece even after her daughter has agreed to it (“By guile unkingly, unworthy Atreus’ son!”[355]). Supported by the Chorus (“Mighty is motherhood, of potent spell:/All mothers for a child’s life will fight hard”[356]), she is even determined to rebel against the gods if they should agree to Agamemnon’s deed:

> O child, he which begat thee murdered thee…
> O surely must we deem the Gods be fools,
> If we wish blessings upon murderers.[357]

In fact, Clytemnestra does not forgive her husband for the loss of her daughter brought about by his decision to sacrifice her. In this respect, the Clytemnestra of Euripides is similar to the Clytemnestra in the play *Agamemnon* by Aeschylus.[358] Here, Clytemnestra conspires to murder Agamemnon upon his return from the Trojan War. Her deed is motivated more by her hate for Agamemnon who sacrificed her daughter than by any interest she may have in maintaining the adulterous relationship with her lover Aegisthos. In a dialogue with the Chorus she says:

> And yet he [Agamemnon], recking no more than if it had been a beast that perished – though sheep were plenty in his fleecy fold – he sacrificed his own child, even her I bore with dearest travail, to charm the blasts of Thrace […]. By Justice, exacted for

353 Ibid., verses 1398–1399.
354 Ibid., verse 1440.
355 Ibid., verse 1457.
356 Ibid., verse 917–918.
357 Ibid., verses 1177, 1188–1189.
358 See Aeschylus, *Agamemnon*, in *Aeschylus in Two Volumes*, trans. Herbert Weir Smyth (1926; reprint, Cambridge, Mass.: Harvard University Press, 1971).

> my child, by Ate, by the Avenging Spirit, unto whom I sacrificed yon man, hope doeth not tread for me the halls of fear.[359]

At the death of Agamemnon also the chorus comments that he is "dying for the dead."[360] Weir Smyth interprets this passage in the sense that Agamemnon "by his own death is to atone for his slaying of Iphigeneia."[361]

Clytemnestra's attitude in fact represents a socially deviant attitude in Greek drama, and, interestingly, she will ultimately lose her cause. In *The Libation-Bearers* by Aeschylus her son Orestes avenges his father Agamemnon by killing her. Subsequently, in the *Eumenides* by Aeschylus, when Orestes is judged, a court composed of both divine and human members ultimately finds this matricide to be justified. The court consists of the Furies, acting as plaintiffs who want to avenge Clytemnestra, Apollo, figuring as Orestes' advocate, selected members of the Aeropag, who form the jury, and Athena, who presents the case. While the Furies argue that it is a supreme crime to violate the mother-child bond, Apollo defends Orestes by saying that the child's affiliation and loyalty to his/her father is more important than the affiliation to his/her mother. Apollo's argument follows the logic of the first symbolic pattern of childbirth presented beforehand in this work. Apollo claims that man possesses the life-giving principle, while women merely receive it in the act of procreation: "The mother of what is called her child is not its parent, but only the nurse of the newly implanted germ. The begetter is the parent, wheras she, as a stranger for a stranger, doth but preserve the sprout, except God shall blight its birth."[362]

With Apollo's victory at the trial, Clytemnestra and the Furies suffer a double defeat. The mother-child bond, which the Furies consider to be primordial, is downgraded in favour of the father-child affiliation. (Apollo, when ordering Orestes to avenge his father, tells him: "But do thou, with good courage, when the part of action comes, cry aloud the name 'Father' when she [Clytemnestra] exclaims 'Son'"[363]). Moreover, Agamemnon having sacrificed Iphigeneia for the sake of the *polis* is retrospectively

359 Ibid., verses 1415–1417…1432–1434.

360 Ibid., verse 1339.

361 Ibid., footnote 3, 119.

362 Aeschylus, *Eumenides*, in *Aeschylus In Two Volumes*, trans. Herbert Weir Smyth (1926; reprint, Cambridge, Mass.: Harvard University Press, 1971), verses 657–662.

363 Aeschylus, *The Libation-Bearers*, in *Aeschylus in Two Volumes*, trans. Herbert Weir Smyth (1926; reprint, Cambridge, Mass.: Harvard University Press, 1971), verses 825–827.

justified. Clytemnestra's reasons for slaying her husband do not gain traction, and, as a result, she is the only one condemned, given that the justification for Orestes' matricide is upheld. Thus from the outcome of the trial it can be concluded that she did not have the right to take revenge on her husband for the loss of her daughter, whereas Agamemnon did have the right to sacrifice his daughter and Orestes is considered as having been morally obliged to avenge his father.

Thus, Clytemnestra's position, which considers the killing of one's own children as the most serious of sins, is defeated. This can be concluded from Agamemnon sacrificing Iphigeneia in the drama by Euripides and from the justification of Orestes' matricide in the *Eumenides* by Aeschylus. Here, a patriarchal law becomes instituted which stresses the father-child bond. Furthermore, the subordination of childbirth to the *polis* as the highest good, which may in its extreme version include the sacrifice of one's child, is depicted as uncontestable.

Up to this point, I have given much attention to the figure of Clytemnestra and the socially deviant behaviour for which she stands. This has been done in order to show that Kierkegaard's comparison between Agamemnon and Abraham – discussed in the previous chapter – needs to be complemented by taking into account Clytemnestra's position in Euripides' *Iphigeneia at Aulis*. Kierkegaard describes Clytemnestra as a very emotional character who questions Agamemnon's decision simply as a result of her motherly devotion.[364] As shown above, Clytemnestra does much more than weep in Euripides' play: She actually challenges the universal, which in Agamemnon's thinking equals the *polis*. Her claim is that there is nothing above absolute duty to one's child, and she is prepared to question the divine authorities and the moral authority of the *polis* if there should be a conflictual situation between the life of her daughter, the gods and the *polis*. Thus, the universal in *Iphigeneia at Aulis* is not such a given, reassuring fact as Kierkegaard presents it as being, when he writes, "every individual who understands him[the tragic hero]in turn understands the universal in him, and both rejoice in the security of the universal."[365]

Contrary to Kierkegaard's reasoning, the tenets of the universal are disputed, by way of the action Clytemnestra takes. Kierkegaard ignores the existence of the conflict most probably because he pays attention almost exlusively to Agamemnon as the winner of the fight about the universal.

364 Kierkegaard, *Fear and Trembling*, 87.
365 Ibid., 76.

The play, nevertheless, takes Clytemnestra's position into account even after she has lost. This becomes obvious through the fact that Iphigeneia, in agreeing to be sacrificed, rightly fears that Clytemnestra's wrath will fall upon Agamemnon: "My father and thine husband hate not thou [...] Sore loth, for Hellas sake, hath he destroyed me."[366]

Here it is important to emphasize that Clytemnestra's behaviour is not to be placed in the category of the Kierkegaardian sinner who is "sinning by asserting himself in his singularity before the universal,"[367] but instead that she advocates for the parent-child relationship as the absolute universal which cannot be reduced in significance. However, Clytemnestra's position is mentioned but not favoured in the plays by Euripides and Aeschylus. Rather unequivocally both plays decide for the *polis* and not for the life of a daughter as the highest good.

6. Christian Devotion versus Childbirth

> *For there are eunuchs who have been so from birth, and there are eunuchs who have been made eunuchs by others, and there are eunuchs who have made themselves eunuchs for the sake of the kingdom of heaven. Let anyone accept this who can.*
>
> Gospel of Matthew, 19:12

> *Fertility is a blessing in marriage,*
> *But integrity in holiness is better.*
>
> Augustine, Nativity Sermons

Matthew 19:12 is the textual basis for all monastic or para-monastic choices made in Christian communities. In the gospel of Matthew an opposition is stated between sexual relations and the leading of a spiritual life devoted to God. This opposition can also extend to spritual life versus the generation of children. For the following chapters some paradigmatic examples have been chosen to illustrate forms of Christian devotion that express contentions between spiritual birth and childbirth. Luke 11: 27–28, the teachings of Gregory of Nyssa and his sister Macrina, and the section on

366 Euripides, *Iphigeneia at Aulis*, verses 1454 and 1456.

367 Kierkegaard, *Fear and Trembling*, 81.

Perpetua and Felicitas in the *Acts of Christian Martyrs* all will be read with this logic in mind.

6.1 Luke 11: 27–28: The Word's Supremacy over the Womb

> *While he was saying this, a woman in the crowd raised her voice and said to him, "Blessed is the womb that bore you and the breasts that nursed you!"*
> *But he said, "Blessed rather are those who hear the word of God and obey it!"*

These sober and clear lines, in the eleventh Book of the Gospel of Luke nearly speak for themselves when read within the context of an investigation into the contrapositions of spiritual birth and childbirth. Jesus is preaching to the crowd, and a woman praises his mother, that is, a woman praises a woman's womb and breasts as the *locus* of origin of Jesus. However, Jesus refuses to honour this origin by contraposing it to the spiritual birth in God, whereby childbirth becomes merely a physical act.[368]

Following this logic Augustine comments in *De Sancta Virginitate* on Luke 11, 27–28. He claims that Mary was made happier by her belief in Christ than by the conception of the flesh of Christ.[369] Clement of Alexandria also comments on the same passage and even more pointedly depicts childbirth as a physical act that is inferior to spiritual birth. He contraposes milk as physical nutrition to the metaphor of the *logos* as divine milk and Christ himself as spiritual nutrition. In Clement of Alexandria's reasoning, breastfeeding becomes a vulgar act he does not want Jesus to be associated with. Therefore Clement of Alexandria develops the

---

368 It is interesting to note that such an opposition between childbirth and spiritual birth in the Gospel of Luke clashes with the relationship between Mary and Jesus as it is depicted in the 19th Sura of the Qur'an. Here Jesus respects Mary as the one who bore him:
"He spake: Lo! I am the slave of Allah. He hath given me the scripture and hath appointed me a Prophet, ….
And (hath made me) dutiful toward her who bore me, and hath not made me arrogant, unblest.
Peace on me the day I was born, and the day I die, and the day I shall be raised alive."
The Glorious Koran, trans., ed., introduction and notes Muhammad Marmaduke Pickthall (1930; reprint Albany: State University of New York Press, 1976), Surah 19, verses 30, 32–33.

369 See Walter Delius, *Geschichte der Marienverehrung* (München and Basel: Ernst Reinhardt Verlag, 1963), 139.

idea that the milk with which Mary was suckling Jesus did not originate from her body but from God.[370] This refined milk is the *logos*, with which God nourishes his son who in turn becomes "spiritual nourishment to the good":

> Further, pregnant women, on becoming mothers, discharge milk. But the Lord Christ, the fruit of the Virgin, did not pronounce the breasts of women blessed, nor selected them to give nourishment; but when the kind and loving Father had rained down the Word, Himself became spiritual nourishment to the good. O mystic marvel![371]

6.2 The Martyrdom of Perpetua and Felicitas

Until the reforms introduced by the second Vatican Council, priests of the Roman Catholic Church included the names of famous martyrs in the canonic prayers of the holy service,[372] since the church had given a special place to those men and women who died for their belief in Christ from the very beginning of Christianity. In this way Perpetua and Felicitas became names which were mentioned in the same breath as Mary and the apostles for many centuries. In the context of the symbolic pattern of childbirth labelled "Theoretical, Spiritual and Political Natality versus Childbirth" the interest in Perpetua and Felicitas lies in the fact that they proved their faith through the sacrifice of abandoning their babies. On the basis of the *Acts of Christian Martyrs*[373] the stories of these two women

370 See for this and a deeper analysis of Clement of Alexandria's conception of Mary's milk as the divine *Logos* and its relationship to the iconography of Mary as the Coptic Galaktotrophousa in Late Egyptian Antiquity Elizabeth S. Bolman, "The Enigmatic Coptic Galaktotrophousa and the Cult of the Virgin Mary in Egypt," in *Images of the Mother of God: Perceptions of the Theotokos in Byzantium,* ed. Maria Vassilaki (Aldershot: Ashgate, 2005), 13–22.

371 Clement of Alexandria, *The Instructor (Paedagogus)*, in *Fathers of the Second Century: Hermas, Tatian, Athenagoras, Theophilus, and Clement of Alexandria*, vol. 2 of *The Ante-Nicene Fathers: Translations of the Writings of the Fathers Down to A.D. 325,* trans. Alexander Roberts and James Donaldson (1867–97; reprint, Grand Rapids, Mich: Eerdmans, 1979) Book I, 142.

372 See *Atti dei Martiri*, Introduzione, traduzione e note di Giuliana Caldarelli (Milano: Edizioni Paoline 1985), 7.

373 I will equally work with the Italian translation by Giuliana Caldarelli (see ibid.) and with the Latin edition and English translation by Herbert Musurillo. See *The Acts of the Christian Martyrs*, Introduction, texts and translations by Herbert Musurillo (Oxford: Clarendon Press, 1972). All English and Latin quotes from the

will be reconstructed with an emphasis on the question of how childbirth figures in the text.

Passio Sanctarum Perpetuae et Felicitatis, the chapter on Perpetua and Felicitas in the *Acts of Christian Martyrs* belongs to those *passiones* which are called *narrative* because they are assumed to have been partially written or dictated by the martyrs themselves.[374] Thus Pepertua's story reads like an "autobiography" to which an anonymous narrator makes an introduction. The "autobiographical" part of Perpetua's story is followed by the narrator's description of her martyrdom. The *Passio Sanctarum Perpetuae et Felicitatis* is an outstanding text in the *Acts of Christian Martyrs* because of its elaborate composition.[375]

Who were these women Perpetua and Felicitas? According to the text Perpetua came from a noble family and several details point to the fact that she most probably lived in Cathargo under the reign of Septimus Severus, that is, at the beginning of the third century.[376] Furthermore, the

---

Passio Sanctarum Perpetuae et Felicitatis in the *Acts of the Christian Martyrs* are from the edition and translation by Musurillo. The section on Perpetua and Felicitas in the *Acts of Christian Martyrs* is composed of the major acts of the *Passio Sanctarum Perpetuae et Felicitatis* and the minor acts of the *Passio Sanctarum Perpetuae et Felicitatis* which in large parts correspond to each other. It is generally assumed that the major acts are older than the minor acts. I will work equally with both sources.

374 See Giuliana Caldarelli, introduction to *Atti dei Martiri*, trans. Giuliana Caldarelli (Milano: Edizioni Paoline 1985), 28–29.

375 See ibid., 30. What is also remarkable about the text is the high degree of historical self-reflexivity on part of the narrator. In the introduction to Perpetua's "autobiography," the anonymous narrator emphasizes the moment of historical change to which Perpetua's and Felicitas' stories belong. S/he states explicitly that s/he is not recounting an event that has become meaningful by tradition but instead, in his/her opinion, will become important in a tradition that is yet to come: "The deeds recounted about the faith in ancient times were a proof of God's favour and achieved the spiritual strengthening of men as well; and they were set forth in writing precisely that honour might be rendered to God and comfort to men by the recollection of the past through the written word. Should not then more recent examples be set down that contribute equally to both ends? For indeed these too will one day become ancient and needful for the ages to come, even though in our own day they may enjoy less prestige because of the prior claim of antiquity" (*Passio Sanctarum Perpetuae et Felicitatis*, I.1–2).

376 For the discussion of the historical setting of the *Passio Sanctarum Perpetuae et Felicitatis* see Giuliana Caldarelli, "La passione delle sante Perpetua e Felicita e dei loro compagni," in *Atti dei Martiri*, trans. Giuliana Caldarelli (Milano: Edizioni Paoline 1985), 185.

narrator gives the information that Perpetua was 22 years old when she was arrested for not sacrificing to the gods or to the Roman emperor, that she had two brothers, had contracted a prestigious marriage, and that she was very well educated. It is said that at the time of the events, she had a baby whom she was still breast-feeding.[377]

This crude list of "facts" acquires a moving liveliness as the text switches from the narrator to Perpetua's "autobiography." For the purpose of examining the symbolic pattern "Theoretical, Spiritual and Political Natality versus Childbirth" woven into the text, here the focus will be on Perpetua's relationship to her child, her judge and her family (especially to her father) while her religious visions and insights are of less importance.

Perpetua describes the conflict between her Christian conviction, on the one hand, and the human relationships that tie her to her baby and her family, on the other. At the heart of this conflict are her father and her baby. When Perpetua is arrested, her father initially tries to make her change her mind by fighting her convictions on an ideological level. Here Perpetua answers with rhetorical skillfulness:

> 'Father,' said I, 'do you see this vase here, for example, or water-pot or whatever?'
> 'Yes, I do', said he.
> And I told him: 'Could it be called by any other name than what it is?'
> And he said: 'No.'
> 'Well, so too I cannot be called anything other than what I am, a Christian.'[378]

At these words Perpetua's father leaves the prison in despair and anger. As the day of the trial approaches, he makes another attempt to save her life by trying to convince her to sacrifice to the Roman gods and to the emperor. This time he uses arguments that will remain the same until the very day of her martyrdom. He says:

> 'Daughter,' he said, 'have pity on my grey head – have pity on me your father, if I deserve to be called your father, if I have favoured you above all your brothers, if I have raised you to reach this prime of your life. Do not abandon me to be the reproach

377 *Passio Sanctarum*, II.1–3.

378 Ibid., III.1–2: "Padre, inquam, uides uerbi gratia uas hoc iacens, urceolum siue aliud? et dixit: Video. 2. et ego dixi ei: Numquid alio nomine uocari potest quam quod est? et ait: Non. sic et ego aliud me dicere non possum nisi quod sum, Christiana."

of men. Think of your brothers, think of your mother and your aunt, think of your child, who will not be able to live once you are gone.[379]

In these lines the reasoning and supplicating by Perpetua's father goes in two directions. First, he emphasizes the meaning that Perpetua's life holds for the older generation. She is at the beginning of her adult life and her death would mean an immense loss to her parents and her aunt.

Another argument made by Perpetua's father concerns her baby. He reminds her of the fact that her child might not be able to live without her. Behind this reasoning may lie the assumption that just as Perpetua's life is of the highest importance to him, her baby's life should be of the highest importance to her. Accordingly, during the trial the father pleads with his daughter with his grandchild in his arms: "Perform the sacrifice – have pity on your baby!"[380] In the minor acts of the *Passio Sanctarum Perpetuae et Felicitatis* the father even throws the baby into his daughter's arms.[381]

The days before Perpetua's execution her father – who cannot understand her behaviour – is full of despair. His life has lost its meaning and he curses it. "Perpetua" writes:

> Now the day of the contest was approaching, and my father came to see me overwhelmed with sorrow. He started tearing the hairs from his beard and threw them on the ground; he then threw himself on the ground and began to curse his old age and to say such words as would move all creation.[382]

Perpetua's judge shares the value system of her father, and by invoking her father and her baby, tries to persuade her to perform the sacrifices: "Have pity on your father's grey head; have pity on your infant son. Offer the sacrifice for the welfare of the emperors."[383] Both Perpetua's father and

379 Ibid. V. 2–3: "Miserere, filia, canis meis; miserere patri, si dignus sum a te pater uocari; si his te manibus ad hunc florem aetatis prouexi, si te praeposui omnibus fratribus tuis: ne me dederis in dedecus hominum. 3. aspice fratres tuos, aspice matrem tuam et materteram, apice filium tuum qui post te uiuere non poterit."

380 Ibid. VI.2: "Supplica. miserere infanti."

381 See the minor acts of the *Passio Sanctarum Perpetuae et Felicitatis*, VI.5.

382 Ibid., IX.2.: "Ut autem proximauit dies muneris, intrat ad me pater meus consumptus taedio, et coepit barbam suam euellere et in terram mittere, et prosternere se in faciem, et inproperare annis suis, et dicere tanta uerba quae mouerent uniuersam creaturam."

383 Ibid., VI.3.: "Parce... canis patris tui, parce infantiae pueri. fac sacrum pro salute imperatorum."

her judge seem to be profoundly puzzled by the fact that Perpetua does not acknowledge her family ties, in particular those to her father and to her baby as the highest good.

How does Perpetua relate to the value system and the people surrounding her? Caldarelli ascribes a profound sensitivity to Perpetua and regards her as having deep affection for her family.[384] In fact, the text pictures Perpetua as a young woman who suffers from seeing her father's despair. This is expressed by sentences like "I was sorry for my father's sake,"[385] "I felt sorry for his unhappy old age,"[386] "I felt sorry for his pathetic old age."[387] Furthermore, Perpetua is closely bound to her baby. Indeed, she is extremely happy, when allowed to breastfeed the baby in prison.[388] Her joy after obtaining permission to keep the child with her in prison is illustrative of the profound love she feels for him: "Then I got permission for my baby to stay with me in prison. At once I recovered my health, relieved as I was of my worry and anxiety over the child. My prison had suddenly become a palace."[389]

Despite the deep affection she feels for both her father and her child, however, Perpetua continues with her decision to die as a martyr. She can act in this way only because she builds up a hierarchy of values in which the mortal immortality that comes with generation – both from the perspective of her father and from her own perspective as a mother – is subordinated to her spiritual natality. Perpetua understands the value system surrounding her, but she refuses to place anything – not even the life of her baby – above her Christian devotion. When her father tries to throw the child into her arms during the trial, she refuses to take the baby in order to avoid any temptation that could keep her from the mortal immortality that comes with faith. She tells her relatives that she cannot consider them and her baby to be more important than God who will lead her to glory.[390]

384 See Caldarelli, *Introduzione,* 38–39 and Caldarelli, "La passione delle sante," 192.

385 Passio *Sanctarum Perpetuae et Felicitatis*, Major Acts, V.6.: "*Et ego dolebam casum patris mei.*"

386 Ibid., IX.3.: "Ego dolebam pro infelici senecta eius."

387 Ibid., VI.5.: "Sic dolui pro senecta eius misera."

388 See ibid. III.8.

389 Ibid., III.9.: "Et usurpaui ut mecum infans in carcere maneret; et statim conualui et releuata sum a labore et sollicitudine infantis, et factus est mihi carcer subito praetorium, ut ibi mallem esse quam alicubi."

390 See ibid., *Minor Acts*, VI.6.

This scene is a lively illustration of the fact that Perpetua sees her family ties and the life of her baby as part of the terrestrial world, which loses any meaning and value when confronted with the Christian faith. "Christiana sum et nominis mei sequor auctoritatem, ut sim Perpetua,"[391] Perpetua says during the trial, making a pun with her name, a proper noun, the perpetuous, and the adjective perpetuous. Following Caldarelli's suggestion one could translate this sentence with "I am a Christian and I follow the significance of my name to become perpetuous." Caldarelli expresses the essence of Perpetua's attitude in the text very well when she writes: "Every thought, every word and every gesture are animated by the desire for eternal life."[392]

In the *Passio Sanctarum Perpetuae et Felicitatis*, Perpetua is given much more space than Felicitas. This may be due to the different social backgrounds of the two women. Perpetua was a noble woman and the education she was given enabled her to write an elaborate "autobiography" (if one follows the assumption that she did indeed partially write the text). Felicitas was a slave and the description of her martyrdom is entirely reliant on the narrator's will and skill to tell her story. Nevertheless, Felicitas' behavior and reasoning truely make her Perpetua's sister: Her story is shorter, but surely not less impressive.

Felicitas is arrested on the same day as Perpetua in Cathargo; she is eight months pregnant. The same judge who tries to persuade Perpetua to sacrifice to the emperor and to carry on living for the sake of her baby and her family also tries to convince Felicitas to place a higher value on her unborn baby than on her Christian faith.[393] In her answer Felicitas makes clear that being a Christian she depreciates the terrestrial world

---

391 Ibid., V.9.

392 Caldarelli, "La passione delle sante," 187: "Ogni pensiero, ogni parola e ogni suo gesto sono animati dal desiderio della vita eterna." What is interesting about Caldarelli's analysis of the *Passio Sanctarum Perpetuae et Felicitatis* is the fact that she morally approves of Perpetua's choice to consider her faith to be more important than her child. Caldarelli speaks of a "faith lived out in its fullness" (See ibid., 187). In another context she speaks of the high human, artistic and spiritual (sic!) value of the text (See ibid., 188). Caldarelli's attitude is a good illustration of an argument yet to be made by the analysis of 20th century sources in the section "Theoretical, Spiritual and Political Natality versus Childbirth": the subordination of the mortal immortality that comes with the birth of children, to the mortal immortality that comes with spirituality, is also part of contemporary culture.

393 See *Passio Sanctarum Perpetuae et Felicitatis*, Minor Acts, V.7.

including her unborn baby.[394] Felicitas' attitude is not unusual, and is supported by the other Christians imprisoned with her. Once the martyrs have been condemned to death, they pray collectively for Felicitas that she would give birth earlier than foreseen. The reason for this lies in the fact that Roman law forbade a pregnant woman to be punished by death and Felicitas wished to die on the same day as the other martyrs.[395]

In Felicitas' story, the sharp distinction drawn between the terrestrial and spiritual worlds extends to a distinction between two different types of pain. Felicitas has very bad labour pains and when one of the guards asks her ironically: "You suffer so much now – what will you do when you are tossed to the beasts? Little did you think of them when you refused to sacrifice?"[396] she answers, "What I am suffering now [...] I suffer by myself. But then another will be inside me who will suffer for me, just as I shall be suffering for him."[397] Labour pain, like the births of children, belongs to the terrestrial world and therefore Felicitas does not expect any divine help in the situation. However, she believes divine intervention will be present in the moment she suffers for her faith.

That giving birth is itself devoid of any spirituality is again illustrated by the narrator's comment on the martyrdom of Felicitas. Here, blood is assigned two different symbolic meanings. As conceived by the narrator, the blood from birthgiving (ie. lochies) is in need of purification, while the blood shed by the martyr belongs to the spiritual world and as such, is purifying. Thus the narrator writes that, in the arena, Felicitas purified herself from giving birth by shedding her blood for her belief and he depicts this as a second baptism: "With them also was Felicitas, glad that she had safely given birth so that now she could fight the beasts, going from one blood bath to another, from the midwife to the gladiator, ready to wash after childbirth in a second baptism."[398]

---

394 Ibid.

395 See *Passio Sanctarum Perpetuae et Felicitatis*, Major Acts, XV.

396 Ibid., XV.5.: "Quae sic modo doles, quid facies obiecta bestiis, quas contempsisti cum sacrificare noluisti?"

397 Ibid., XV.6.: "Modo ego quod patior; illic autem alius erit in me qui patietur pro me, quia et ego pro illo passura sum."

398 *Passio Sanctarum Perpetuae et Felicitatis*, Major Acts, XVIII.3: "Item Felicitas, saluam se peperisse gaudens ut ad bestias pugnaret, a sanguine ad sanguinem, ab obstetrice ad retiarium, lotura post partum baptismo secundo." The blood of the martyr not only in Felicitas' case but also in general is considered to be holy blood.

The description of the martyrdom of Felicitas is perhaps one of the most "extreme" examples of the opposition between spiritual birth and childbirth in Christian texts. In the following chapter on Gregory of Nyssa this opposition will again be encountered. However, here it appears in the form of Christian thinking fused with Platonism.

6.3 Birth as deriving "from the Skins of Brutes": Gregory of Nyssa's Understanding of Marriage and Virginity as Different Conditions of the Soul

In Eastern Anatolia during the second half of the fourth century C.E., Christian ascetic communities were steadily growing, creating a world that ran parallel to the life of urban Christian families of the time.[399] Basileus, the older brother of Gregory of Nyssa in 370 became bishop of Cesarea. He dedicated himself to founding monastic confraternities which would form economic units who gave to the poor what they did not need for their own survival. With his ideas promoting an ascetic Christian life, Basileus met the resistance of urban elites. It is in this context that Gregory of Nyssa set out to write his first work *On Virginity* between 370 and 379 C.E. With his elaborate praise of virgin life he wanted to support his older brother's effort to gain broader social acceptance of asceticism. *On Virginity* uses their sister Macrina's life as an implicit model, though her name is never mentioned.[400] Contrary to Gregory – who had been married to a woman named Theosebia – she chose to refrain from marriage and to lead an ascetic life together with other women on a farm in the region of Annesi.[401]

As will be shown in the following, *On Virginity* is a most interesting work for the context of a symbolic pattern of childbirth opposing spiritual birth and the birth of children. Here, Gregory of Nyssa, in his quest for a mortal immortality, develops the idea that the life of a virgin leads to a different condition of the soul than the life of a married person. In his work

For example, the martyr Saturo bathes the ring of a soldier whom he had just converted to Christianity in his blood, leaving him a "holy heritage" (See ibid., XXI.3–5).

399 See for this and the following Peter Brown, *The Body and Society: Men, Women and Sexual Renunciation in Early Christianity* (London: faber and faber, 1988), 290–292.

400 See Mariella Carpinello, *Libere donne di Dio: Figure femminili nei primi secoli cristiani* (Milano: Mondadori, 1997), 25.

401 See Brown, *The Body and Society*, 298.

he emphasizes that he does not intend to depreciate marriage as an institution but rather wants to give an incentive to make the choice for an ascetic life, as most people opt for getting married anyhow.[402] However, Gregory of Nyssa depicts marriage in dominantly darkish colours, as he conceives of life from the perspective of death. He identifies marriage with having children and founding a family. Even under ideal circiumstances death and the fear of death are continuous companions of family life. Therefore, the wife lives in fear that something might happen to her husband[403]; the sorrows of widowhood and orphanhood are most painful[404] and "death [is] always hanging by expectation over the children that are born, and putting a finger upon each of the sweetest joys."[405]

Gregory of Nyssa sees marriage as an indirect consequence of original sin. Death came into the world because of sin[406] and marriage, by divine providence, functions as a means to mitigate death.[407] It is from this reasoning that Gregory of Nyssa's advocacy for a virgin life departs: "Marriage, then, is the last stage of our separation from the life that was led in Paradise; marriage therefore, as our discourse has been suggesting, is the first thing to be left."[408] Thus, as it were, the virgin, by refraining from marriage, reapproaches paradise by "going the way back" to God. In a similar vein, Gregory of Nyssa argues that an ascetic life gives a pretaste of the life after resurrection. Life in the afterworld, according to the Scriptures, is supposed to be of an angelic nature, the main characteristic of angels being that "they are strangers to marriage."[409] Therefore to lead an ascetic life means to approach the world of the resurrection and the angels.

In the same measure, as virginity becomes the "practical method in the science of the Divine life"[410], to Gregory of Nyssa, marriage standing

---

402 See Gregory of Nyssa, *On Virginity*, trans. William Moore and Henry Austin Wilson, vol. 5 of A Select Library of Nicene and post-Nicene Fathers of the Christian Church: Gregory of Nyssa, ed. Philip Schaff and Henry Wace (1892; reprint, Grand Rapids, Michigan: Eerdmans, 1988), chap. VIII, p. 352.

403 See ibid., chap. III, p. 347.

404 See ibid.

405 Ibid., chap. III, p. 346.

406 Ibid., chap. XIII, p. 359: "The flesh is subject to death because of sin."

407 Ibid., chap. XII, p. 358: "As the compensation for having to die, marriage was instituted."

408 Ibid., chap. XII, p. 358.

409 Ibid., chap. XIII, p. 360.

410 Ibid., chap. V, p. 351.

for sexual intercourse and the generation of children becomes an obstacle for approaching the divine. The manner in which Gregory of Nyssa expresses the superiority of spiritual birth over childbirth is highly reminiscent of Plato's *Symposium*. Both the philosopher and the bishop use pregnancy, procreation, conception and birth as metaphors to designate a spiritual transformation.They both see spiritual birth as the only way to immortality. Furthermore, Gregory of Nyssa – just like Plato – opposes spiritual birth to the birth of children: "Every one knows that the propagation of mortal frames is the work which the intercourse of the sexes has to do; whereas for those who are joined to the Spirit, life and immortality instead of children are produced by this latter intercourse."[411]

Instead of a child, the Christian virgin, as a model for a Christian life, "by the operation of the spirit conceives the deathless children."[412] Instead of the mortal children of marriage, virginity "has the offspring of devotion always to rejoice in."[413]

Gregory of Nyssa, seeing life exclusively through the prism of death, goes as far as attributing a somehow physical capacity to virginity that enables her to defeat death and to attain a mortal immortality. By refraining from giving birth, the virgin breaks the chain of generations succeeding one another and dying one after the other. Thereby her body is invested with the touch of immortality: "That body is rightly named undying which does not lend its service to a dying world, nor brooks to become the instrument of a succession of dying creatures."[414]

I wish to conclude this section on Gregory of Nyssa with what is perhaps the harshest passage of his works concerning the mutual exclusion of birth and spiritual birth. This passage does not come from *On Virginity* but from his work *On the Soul and the Resurrection,*[415] which consists of a dialogue between Gregory of Nyssa and a female teacher, described as a virgin. Though not explicitly mentioned, it is Gregory's sister Macrina

411 Ibid., chap. XIII, p. 359.
412 Ibid., chap. XIII, p. 359.
413 Ibid., chap. III, p. 347.
414 Ibid., chap. XIII, 359.
415 See Gregory of Nyssa, *On the Soul and the Resurrection*, trans. William Moore and Henry Austin Wilson, vol. 5 of A Select Library of Nicene and post-Nicene Fathers of the Christian Church: Gregory of Nyssa, ed. Philip Schaff and Henry Wace (1892; reprint, Grand Rapids, Michigan: Eerdmans, 1988).

with lullabies, and all the noisy coming and going of men and women about the house? Will he put up with the constant muddle and squalor which small children bring into the home? The wealthy can do so, you will say, for their mansions and large houses can provide privacy and, being rich, they do not have to count the cost nor be tormented by daily cares. But philosophers lead a very different life from rich men, and those who are concerned with wealth or are involved in mundane matters will not have time for the claims of Scripture or philosophy.[422]

This statement of Héloise describes the conception of two different worlds which cannot be reconciled with one another. In her eyes one has to choose between desks and cradles, pens and spindles – in other words, philosophy and theology on the one hand and a family on the other. Her reasoning brings with it a whole construction of childbirth that goes far beyond the practical aspects regarding the impediments brought about by having children in the house of a philosopher. Children, within the frame of her logic stand in opposition to the spirit. They can only constitute a threat to practising philosophy, which is valued so highly, that Héloise thinks of refusing to marry Abélard because she does not want to endanger his status as a philosopher.[423]

Interestingly, at a distance of something like two decades, Abélard, in a letter to his now grown-up son Astralabius, expresses a similar attitude in that he assigns a very high value to philosophy and poetry. He explicitly tells his son to use the world of the mind to reach immortality:

Qui pereunt in se, vivunt per scripta poetae;
Quam natura negat, vita per ista manet.
Per famam vivit defuncto corpore doctus,
Et plus natura philosophia potest.[424]

---

422 *The Letters of Abélard and Héloise*, trans. B. Radice (Harmondsworth: Penguin, 1974), 71–72.

423 This perception of an incompatibility between philosophy and children in the letter of Héloise somehow hilariously contrasts with the description of the family life of the philosophers Elizabeth Anscombe and Peter Geach in Paul Feyerabend's autobiography *Killing Time*: "The morning started with a bang: the children invaded my bedroom and played war. "Peach," as Elizabeth calls her husband, moved around forlornly – until he had his daily fit of anger. .... Jam, coins, pages of manuscripts could be found in the most unlikely places; amid all this was Elizabeth – distant, smoking like a chimney. Visitors dropped in, looked around, left again" (Feyerabend, *Killing Time*, 92).

424 Abélard, quoted in Curtius, *Europäische Literatur und lateinisches Mittelalter*, 470.

["Those who perish in themselves live on through the writings of poets
As nature denies, life through that abides.
Through report the learned man lives with a dead body.
And philosophy is able to do more than nature."[425]]

8. *A World Where Saps Will Have Their Way*: The Opposition of Life and Art in Rainer Maria Rilke's *Requiem for a Friend*

Still another variation of the symbolic pattern of childbirth labelled "Theoretical, Spiritual and Political Natality versus Childbirth" can be encountered in Rainer Maria Rilke's poem *Requiem for a Friend*.[426] Here, it is not the *polis*, faith, philosophy or the study of the Holy Scriptures that stand in opposition to childbirth but rather, a conception of art demanding the utmost dedication from the artist comes into tension with childbirth.

Rilke wrote *Requiem for a Friend* in memory of the painter Paula Modersohn-Becker, who had died in 1907, a fortnight after she had given birth to her daughter Mathilde.[427] In the opening stanza of the poem, a fictitious speaker is sitting in his room thinking of his friend, or rather, feeling haunted by the spirit of his dead friend who does not seem to find any peace in being dead. Thus, he starts a long monologue, addressing

425 Abélard, quoted and translated in Gerald Seaman, "Signs of a New Literary Paradigm: The 'Christian' Figures of Chrétien de Troyes," in *Nominalism and Literary Discourse: New Perspectives,* ed. Hugo Keiper, Christoph Bod, and Richard J. Utz (Amsterdam, Atlanta, GA: Editions Rodopi B.V., 1997), 95.

426 See for the following quotes from *Requiem for a Friend* Rainer Maria Rilke, "Requiem für eine Freundin," in Rainer Maria Rilke, *Sämtliche Werke*, ed. Rilke-Archiv in collaboration with Ruth Sieber-Rilke (Frankfurt/M: Insel, 1987), 1:645–656 and Rainer Maria Rilke, "Requiem for a Friend," in Rainer Maria Rilke: *Requiem and Other Poems*, trans. with an intr. and notes J.B. Leishman (London: Hogarth Press, 1949), 129–136.

427 Strangely enough, as much as the Rilkean construction of childbirth in the *Requiem* belongs to the symbolic pattern of childbirth which opposes a spiritual identity (artistic, philosophic or religious) to the birth of children the pictures by Modersohn-Becker belong to the fourth symbolic order of childbirth, as will be shown in section III.4. of this work. See also Anja Hänsch, "The Body of the Woman Artist: Rainer-Maria Rilke and Paula Modersohn-Becker on Giving Birth and Art," *European Journal of Women's Studies*, no. 4 (1997): 435–449.

his friend, trying to discover what is making her so restless. What is very special about this monologue is the fact that the distance between the fictitious speaker and Rilke, the author, projecting his ideas on the lyrical "I" is narrowed considerably by what Freud calls *Trauerarbeit*.[428] It is in the process of going through this kind of mourning that Rilke, in the guise of the fictitious speaker, tries to come to terms with his friend's death. As part of a *Trauerarbeit,* the *Requiem* connects Paula Modersohn-Becker's death to the more general problem of death, seen from a pre-existentialist perspective. The reason the poem gives for the imagined restlessness of Modersohn-Becker's spirit lies with the Rilkean idea that she did not experience her "own" death. What does this mean?

The problem of one's own death appears frequently in Rilke's work. It refers to the idea that dying should be connected to the life of an individual. Thus, in this sense, living one's own life, taking one's own existence upon oneself also means dying one's own death. In Rilke's understanding, death should ideally be generated by each individual life. In a way, death thus becomes the carrier of individuality, which Rilke feels is threatened by the mass existence of men in over-crowded towns. In the *Aufzeichnungen des Malte Laurids-Brigge* Rilke writes:

> The desire to have one's own death becomes more and more rare. Soon it will be as rare as having one's own life. My God, all this is happening. You come, you find a life ready, you only have to put it on. You want to go or you are obliged to do so: no effort: Voilà votre mort, monsieur. You take death as it comes.[429]

The questions to be posed are, why is it then that Modersohn-Becker, according to Rilke, did not die her "own" death, even though she did not die as people in a large metropolis die? Why does Rilke, in the guise of the fictitious speaker, transfigure his own inability to come to terms with her death into a feeling of being persecuted by his friend? One answer, which

---

428 Many thanks to Vladimir Gradev, who pointed out the link between the *Requiem* and the process of *Trauerarbeit* to me.

429 Rainer Maria Rilke, *Die Aufzeichnungen des Malte Laurids Brigge* (Frankfurt/M: Insel, 1982), 13: "Der Wunsch einen eigenen Tod zu haben wird immer seltener. Eine Weile noch, und er wird ebenso selten sein wie ein eigenes Leben. Gott, das ist alles da. Man kommt, man findet ein Leben, fertig, man hat es nur anzuziehen. Man will gehen oder man ist dazu gezwungen: nun, keine Anstrengung: Voilà votre mort, monsieur. Man stirbt, wie es gerade kommt."
I would like to thank Barbara MacLennan for helping me to translate this passage and several other passages of this section from German into English.

can be suggested, is that the problem lies in the fact that the artist died after giving birth. Rilke blames his friend for not having died the death of an artist, a death which would have been more intrinsically linked to her life. He argues that by having been pregnant and giving birth to a child, Paula Modersohn-Becker became the protagonist of a series of events which were in dramatic contrast with her existence as an artist, and thus also with her potential death as one. That is to say, she destroyed her future as an artist by directing all her creative forces towards the child ("Hours you used to sit in silence, bending/ the boundless forces of your boundless future/ out of their course to the new germination,/ that became fate once more. O painful labour"[430]). Therefore she could not experience her "own," individual death; metaphorically speaking, she ate the "green seeds" from which her own death would have then grown:

> And then
> you took yourself away and from your heart's
> warm, night-warm, soil you dug the yet green seeds
> your death was going to spring from: your own death,
> the death appropriate to your own life.
> And then you ate those grains of your own death.[431]

In Rilkean thought, death is a means to achieve the maximum expression of individuality, which equals self-fulfillment as a human being.[432]

430 "Da du saßest und
die vielen Kräfte deiner vielen Zukunft
schweigend herabbogst zu dem neuen Kindkeim,
der wieder Schicksal war. Oh wehe Arbeit."

431 "Und grubst aus deines Herzens
nachtwarmem Erdreich die noch grünen Samen,
daraus dein Tod aufkeimen sollte: deiner,
dein eigner Tod zu deinem eignen Leben.
Und aßest sie, die Körner deines Todes."

432 In *Florenzer Tagebuch* the poet writes: "Je menschlicher wir werden, desto verschiedener werden wir. Es ist, als würden plötzlich die Wesen sich vertausendfachen; denn ein Kollektivname, der früher über Tausende reichte, wird bald schon für zehn Menschen zu eng, und man wird gezwungen, jeden einzelnen zu betrachten. Man denke: Wenn wir statt Völkern, Menschen, Nationen, Familien und Gesellschaften mal Menschen haben werden, wenn man selbst drei nicht mehr in einem Namen vereinen kann! Wird dann die Welt nicht größer werden müssen?" Rainer Maria Rilke, *Das Florenzer Tagebuch*, ed. Ruth Sieber-Rilke and Carl Sieber (Frankfurt/M and Leipzig: Insel, 1994), 97.

According to Rilke, Modersohn-Becker did not appropriate her death to herself, instead, she died the death of women after labour:

> And so you died like women long ago,
> died in the old warm house, old-fashionedly,
> the death of those in child-bed.[433]

Underlying these verses is a quite subtle but nervertheless important opposition. Death from childbirth is pictured as the death of "ordinary" women and not of women artists. An artist's dying in childbed is considered an inappropriate death, because birthgiving and pregnancy for Rilke belong to the sphere of life (and matter) as opposed to art. In the *Requiem*, Rilke writes: "For somewhere there's an old hostility/ between our human life and greatest work."[434] Pregnancy is labelled a coincidence[435] (*Zufall*) which pulls his friend, who has already transcended the world of matter by being an artist, violently back into this world where – as Rilke puts it – "saps will have their way":

> Then, for the last time, chance got hold of you,
> and snatched you back out of your farthest progress,
> back to a world where saps will have their way.[436]

The result is that the artist Paula Modersohn-Becker, by giving birth and subsequently dying, becomes an ordinary woman, connected to a sphere of immanence. With this judgement, the poet measures his friend according to his own ideals; in his own life, he perceived there to be a dichotomy between life and art and was convinced that in the case of a conflict between the two, the real artist should choose art in order to be true to himself.[437] In Rilkean thought, art functions as a means to transcend one's existence and thus becomes a means of self-redemption. The fact that

433 "So starbst du, wie die Frauen früher starben,
altmodisch starbst du in dem warmen Hause
den Tod der Wöchnerinnen."

434 "Denn irgendwo ist eine alte Feindschaft/zwischen dem Leben und der großen Arbeit."

435 Probably the word coincidence is a more exact translation for the German word "*Zufall*" than the word chance used by the translator.

436 "Da riß ein Zufall dich.../ riß dich zurück aus deinem fernsten Fortschritt/ in eine Welt zurück, wo Säfte wollen".

437 See Seon-Ae Eom, *Todesvertrautheit: Deutungen der Orpheus-Gestalt in Rilkes Dichtung* (Frankfurt/M: Lang, 1988), 82.

Paula Modersohn-Becker had actually chosen to give birth to a child was for Rilke a decision which went against the essence of her being, given that he defined this in terms of art and not in terms of "life." In this context it is important to understand the significance of the fact that in the *Requiem* Modersohn-Becker's pregnancy is called a coincidence ("Zufall"). Rilke was a close friend of hers and thus would have known how much she desired to have a child. If he, in the guise of the fictitious speaker, pictures Modersohn-Becker's pregnancy as a coincidence, this means that he turns her into a victim of female fertility, that is, a victim of the laws of "life" which – in Rilke's eyes – the woman artist did not escape.

In summary, the poem antagonizes the artist Paula Modersohn-Becker and the "woman" Paula Modersohn-Becker. Female fertility cannot be part of the identity of a woman artist because the whole sphere of birthgiving is connected to immanence while the whole sphere of art is connected to transcendence.[438]

---

438 As Adelheid Hausen has pointed out to me, reflections on the woman artist and the birthgiving artist are also included in Rilke's *Florenzer Tagebuch* ("Florentine Diary") from 1898. Even ten years before the *Requiem,* he thought of motherhood and art as incompatible with one another. In this context he conceives of birthgiving as an artistic act, a kind of creation, and excludes the possibility that for the woman there could be two moments of creativity, only championing one of them, namely motherhood, replacing art:
"Die Mütter freilich sind wie die Künstler. Des Künstlers Mühe ist, sich selbst zu finden. Das Weib erfüllt sich im Kinde. Und was der Künstler stückweise sich entringt, das hebt das Weib wie eine Welt voll von Mächten und Möglichkeiten, aus ihrem Schoß. … Eine Frau, welche Künstlerin ist, muß nicht mehr schaffen, wenn sie Mutter wurde." ("Mothers are like artists. The artist takes pains to find himself. Woman fulfils herself in the child. And what the artist piece by piece wrests from himself, the woman lifts up like a world of powers and possibilities from her womb. … A woman who is an artist no longer has to create, when she becomes a mother"). Rilke, *Florenzer Tagebuch*, 95–96.
I wish to warmly thank Barbara MacLennan for helping me with the translation of this passage from *Florenzer Tagebuch*.
In order to do justice to the complexity of Rilkean thoughts about childbirth and also to the different emotional tensions which obviously lie beneath them, here it has to be emphasized that the dichotomy of the woman artist and the mother are of a different nature in the *Florenzer Tagebuch* than in the *Requiem*. While in the Requiem it is the vocation of the artist which stands above life, in the *Florenzer Tagebuch*, the birthgiving mother herself appears as an artist whose creative act is superior to that of a poet, or a painter.

In Rilkean reasoning, the artistic identity stands in direct opposition to childbirth. Carrying a child in one's womb and giving birth to it cannot be integrated into the artist's will to the *farthest progress.* This is why Rilke pictures Modersohn-Becker's pregnancy as fundamentally alien to her artistic self. With regard to one of her self-portraits, most probably *Selbstbildnis am 6. Hochzeitstag,*[439] he writes:

> And finally you saw yourself as fruit,
> lifted yourself out of your clothes and carried
> that self before the mirror, let it in
> up to your gaze; which remained large, in front,
> and did not say; that's me; no, but: this is.[440]

In these verses Rilke – in accordance with his perception of Modersohn-Becker's pregnancy as a coincidence – suggests a deep alienation of the artist from her pregnancy. The fictive artist does not identify with pregnancy as an expression of herself but, on the contrary, is overwhelmed by the forces of nature, matter, destiny: "And did not say; that's me; no, but: this is."

As has been shown, in *Aufzeichnungen des Malte Laurids Brigge* and *Requiem,* Rilke sees death as a potentially highly individualizing event. Birth, however, is disconnected from individuality. Death can become "one's own" death, but birthgiving cannot become "one's own." This is because, in Rilke's understanding, thc birthgiving woman belongs to the realms of life and immanence. For the Rilke of the *Requiem*, there cannot be any transcendance for a woman artist rooted in pregnancy/birthgiving, as these events belong to "a world where saps will have their way." The "proper" way for an artist to transcend his/her existence remains that of art (as opposed to life).

Rilke's approach to childbirth in the *Requiem* does not seem to be completely isolated. Apart from the fact that it forms part of a tradition which subordinates childbirth to some higher good (in this case, art) the

---

439 See Gillian Perry, *Paula Modersohn-Becker: Her Life and Work* (London: Women's Press, 1981), 54.

440 "Und sahst dich selbst zuletzt wie eine Frucht,
nahmst dich heraus aus deinen Kleidern, trugst
dich vor den Spiegel, ließest dich hinein
bis auf dein Schauen; das blieb groß davor
und sagte nicht: das bin ich; nein: dies ist."

Rilkean attitude also reflects a specific definition of art which, according to David D. Gilmore, functions as a means of creating a male identity:

> There is a venerable literary tradition that identifies masculinity with the act of artistic creation, the process that forges beauty from an unyielding raw material. Among those following this view, a definition of masculinity is bound up with purposive construction. Manhood is seen as the conjoining of disperate elements into an ordered whole, the imposition of form upon chaos – a kind of aesthetic confabulation obviously the counterpart to motherhood.[441]

If it is both true that the Rilkean approach to art can be read as a counterpart to motherhood (as he states in the *Florenzer Tagebuch*) and also that motherhood and birthgiving are "materialized" in his conception of life, this may give a further insight into the construction of childbirth in the *Requiem*. The opposition of childbirth, motherhood, woman, life versus artistic creation, artist, man, art, may also be interpreted as a certain construction of masculinity. The *Requiem* relies on this opposition in that Rilke constructs the identity of the fictive Modersohn-Becker in analogy to his own "male" identity as an artist. By placing the fictive Modersohn-Becker on the side of "artistic creation, artist, man, art," Rilke forces her into an opposition with "childbirth, motherhood, woman, life": the two parts of the opposition remain mutually exclusive. Thus the fictive artist betrays the Rilkean construction of an artistic identity which is constituted by perceiving childbirth as a point of non-identification in the contrast between life and art.

9. "The Ejaculation is a Promise of Death": Simone de Beauvoir's Conception of Individuality as Being Opposed to the Human Species

With the following investigation of Simone de Beauvoir's feminist classic *The Second Sex* from the perspective of childbirth, we will move from the Rilkean contrast between childbirth and art back to contentions between the realm of the mind and childbirth. However, Simone de Beauvoir's

441 Gilmore, *Manhood in the Making,* 113.

work displays quite a peculiar version of this theme. In her writing, it is not poetry, virtues and laws that are opposed to childbirth, as in Plato's *Symposium*, but rather it is an existentialist conception of individuality linked to reason that comes into tension with childbirth and procreation.

In her pioneering work *The Second Sex*, Simone de Beauvoir argues for a separation of the biological woman from the cultural woman. She explores transformations of what she sees as biologically given facts into cultural constructions of women. With this step she paved the way for contemporary thinkers such as Judith Butler and Donna Haraway to suggest, decades later, that there are no biological "facts" as such and that not only gender but also sex is a construction.[442] However, in Simone de Beauvoir's writings, biology – to quite a degree – is still a fixed point of reference. Furthermore, her deconstruction of woman as an idea also brings with it the construction of woman as an idea. This will be examined with regard to De Beauvoir's conception of the relationship between woman and childbirth. De Beauvoir mainly touches upon this issue in an extended chapter about motherhood entitled *Destiny* which deals with what she perceives as biological "facts." Additionally, she comments on women and childbirth in various passages throughout the whole book. In the following I will comment on De Beauvoir's conception of childbirth and procreation in the light of the symbolic register of childbirth perpetuating an opposition between theoretical natality and birth.

De Beauvoir sees the fertile female body as a living battlefield where a conflict between the species and the individual[443] (*"conflit espèce-individu"*[444]) is fought. Analysing the biologically given "facts" about woman, De Beauvoir comes to the conclusion that pregnancy and birthgiving, from a purely physical perspective, go against the woman

442 See e.g. Butler, *Bodies That Matter*; Butler, *Gender Trouble*; Donna Haraway, *Simians, Cyborgs, and Women: The Reinvention of Nature* (London: Free Association Books, 1991). An interesting work on the constructedness of a bipolar gender model in biology and medicine is a study by Heinz-Jürgen Voß. He argues that from a biological perspective there is an evidence for a plurality of gender which due to cultural reasons is not perceived as such. See Heinz-Jürgen Voß, *Making Sex Revisited: Dekonstruktion des Geschlechts aus biologisch-medizinischer Perspektive* (Bielefeld: transcript Verlag, 2010).

443 De Beauvoir, *The Second Sex*, trans. and ed. H. M. Parshley (London: Vintage, 1997), 63.

444 Simone de Beauvoir, *Les faits et les mythes*, vol. 1 of *Le deuxième sexe* (1949; renouvelé en 1976, reprint, Paris: Éditions Gallimard, 1989), 68.

as an individual. The child, even in the form of a fertilized ovulum, is seen as an invader of female individuality: "Woman experiences a more profound alienation when fertilization has occurred and the dividing egg passes down into the uterus and proceeds to develop there."[445] Likewise, De Beauvoir sees a deep cleavage between the woman and the child, (the individual and the species) during the moment of birthgiving because of the fact that the mother's life may be at risk: "Childbirth itself is painful and dangerous. In this crisis it is most clearly evident that the body does not always work to the advantage of both species and the individual."[446] It is emphasized that pregnancy for the woman does not bring with it any benefits for her as an individual: "Gestation is a fatiguing task of no individual benefit to the woman."[447] Although De Beauvoir, in this context, does admit in a footnote that motherhood may bring with it psychic benefits (as well as psychic disasters), in the following analysis of her chapter on motherhood, it will become clear that the contrast between individuality and species persists in her construction of childbirth.

In De Beauvoir's view, artistic or spiritual activities may contribute to the formation of woman as an individual, whereas childbirth only brings her down to the species level and hinders her individual development. The pregnant body is described with dark metaphors. With regard to this point, De Beauvoir belongs to a tradition of philosophical thought that constructs the body as being in a dichotomous relationship with the mind. She writes: "Day after day a growth arising from her flesh but foreign to it is going to enlarge within her; she is the prey of the species, which imposes its mysterious laws upon her."[448] In a sense, De Beauvoir sees the corporeality of woman as being accentuated through pregnancy and childbirth. Because

445 De Beauvoir, *The Second Sex*, 62. De Beauvoir, *Les faits*, 67: "La femme connaît une aliénation plus profonde quand l'oeuf fécondé descend dans l'utérus et s'y développe."

446 De Beauvoir, *The Second Sex*, 62. De Beauvoir, *Les faits*, 68 : "L'accouchement lui-même est douloureux; il est dangereux. C'est dans cette crise qu'on voit avec le plus d'évidence que le corps ne satisfait pas toujours l'éspèce et l'individu ensemble."

447 De Beauvoir, *The Second Sex*, 62. De Beauvoir, *Les faits*, 67: "La gestation est un travail fatigant qui ne présente pas pour la femme un bénéfice individuel."

448 De Beauvoir, *The Second Sex*, 515. De Beauvoir, *L'expérience vécue*, vol. 2 of *Le deuxième sexe* (1949; renouvelé en 1976, reprint, Paris: Éditions Gallimard, 1989), 353: "Jour après jour, un polype né de sa chair et étranger à sa chair va s'engraisser en elle; elle est la proie de l'espèce qui lui impose ses mystérieuses lois."

she conceives of the body as of the opposite pole of the "mind," such an accentuated corporeality cannot be but negative:

> Her flesh engenders flesh only, and she is quite incapable of establishing an existence that will have to establich itself. .... every mother entertains the idea that her child will be a hero, thus showing her wonderment at the thought of engendering a being with consciousness and freedom; but she is also in dread of giving birth to a defective or a monster, because she is aware of the frightening hazards of the flesh – and this embryo dwelling within her is only flesh.[449]

Although De Beauvoir mainly conceptualizes woman as a victim of the species in the period of pregnancy and birthgiving, she also sees a connection between childbirth and a mortal immortality: "Caught up in the great cycle of the species, she affirms life in the teeth of time and death: in this she glimpses immortality."[450] Nevertheless, the mortal immortality that comes with children is immediately devalued by two different ideas. One is that childbirth reminds parents of the finiteness of their own life. Here she quotes Hegel's saying "The birth of children is the death of parents."[451]

Secondly, the mortal immortality that comes with childbirth is devalued by opposing it to activities of the mind. Childbirth cannot be a means of individualization ("she engenders him [the child] as a product of her generalized body, not of her individualized existence"[452]). However, a woman becomes a heroine if she can keep her individuality in spite of pregnancy and birthgiving. This idea becomes clear by some examples De Beauvoir gives of women who firmly insisted on their intellectual/artistic identities, which they felt to be threatened by pregnancy and childbirth. Women, according to De Beauvoir, are brave if they gain control over their bodies and if they defend their theoretical natality against childbirth which

---

449 De Beauvoir, *The Second Sex*, 513–514. De Beauvoir, *L'expérience vécue*, 351–352: "Sa chair engendre seulement de la chair: elle est incapable de fonder une existence qui aura à se fonder elle-même. … Toute mère a l'idée que son enfant sera un héros; elle exprime ainsi son émerveillement à l'idée d'engendrer une coscience et une liberté; mais elle redoute aussi d'accoucher d'un infirme, d'un monstre, parce qu'elle connaît l'affreuse contingence de la chair, et cet embryon est seulement chair."

450 De Beauvoir, *The Second Sex*, 514. De Beauvoir, *L'expérience vécue*, 352: "Prise dans le grand cycle de l'espèce, elle affirme la vie contre le temps et la mort: par là elle est promise à l'immortalité."

451 Ibid.

452 De Beauvoir, *The Second Sex*, 514. De Beauvoir, *L'expérience vécue*, 351 : "Elle […] engendre [l'enfant] dans la généralité de son corps, non dans la singularité de son existence."

she mainly considers to be a burden of the species, an "enslavement of the female to the species" ("*asservissement de la femme à l'espèce*"[453]). The examples she gives for this kind of heroic behavior, of which she clearly approves, are Mme de Staël and Colette. Of Mme de Staël she writes: "Mme de Staël carried on a pregnancy as readily as a conversation."[454]

From statements like this one gains the impression that it is a matter of honour for the intellectual/artistic woman to have control over her pregnant/birthgiving body and not to let it dominate over the self, conceived of as completely detached from the body. Such an idea of the ideal behaviour of the pregnant, intellectual woman is also contained in De Beauvoir's comment on the writer Colette, who apparently lived up to this model: "And in fact she seems typical of those women who bear their condition valiantly because they are not absorbed in it. At the same time she continued her work as a writer."[455]

In *The Second Sex* women like Mme de Staël and Colette who contribute to the maintenance of honour of intellectual women by controlling their bodies and subordinating childbirth to their intellectual life are sharply contrasted to intellectual women who take a different attitude to childbirth. The poet Cécile Sauvage who wrote about childbirth in her collection of poems *L'Âme en bourgeon* and in a letter to her husband comes under heavy attack here. In order to understand De Beauvoir's critique of Sauvage, which, in essence, is a critique of a different construction of childbirth than the one preferred by herself, it is important to reproduce both the texts by Sauvage and the comments by De Beauvoir. During her pregnancy the poet Cécile Sauvage wrote to her husband:

> It's queer, I feel as if I were in attendance at the formation of a very tiny planet and were shaping the fragile orb. I have never been so close to life. Never have I so clearly felt that I am sister to the earth, with its vegetation and vital sap. My feet tread on the earth as if it were a living thing. I dream in broad daylight of flutes, awakened bees, and dew, for now he kicks and stirs within me. Could you but know how this building soul fills my heart with the freshness of springtime and with youth! And to think that

453 De Beauvoir, *The Second Sex*, 69. De Beauvoir, *Les faits*, Vol. I., 75.

454 De Beauvoir, *The Second Sex*, 517. De Beauvoir, *L'expérience vécue*, 356: "Mme de Staël menait une grossesse aussi rondement qu'une conversation."

455 De Beauvoir, *The Second Sex*, 519. De Beauvoir, *L'expérience vécue*, 358: "Et elle apparaît en effet comme le type de ces femmes qui supportent vaillament leur état parce qu'elles ne s'absorbent pas en lui. Elle poursuivait en même temps son travail d'écrivain."

it is the infant soul of Pierrot, and that in the darkness inside me this soul is perfecting two great eyes of infinite depth like his.[456]

What Cécile Sauvage here expressed in prose, in *L'Âme en Bourgeon*, she put in poetry as follows:

You belong to me as the dawn to the plain
Around you my life is like warm wool
In which your delicate members grow in secret
…
Little soul in bud joined to my flower
Your heart I fashion from a bit of mine.[457]

In De Beauvoir's eyes, Cécile Sauvage forms part of a group of women who – in contrast to the heroines Mme de Staël and Colette – give unjustified importance to their pregnancies:

Other women feel the weight of it more; they muse endlessly on their new importance. With the slightest encouragement they revive in their own cases the masculine myths: against the light of the mind they oppose the fecund darkness of Life; against the clarity of consciousness, the mysteries of inwardness; against productive liberty, the weight of this belly growing there enormously without human will. The mother-to-be feels herself one with the soil and sod, stock and root; when she drowses off, her sleep is like that of brooding chaos with worlds in ferment. Some, those more

456 De Beauvoir, *The Second Sex*, 520. De Beauvoir, *L'expérience vécue*, 359: "C'est drôle, il me semble que j'assiste à la formation d'une infirme planète et que j'en pétris le globe frêle. Je n'ai jamais été si près de la vie. Je n'ai jamais si bien senti que je suis soeur de la terre avec les végétations et les sèves. Mes pieds marchent sur la terre comme sur une bête vivante. Je songe au jour plein de flûtes, d'abeilles réveillées, de rosée car voici qu'il se cabre et s'agite en moi. Si tu savais qu'elle fraîcheur de printemps et quelle jeunesse cette âme en bourgeon met dans mon coeur. Et dire que c'est là l'âme enfantine de Pierrot et qu'elle élabore dans la nuit de mon être deux grands yeux d'infini pareils aux siens."

457 Cécile Sauvage, *L'Âme en Bourgeon*, quoted in De Beauvoir, *The Second Sex*, 519–520. Cécile Sauvage, *L'Âme en Bourgeon*, quoted in De Beauvoir, *L'expérience vécue*, 359 : "Tu m'appartiens ainsi que l'aurore à la plaine/ Autour de toi ma vie est une chaude laine/ Où tes membres frileux poussent dans le secret/ … O toi que je cajole avec crainte dans l'ouate/ Petite âme en bourgeon attachée à ma fleur/ D'un morceau de mon coeur je façonne ton coeur/ O mon fruit cotonneux, petite bouche moite."

forgetful in self, are delighted above all with the living treasure growing within them. This delight is given expression in Cécile Sauvage's poems, L'Âme en bourgeon.[458]

Taking a closer look at both the texts of Sauvage and the implicit critiques of De Beauvoir, it becomes obvious that De Beauvoir herself does not escape perpetuating what she calls the *masculine myths* to which women like Sauvage, in her eyes, are falling prey. In fact, it is De Beauvoir herself who perpetuates these myths by maintaining the juxtaposition between the body and mind, applying it to the pregnant body and the female mind. By siding the pregnant woman with the positively connoted parts of the *masculine myths* ("light of the mind," "the clarity of consciousness") in case she subordinates her pregnant body to the mind, the dichotomy is preserved nevertheless.

However, Sauvage herself has an attitude towards childbirth which differs from the dichotomies put forth by De Beauvoir. The difference between De Beauvoir and her perception of childbirth is mainly a difference in the construction of nature. For Sauvage, her pregnant body is part of nature, which she sees as animated. The earth seems to be a living creature and the child is perceived as a small soul. It is rather obvious that to De Beauvoir such a fusion with animated nature is threatening when we remember her conception of female individuality. Woman has to be protected against the species and nature, which may bring her down to the level of matter.

Nevertheless, it is not only in relation to women that De Beauvoir speaks of an opposition between individuality and the human species. She takes a similar position on how men relate to childbirth through procreation, which in her reasoning, like pregnancy and giving birth, remains without any type of spirituality. Like the woman giving birth, the procreating

458 De Beauvoir, *The Second Sex*, 519. De Beauvoir, *L'expérience vécue*, 358: "D'autres femmes s'appesantissent davantage; elles ruminent indéfiniment leur importance neuve. Pour peu qu'on les y encourage, elles reprennent à leur compte les mythes masculins: elles opposent à la lucidité de l'esprit la nuit féconde de la Vie, à la conscience claire les mystères de l'interiorité, à la liberté fertile, le poids de ce ventre qui est là dans son énorme facticité; la future mère se sent humus et glèbe, source, racine; quand elle s'assoupit, son sommeil est celui du chaos où fermentent les mondes. Il y en a qui plus oublieuses de soi s'enchantent surtout du trésor de vie qui grandit en elles. C'est cette joie qu'exprime Cécile Sauvage au long de ses poèmes l'Âme en bourgeon."

man is in danger of being annihilated as an individual and of becoming a victim of the species:

> As subject, he [man] poses the world, and remaining outside this posed universe, he makes himself ruler of it; if he views himself as flesh, as sex, he is no longer an independent consciousness, a clear, free being: he is involved with the world, he is a limited and perishable object. And no doubt the generative act passes beyond the frontiers of the body; but at the same moment it establishes them. The penis, father of generations, corresponds to the maternal womb; arising from a germ that grew in woman's body, man is himself a carrier of germs, and through the sowing which gives life, it is his own life that is renounced. [...] The ejaculation is a promise of death, it is an assertion of the species against the individual.[459]

De Beauvoir here seems to stand in the tradition of Greek philosophy, advocating for a supremacy of *theorein* over doing.[460] In an existentialist turn, however, she sides *theorein* with individuality. Subjectivity is constituted by remaining distant from the world: "As subject, he [man] poses the world, and remaining outside this posed universe, he makes himself ruler of it." However, to get mingled with the world by procreation means to lose individuality and to be reduced to the species: "The ejaculation is a promise of death, it is an assertion of the species against the individual." As has been shown above, Simone de Beauvoir's conception of both childbirth and procreation works with the opposition between individuality and the human species which can be read as an opposition between theoretical natality and childbirth. This kind of pattern is intertwined with the question of equality between men and women. In *The Second Sex,* Simone de Beauvoir attempts to wrest the space of the mind for women. She explores

---

459 De Beauvoir, *The Second Sex*, 194. De Beauvoir, *Les faits*, 112: "En tant que sujet, il [l'homme] pose le monde et, restant hors de l'univers qu'il pose, il s'en fait le souverain; s'il se saisit comme chair, comme sexe, il n'est plus conscience autonome, liberté transparente: il est engagé dans le monde, un objet limité et périssable. Et sans doute l'acte générateur dépasse les frontières du corps: mais dans le même instant il les constitue. Le pénis, père des générations, est symétrique de la matrice maternelle; sorti d'un germe engraissé dans le ventre de la femme, l'homme est lui-même porteur de germes et, par cette semence qui donne la vie, c'est aussi sa propre vie qui se renie. ... L'éjaculation est promesse de mort, elle affirme l'espèce contre l'individu." In this quote there also seem to be some reminiscences of the Aristotelian idea of male semen developing into a child with the help of female matter (see section III.1.7.) when De Beauvoir writes that "arising from a germ that grew in woman's body, man is himself a carrier of germs."

460 See the discussion "Reflections on *Theorein*, Doing and Childbirth" in section III.2.2.

how women – on the basis of a special construction of their bodies – have been largely excluded from this space. To attribute the same intellectual capacities to women as to men, she takes a special attitude toward the body in general and specifically to the body involved with childbirth and procreation: Both female and male bodies are seen as subordinate to the mind which determines individuality. With this assertion, the differences between the male and female body lose any substantial importance. In this sense, the equality of men and women depends on their equal share in the activity of the mind. Thus in conclusion, both male and female bodies in Simone de Beauvoir's writing are seen as unanimated flesh operating on the level of the species when it comes to procreation and childbirth, while the supremacy of the mind, creating individuality, bestows equality onto women and men.

10. Against the Tyranny of the Fates: Joseph Fletcher's Plea for Rational Procreation as Opposed to Childbirth by Raw Nature

In 1988 Joseph Fletcher, who was in 1994 still called the "esteemed patriarch of bioethics,"[461] re-published his book *The Ethics of Genetic Control: Ending Reproductive Roulette*. Here Fletcher portrays himself as a moral philosopher dealing with "human babymaking,"[462] or more precisely, the question of which attitude to take towards the (potential) medical techniques of conception and birth. As will be shown in the following, Fletcher maintains a construction of childbirth that has been encountered all along in the symbolic pattern labeled "Theoretical, Spiritual and Political Natality versus Childbirth." In Simone de Beauvoir's writings childbirth belonged to the realm of "flesh." For Rilke the birth of children belonged to "a world where saps will have their way" and Gregory of Nyssa saw it as deriving

461 Albert R. Jonsen, *Reproduction and Rationality*. Paper presented at the International Bioethics Institute Conference on Designs on Life, San Francisco, CA, April 15, 1994, 1. Many thanks to Francesco de Martis who pointed the work of Fletcher out to me.

462 Joseph Fletcher, *The Ethics of Genetic Control: Ending Reproductive Roulette* (New York: Prometheus Books, 1988), xiii.

from the "skins of brutes." Fletcher fits perfectly in line when he writes of generation as of being part of "raw nature."[463] He also continues with the by now familiar opposition of childbirth and reason/mind.[464] However, in Fletcher's writing, this opposition translates into a rather peculiar form in that he creates a contrast between "random sexual reproduction"[465] and rational procreation. Thus different forms of childbirth, one associated with raw nature and one identified with reason and modern medicine are valued in different ways. How does this come about?

Fletcher using the logic of eugenics sets out to challenge the "traditional morality of babymaking […] based on heterosexual intercourse or coital conception, and on uterine gestation or fetal nurture in the human womb."[466] In the name of human well-being, he argues for the attempt to eliminate diseases through the control of genetic patrimony, that is of the "quality" of future children:

> Moral responsability (response ability) in human reproduction may be shifted from the simple matter of controlling the number of children we have to the trickier business of controlling the genetic or physical quality of our children. It would be quite a jump to go from the blind chance of sexual roulette or "taking what you get" in babymaking to the careful production of a baby by design.[467]

What Fletcher is expressing here in the introduction, runs continuously throughout the whole book. There is a strong fascination with a scenario in which childbirth should ideally come under complete control of the medical mind. His ideas trace the lines of a perceived conflict between contingency (linked to "raw nature") and medical rationality. In his view, the contingency of nature inherent in childbirth, "sexual roulette" as he calls it, should be abolished in favour of "rational procreation" utilizing the new (potential) techniques of conception and birth. In many instances found throughout the text, Fletcher's vocabulary points to the importance he places upon the mind's control over human life. "Control of our human condition,"[468] "manageable reality,"[469] "quality control,"[470] "our human

463 Ibid., 36.
464 See e.g. the chapters on Plato, Gregory of Nyssa and Simone de Beauvoir.
465 Fletcher, *The Ethics*, 29.
466 Ibid., xiv.
467 Ibid., xiv–xv.
468 Ibid., 6.
469 Ibid., 7–8.
470 Ibid., 16.

capacity to make choices and contrive controls,"[471] "control of man's physical structure genetically"[472] … on almost every second page there is an expression which makes Fletcher's advocacy for the regulating and planning function of reason tangible. "In the twentieth century," Fletcher writes, "there has been a conversion of the scientific motive from 'just to know' to 'how to control with what we know.'"[473]

Fletcher's conception of rational procreation relies on placing medical reason as a principle of control leading to "a baby by design"[474] above childbirth by "raw nature." In a way he applies a mind-body hierarchy to genetics by promoting the idea that procreation outside the body, with the help of new technologies, is more rational and therefore more desirable than bodily procreation. From his perspective childbirth, for the sake of medical control, should ideally be "de-corporealized" by the substitution of the body during conception and gestation. The aim of gaining control "over the quality of the infants to be born"[475] should be reached by the elimination of sexual intercourse for procreation:

> We first found out how to have sex without babies, and now we are finding out how to have babies without sex. No longer is human reproduction centered in the genitalia or even dependent on them. Even the gonads, testicles and ovaries are no longer necessary. In fact, we have bypassed in theory even the "gametes" or germ cells (eggs and sperm) supplied by the gonads, since theoretically they can be articicially synthesized – that is, constructed chemically without the biological process of forming them. […] Sex in the sense of coital intercourse is no longer necessary for human reproduction.[476]

This kind of utopian reproduction, freed from the body, especially the sexual body would in Fletcher's thinking prevent "random sexual reproduction,"[477] which equals "trusting to the blind worship of raw

471 Ibid., 21.

472 Ibid., 22.

473 Ibid., 8. Even to determine what is human, Fletcher makes *ratio* the decisive element: "The essence of a person is reason, the rational function, the ratio. On this view everything depends on the mental capability of the individual. This is not to say that reason is everything; feeling is an important part of mental function too. But without intelligence the feeling alone is subhuman. The cerebral has to undergird the visceral" Ibid., 136.

474 Ibid., XV.

475 Ibid., 9.

476 Ibid., 10.

477 Ibid., 29.

nature,"[478] or living "under the tyranny of the Fates, the three daughters of Darkness."[479] By using these metaphors Fletcher clearly devalues childbirth in case that it takes place without medical intervention. In his thinking, such a way of giving birth is marked by the contingencies inherent in "raw nature." To get rid of this contingency, Fletcher not only advocates for conception in test tubes to replace sexual intercourse, but he also hopes for a future where glass wombs substitute the human uterus. This is because he sees the female womb as a dangerous place beyond control: "We realize that the womb is a dark and dangerous place, a hazardous environment."[480] It is obvious that in this picture Fletcher is projecting onto the womb the sexist imagery of women belonging to a sphere of darkness and irrationality. In Fletcher's advocacy for the glass womb, the female womb seems to be the *locus* of darkness, which needs to be made transparent for the sake of rational procreation:

> The glass womb will offer a much safer and more easily monitored container for fetuses, a place where they can be more easily manipulated for treatment and salvation.[481]

> The prospect of having an open window on a growing fetus is welcomed by most of those in responsible roles – embryologists, placentologists, fetologists. Their chance to monitor fetal life in the light, out of the darkness and obscurity of the womb, will add enormously to our knowledge and help us reduce the hazards that face obstetricians and their patients. We realize that the womb is a dark and dangerous place, a hazardous environment. We should want our potential children to be where they can be watched and protected as much as possible.[482]

With Fletcher's utopian glass womb as the utmost expression of rational procreation, sight, the sense which is commonly associated with the brain, and also used as a metaphor for the mind, will thus be able to penetrate the darkness of the body – dark human tissue substituted by transparent glass. Thus the designed child would not have to come out of the darkness by means of the birthing process any longer, like the child of raw nature must,

478 Ibid., 36.

479 Ibid., 129.

480 Ibid., 103. In a similar vein Fletcher states: "Now that we know something about it we realize that contrary to popular sentiment the womb is a very dangerous place – a hazardous environment" (Ibid., 129).

481 Ibid., 109.

482 Ibid., 103.

but instead would grow inside the artificial womb, a product of the mind, watched and controlled by the eyes of scientists, rather than being felt by the woman. In Fletcher's utopian thinking women's wombs and women giving birth are rather seen as obstacles standing in the way of rational procreation. This becomes clearer still by yet another argument for the glass womb, as Fletcher hopes this technology will allow the brain cells of the foetus to increase:

> At present the human brain reaches nine billion cells in the fetal cerebral cortex with thirty-three divisions, but with a thirty-fourth division the brain power would be tremendous. But since this would make the head too big at birth for the birth canal (it is already too big for comfortable delivery), the only answer would be the glass womb. All that limits I.Q. now, as far as its neurologic apparatus is concerned, is the size of the pelvis.[483]

Thus in Fletcher's reasoning the female womb is seen as a dangerous place. The pelvis is pictured as a corporeal obstacle to the increase of the brain volume and to the medical quality control of the embryo/fetus.[484] This is why the glass womb should ideally substitute the female womb. These ideas poignantly demonstrate that Fletcher's conception of rational procreation relies upon the supremacy of reason (identified with medicine) over childbirth. In his utopian thinking, women's function with regard to childbirth and gestation is transferred to medical experts by replacing the female womb with the glass womb.

This type of advocacy for the supremacy of reason, in the guise of medicine, over childbirth makes Fletcher's philosophy stick out from the other examples, which so far, have been given for the second symbolic pattern of childbirth. The supremacy of the mind over the birth of children here finds its rather peculiar expression through a hierarchization and an opposition of different forms of childbirth itself: "Random sexual reproduction" and the children of "raw nature" are subordinated to rational procreation and babies by design.

---

483 Ibid., 75.

484 The supremacy of reason in the guise of medicine over childbirth also figures prominently in Hemingway's short story *Indian Camp* (see section III.1.11.2.). However, in Hemingway's short story such a supremacy of medicine is linked to a male identity construction. As far as Fletcher is concerned medicine standing for rationality becomes much more abstract, though here too, one may see a male identity construction at work with his conception of rational procreation.

11. From the Supremacy of *Theorein* over Childbirth to Childbirth in Theory?

In the analysis of the previous symbolic pattern of childbirth it was shown that up to the 20th century, the subordination of the birth of children to theoretical, political or spiritual natality (connected to philosophy, faith, the arts, the *polis*, or the *ratio*) has continued to be a feasible attitude to have towards childbirth. The following reflections touch upon another potential link between childbirth and an absolute supremacy of the mind which may be the result of modern rationalization processes. Two literary works to be presented in the following, namely *Headbirths* by Günter Grass and *Who's Afraid of Virginia Woolf?* by Edward Albee deal with the peculiar phenomenon of childbirth moving itself into the realm of thought by children remaining fictional, or potential children. The main characters of the novel *Headbirths,* endlessly discuss about whether to have, or not to have children and the protagonists of Albee's play invent the existence of a son who grows up with them as the years go by. It could be that the tradition of opposing theoretical, political or spiritual natality to childbirth is connected to the development of children becoming a product of the mind.

11.1 Günter Grass: Headbirths

In 1979 Günter Grass wrote the novel *Headbirths* ("Kopfgeburten"). It is an experimental novel belonging to the "book in the book" genre. The author becomes a figure in his own work and thereby questions its fictional unity. Günter Grass reflects on the upcoming German elections, the divisions between the East and West literatures of the still divided Germany and on the plot of his novel *Headbirths,* which he would like to be turned into a film, and all this while he is on a trip to China.

Analogous to his experiences in China, Grass sends the main characters of his novel, the couple Harm and Dörte Peters, both high school teachers in their thirties, on a trip to Southern Asia. However, as intellectual baggage, they take with them their endless discussions about whether or whether not, to have a child:[485] "They dragged their quarrel about the negated and affirmed baby from Bombay via Bangkok to Bali." The child becomes a constant topic ("The child is always present"[486]) and its potential coming into existence starts to depend on a number of private and political issues. There is Harm's old mother, whom he thinks of taking into the household. Here the question is whether the flat would be big enough for both a child and a grandmother. Harm and Dörte are not capable of reaching agreement on this point: "But they never get beyond the whatif or supposingthat stage, and Harm's mother (as surrogate child) is alternately moved to their apartment and shipped to an old-people's home, until some forenoon shock derails their single-tracked dialogue."[487]

The political reasons for not having a child are numerous. Harm and Dörte belong to the '68 generation and therefore consciously see their lives as being embedded in a socio-political context. Over-population, the unclear outcome of the German elections and the building of nuclear power stations all work against the coming-into-existence of their child. Since Dörte teaches about India in her geography lessons, she feels obliged to renounce her own wish to have a child: "She, who is basically committed to motherhood, believes herself, now that her geography program is burdened with the Indian subcontinent, in duty bound to forgo children."[488] Given that Dörte did not want a child of hers to be born into a world increasingly polluted by nuclear energy, she had already once aborted a pregnancy,[489] after which the couple had started psychotherapy.[490] However, the expected result of solving the problem of "Yes-to-baby No-to-baby" was not achieved.

485 Günter Grass, *Headbirths or The Germans Are Dying Out*, trans. Ralph Manheim (New York: Harcourt, 1990), 119. Günter Grass, *Kopfgeburten* (1980; reprint, Frankfurt/M: Luchterhand, 1982), 116: "Sie [verschleppen] den Streit über das verneinte, bejahte Kind von Bombay über Bangkok bis nach Bali."

486 Grass, *Headbirths*, 12. Grass, *Kopfgeburten*, 15: "Das Kind bleibt Thema."

487 Grass, *Headbirths*, 12. Grass, *Kopfgeburten*, 15: "Doch es bleibt bleibt beim Alsob und Angenommen, wobei Harms Mutter (als Ersatzkind) mal in die Lehrerwohnung aufgenommen, dann wieder in ein Altersheim abgeschoben wird."

488 Grass, *Headbirths*, 12. Grass, *Kopfgeburten*, 15: "Sie, die prinzipiell auf Mutterschaft fixiert ist, sieht sich, seitdem der indische Subkontinent ihren Geografie-Unterricht belastet, wieder einmal dem Verzicht auf das Kind verpflichtet."

489 See Grass, *Headbirths*, 22 and Grass, *Kopfgeburten*, 25.

490 See Grass, *Headbirths*, 58 and Grass, *Kopfgeburten*, 59–60.

Two months before their trip to Asia, Dörte promised that she would stop taking the birth control pill as soon as they got on the plane.[491] Then, just before landing, she takes it again:[492] "Now, shortly before the landing, she contrary to her sworn intention – Yes-to-baby! – takes the pill – No-to-baby!"

Then on Bali, comes a sudden change: Dörte wants a child. She participates in a local fertility cult, carries bowls of rice to some temples and goes through a period of abstinence for purification.[493] However, Harm is not convinced by this new approach to childbirth, sticking firmly to his own "rationality cult": "When you finally want it, I won't want it. This temple shit! I don't want an irrational child!"[494] Suddenly it is not only the question of socio-political and environmental conditions but also the meaning of childbirth, its connectedness, or non-connectedness to a transcendental moment, which enters the debate. Harm argues:[495] "If I make a child, I want to do it consciously. Do you hear? Not the Hindu way!" Dörte – before throwing three boxes of pills into a magic Hindu cavern – replies passionately: "I can't make it with our shitty reason! I have to break free, to let go. I need something different, the force that comes from inside, no, from outside, all right, laugh, something supersensory, a divine power, whatever."[496]

Dörte's statements, show how God, or the religious sphere, can become a symbol of anti-structure. Victor Turner has argued against the Durkheimian conception of God as a symbol of society in the following way:

> Durkheim considered God to be the symbol of society. But if one distinguishes social structure from communitas, this symbol may be seen as having two senses which are at opposite semantic poles. God may be regarded a "symbol of structure", by which is meant everything that has to do with social differentiation and

491 See Grass, *Headbirths*, 24 and Grass, *Kopfgeburten*, 27.

492 Grass, *Headbirths*, 31. Grass, *Kopfgeburten*, 34: "Jetzt kurz vor der Landung, nimmt sie, wider alle beschworene Absicht: das Kind Ja, – die Pille: das Kind Nein!".

493 See Grass, *Headbirths*, 48–49 and Grass, *Kopfgeburten*, 50–51.

494 Grass, *Headbirths*, 49. Grass, *Kopfgeburten*, 51: "Wenn du endlich willst, werde ich nicht wollen. Diese Tempelscheiße! Ich will kein irrationales Kind."

495 Grass, *Headbirths*, 52. Grass, *Kopfgeburten*, 54: "Ich will bewußt ein Kind machen. Hörst du. Nicht auf die hinduistische Tour."

496 Grass, *Headbirths*, 52. Grass, *Kopfgeburten*, 54: "Und ich krieg das nicht hin mit unserer Scheiß-Vernunft! Ich muß mich lösen, muß mich fallenlassen. Ich will das andere, das mir von innen, nein, von außen, ja, lach doch, das Übersinnliche, ich meine, ich muß sie spüren, die göttliche Kraft."

> with the authorative ordering of that differentiation. Per contra, God may be the symbol of antistructure or the negation, hereditarily ascribed, of hierarchical and segmentary differentiation.[497]

With the figure of Dörte in *Headbirths*, the religious sphere becomes a symbol of rebellion against the supremacy of the mind and rational society which actually "prevent her" from having a child.

However, once back to the familiar structures in Northern Germany, Dörte affirms that she cannot have a child if the conservative politician Strauß should win the elections. "I will not bring a child into the world under Strauss,"[498] she says. Harm, on the other hand, finally wants to become a father. Southern Asia thus did not work as therapy for the German couple trapped by a culture of rationality and rationalization. In the end it is not Harm and Dörte but their cat that procreates: it manages to have five kittens during their absence! In a tragicomic reaction, Dörte breaks into tears at the sight of the kittens.[499]

What remains are the *headbirths* "without ovulation or effusion of sperm,"[500] while the only real birth is subjected to rational concerns: the difficulty of finding homes for all the kittens. Thus Harm discretely kills four of the kittens in the bath-tub. In the aftermath of this, back at the "headbirths," Dörte is overcome with fear: "I'm afraid, Harm. Of us, of everything."[501]

However, Grass leaves space for some hope. In a world dominated by rationalization processes, the cold war, inequality and ecological problems, childbirth can figure as a potential act of resistance. Grass writes: "We will want to chuck it all and reproduce,"[502] and he adds ironically: "And in the end (when the film is over) so will Dörte and Harm."

497 Victor Turner, *Blazing the Trail: Way Marks in the Exploration of Symbols*, ed. Edith Turner (Tucson, Arizona and London: The University of Arizona Press), 1992, 140.

498 Grass, *Headbirths*, 45. Grass, *Kopfgeburten*, 48: "Unter Strauß setz ich kein Kind in die Welt."

499 Grass, *Headbirths*, 128. Grass, *Kopfgeburten*, 117.

500 Grass, *Headbirths*, 129. Grass, *Kopfgeburten*, 126: "Ohne Eisprung und Samenguß."

501 Grass, *Headbirths*, 128. Grass, *Kopfgeburten*, 125: "Ich hab Angst, Harm. Vor uns, vor allem."

502 Grass, *Headbirths*, 120. Grass, *Kopfgeburten*, 118: "Wir werden aussteigen wollen und uns fortpflanzen; am Ende (nach Filmschluß) auch Dörte und Harm."

11.2 Edward Albee: Who's Afraid of Virginia Woolf?

In 1962 Edward Albee published his three-act play *Who's Afraid of Virginia Woolf?* At its heart is the marriage crisis of a couple brought about by their incapacity to conform to the ideal American family life of having children and having a high social status. The main characters, Martha and George are childless and George did not achieve the social status his wife would have wished for. Thus in the living-room of a house on the campus of a small New England College a psycho-drama takes place.

In Act One, *Fun and Games*, Martha, the 52-year-old daughter of a college president and her husband George, aged 46, associate professor in the history department of the same college, come home from a party where they have learnt a song with the words "Who's afraid of Virginia Woolf?" The relationship between the two is one of hate and distrust. Martha, who grew up with her adored father, married George in order to secure a successor for him. George was supposed to have become dean of the history department and to have carried out public relations for the college in order to become its president later on. Once George rejected that role, Martha's and her father's disappointment with him turned into hate.

After coming home from the party Martha tells George that she has invited guests for a drink. The bell rings and Nick, a successful 30-year-old biologist working on genetic engineering and his wife Honey, 26-years old and somewhat naive, enter the scene. In Act One, the theme of the birth of children in theory is first taken up in relation to Nick's work. George criticizes the unification and selection process to which genetic engineering could lead. Interestingly, he refers only to the male genetic patrimony. This is slightly reminiscent of the Aristotelian idea–already discussed in the context of the first symbolic pattern of childbirth–that only man is in possession of a soul-giving principle:

> It's very simple, Martha, this young man is working on a system whereby chromosomes can be altered [...] the genetic make-up of a sperm cell changed, reordered... to order actually... for hair and eye colour, stature, potency ... I imagine ... hairiness, features, health ... and mind. Most important... Mind. All imbalances will be corrected, sifted out ... propensity for various diseases will be gone, longevity assured. We will have a race of men ... test-tube-bred... incubator-born... superb and sublime.[503]

503 Edward Albee, *Who's Afraid of Virginia Woolf? : A Play*. New York: Atheneum, 1962, 45.

The discussion about genetic engineering, childbirth in theory as conceptualized by the sciences, is very rapidly intertwined with the theme of the fictitious birth of children. Honey asks:[504] "When is… where is your son… coming home?" Although it is not revealed until the last act ("The Exorcism") that the son of Martha and George is actually a twenty-year old invention, Honey's question is most meaningful here. Both Nick's work on genetic engineering and the invention of a son to remedy childlessness, turn children into fictional children, or rather: in both cases fictional children replace "real" children while the border-lines between fiction and reality are blurred. In Act Three, George says: "Truth and illusion. Who knows the difference, eh, toots? Eh?," and some sentences further on he exchanges the following words with Martha:

> Martha [pleading]: Truth and illusion, George; you don't know the difference.
> George: No; but we must carry on as though we did.[505]

The fictional children even acquire a status of reality that is superior to that of a child in flesh and blood. George affirms that the only thing of which he is sure is that it is he who fathered his son:

> There are very few things in this world that I am sure of… national boundaries, the level of the ocean, political allegiances, practical morality… none of these would I stick on any more… but the one thing in this whole sinking world that I am sure of is my partnership, my chromosomical partnership in the… creation of our… blond-eyed, blue-haired… son.[506]

The only children born in *Who's Afraid of Virginia Woolf?* are fictional children, products of the mind, while the births of "real" children end up in abortions. Honey, a healthy young woman, is so afraid of childbirth that she secretly takes pills to abort her pregnancies. It is George who discovers her secret. In front of him she breaks down: "No!… I don't want any… I don't want them…. Go 'way….[Begins to cry] I don't want… any… children…. I… don't… want… any… children. I'm afraid! I don't

504 Ibid., 48.
505 Ibid. 119.
506 Ibid., 49.

want to be hurt.... Please!"[507] It is only after hearing about the childhood of George's and Martha's invented son that Honey undergoes a change of mind. She repeats in tears: "I want a child. I want a baby."[508] George immediately doubts her sincerity, he sees a change taking place purely in the mind but without any effects. "On principle?", he asks Honey after her exclamations.

As in the novel *Headbirths*, where Dörte says to Harm: "I'm afraid, Harm. Of us, of everything,"[509] Albee's play too sees the transformation of children into fictional children accompanied by fear. Interestingly, in both the novel and the play, a female character expresses that fear. The final dialogue in *Who's Afraid of Virginia Woolf?* takes place after George has taken terrible revenge on Martha. The couple had once agreed that their "son" would always be kept secret from the public. After Martha has violated this taboo by talking about her son to her guests, George pretends to have received a telegramme informing them about the death of their son in a car accident. Martha is as shocked by this as if a real son of flesh and blood had died. She does not want to accept the end of the fictional child:

> George: *It's late.*
> Martha: *Yes.*
> George [*long silence*]: *It will be better.*
> Martha [*long silence*]: *I don't... know.*
> George: *It will be... maybe.*
> Martha: *I'm... not... sure.*
> George: *No.*
> Martha: *Just... us?*
> George: *Yes.*
> Martha: *I don't suppose, maybe, we could...*
> George: *No, Martha.*
> Martha: *Yes. No.*
> George: *Are you all right?*
> Martha: *Yes. No.*

---

507 Ibid., 105.

508 Ibid., 130.

509 Grass, *Headbirths*, 128. Grass, *Kopfgeburten*, 125: "Ich hab Angst, Harm. Vor uns, vor allem."

George, to comfort his wife, sings the party song "Who's afraid of Virginia Woolf?" to her. However, the play ends with Martha's fear and despair[510]:

Martha: *I… am… George….*
George: *Who's afraid of Virginia Woolf….*
Martha: *I… am… George… I… am….*[511]

510 Ibid., 140.
511 Albee, *Who's Afraid,* 139–140.

III.3 The Supremacy of the Female

Women can be pictured as being more important for the coming into existence of children than men. This is what I label "The Supremacy of the Female." At first sight one could easily think that this symbolic pattern of childbirth reflects the "fact" that the female body is more involved in the process of generation than the male body. Nevertheless, as has been shown by the sections "The Supremacy of the Male" and "Theoretical, Spiritual and Political Natality versus Childbirth" this is but one potentiality of meaning of childbirth though it may be considered to be the "closest at hand." "The Supremacy of the Female" here will be mostly illustrated by myths and cults of several goddesses of antiquity among whom the Egyptian goddess Isis figures prominently.

The worship of Isis deeply influenced the transformation of Christian Mary into a goddess-like figure who equally testifies to the supremacy of the female over the male in matters of childbirth. The cults of Isis and Mary are not only closely connected to but also virtually inseparable from the fourth symbolic pattern of childbirth that is concerned with the idea of a harmony between spiritual birth, theoretical natality and childbirth. Thus it is preferable to refer to Isis and Mary at a later stage as they stand for a long lasting combination of the ideas of the supremacy of the female in relation to childbirth and harmony between spiritual birth and childbirth.

Analogous to some expressions of "The Supremacy of the Male," "The Supremacy of the Female" too can assume a rather "dubious" character. As has been shown, in the writings of Christian thinkers such as Tertullian, Augustine and Thomas Aquinas the supremacy of the male in matters of childbirth became a rather tricky affair because male semen was seen as a transmitter of original sin. Analogously, the symbolic pattern to be analysed in the following, includes what could be labeled a "dubious supremacy of the female." For this I propose the gnostic myth of the creation of the world by Sophia, the "fallen wisdom," as an example.

1. The First Birthgiving: Goddesses as Mothers of the Gods and as the Origin of the World

In Greek myth, the beginning of the (divine) world is pictured as relying on a female divinity. Gaia, the earth goddess, generates the world in a parthenogenic act. In his *Theogony*, Hesiod describes Gaia as the origin of the gods:

> First of all there came Chaos,
> and after him came
> Gaia of the broad breast,
> to be the unshakable foundation
> of all the immortals
> who keep the crests
> of snowy Olympos[512]

In the *Theogony*, the first childbirth is that of Gaia giving birth to her son, the sky god Uranos, the mountains, and the sea. Due to the union with her son she then gives birth to the divine children who are at the origin of the Greek pantheon:

> Earth first of all bore starry Sky, equal to herself,
> to cover her on every side, so that she would be the ever
> immovable seat for the blessed gods; and she bore the high
> mountains the graceful haunts of the goddesses, Nymphs
> who dwell on the wooded mountains; and she also bore the
> barren sea seething with its swell, Pontus – all of them
> without delightful love; and then, having bedded with Sky,
> she bore deep – eddying Ocean and Coeus and Crius and
> Hyperion and Iapetus and Theia and Rhea and Themis
> and Mnemosyne and golden-crowned Phoebe and lovely
> Tethys.[513]

Also in Sumerian myth the origin of the divine world seems to have been imagined as female and rooted in giving birth. Here Nammu, the goddess

512 Hesiod, *Theogony*, trans. Richmond Lattimore, 116–118.

513 Hesiod, *Theogony*, ed. and trans. Glenn W. Most (Cambridge, Mass.: Harvard University Press, 2006), 126–136.

of the sea, could be called the "mother who bore the sky and the earth," or the "mother who bore all the gods."[514]

Another example of a goddess as the first life giving principle may be the "Pelasgian creation myth." Robert Graves in his *The Greek Myths* assumes the existence of such a pre-Hellenic myth which he imagines and pieces together from various sources.[515] In his rather poetic version, the myth would run as follows:

> In the beginning, Eurynome, the Goddess of All Things, rose naked from Chaos, but found nothing substantial for her feet to rest upon, and therefore divided the sea from the sky, dancing lonely upon its waves. She danced towards the south, and the wind set in motion behind her seemed something new and apart with which to begin a work of creation. Wheeling about, she caught hold of this North wind, rubbed it between her hands, and behold! The great serpent Ophion. Eurynome danced to warm herself, wildly and more wildly, until Ophion, grown lustful, coiled about those divine limbs and was moved to couple with her. .... Next she assumed the form of a dove, brooding on the waves and, in due process of time, laid the Universal Egg. At her bidding, Ophion coiled seven times about this egg, until it hatched and split in two. Out tumbled all things that exist, her children: sun, moon, planets, stars, the earth with its mountains and rivers, its trees, herbs and living creatures.
>
> Eurynome and Ophion made their home on mount Olympus, where he vexed her by claiming to be the author of the Universe. Forthwith she bruised his head with her heel, kicked out his teeth, and banished him to the dark caves below the earth.[516]

The Pelasgian creation myth centers on the goddess as creatress. The agency of creation almost exclusively lies with the female sex. Eurynome transforms the North Wind into a male counterpart to conceive the Universal Egg and she jealously watches over her privilege as creatrix: Ophion is severely punished when he claims to be the creator of the universe. Eurynome not only controls the act of conception, but conceiving and birthgiving appear as more important for the beginning of life than procreation and the obstetrician-like function of the man (Ophion's coiling around the egg).

However, the goddess as creatress as one symbolic expression of the supremacy of the female in matters of childbirth is not always positively connoted. The following chapter on the gnostic myth of Sophia shows that

---

514 See Samuel Noah Kramer, *From the Poetry of Sumer: Creation, Glorification, Adoration* (Berkeley, Los Angeles, London: University of California Press, 1979), 26–29.

515 See Robert Graves, *The Greek Myths* (London: Penguin Books, 1992), 27–28.

516 Ibid., 27.

the supremacy of the female over the male in matters of childbirth and creation can become a highly dubious enterprise.

2. The Creation of the World by Sophia the "Fallen Wisdom": A Gnostic Myth

The myth of Sophia giving birth to an ignorant son, the Demiurge, who becomes the creator of the world, has been chosen here as an example of how the supremacy of the female over the male in matters of childbirth can assume rather dubious characteristics.

However, before coming to the different versions of the Sophia myth, it should be pointed out that the story of Sophia finds its place in the general logic of gnostic thinking in the first centuries C.E.[517] Gnosticism rejects the assumptions of Judaism, Platonism, and Christianity that "an intelligent and good cause [...] created the world."[518] It furthermore tends to deny the "anthropic principle," that is, the idea that humanity and the world were created for each other and belong to each other. Gnosticism sees humanity as lost in an alien world. This type of worldview finds its mythical expression in the story of Sophia. Here so-called hypostatizations – typical of Gnostic thought – play an important role. In the *Reallexikon für Antike und Christentum*, H. S. Wiesner defines hypostatization ("Hypostasierung") as "the deification/personification of abstract concepts, the elaboration of divine parts or powers into active entities, or the postulation and systematization of abstract, generative entities which function as *arkhai*, constituents, or governors for our cosmos and its ontology."[519]

The idea of gnostic hypostases has to be understood in connection with the idea of the so-called *Pleroma* or Fullness. Pleroma is formed by the multiplication of hypostases or aeons:

517 For this and the following see Couliano, *The Tree of Gnosis*, 56–73.

518 Ibid., 56.

519 H. S. Wiesner, quoted in Couliano, *The Tree of Gnosis*, 70.

> Pleroma is opposed to Kenoma (emptiness), the chaotic space 'underneath'; Fullness is opposed to the Void. To give just one example, the Valentinian Pleroma is particularly rich in hypostases, usually in the number of thirty aeons forming an Ogdoad (The Eight), a Decad (The Ten), and a Dodecad (The Twelve).[520]

In his version of the Sophia myth, the gnostic thinker Valentine sees Sophia as the last aeon of the Dodecad. Until the discovery of the Nag Hammadi Library in Egypt in 1945, gnostic thought, including the different versions of the myth of Sophia, was mostly reconstructed by Christian polemics against the gnostics who were stigmatized as heretics. Until 1945, regarding the Sophia myth, Irenaeus' work *Against Heresies* and Hippolytus' *Refutatio Omnium Haeresium* were considered to be the main sources of information. However, the discovery of the Nag Hammadi Library brought to light authentic gnostic sources for the myth of Sophia. The Nag Hammadi texts which will be used to illustrate the Sophia myth are *The Apocryphon of John*, *The Sophia of Jesus Christ*, *The Hypostasis of the Archons*, *On the Origin of the World* and *The Letter of Peter to Philip.*

The Apocryphon of John is dated before 185 C. E.[521], and it was still used in the eighth century by the Audians of Mesopotamia.[522] One of the most important questions of *The Apocryphon of John*, according to Frederick Wisse, is the question about the origin of evil.[523] In fact, gnostic theodicy is thoroughly interwoven with the figure of Sophia. *The Apocryphon of John* pictures Sophia as an aeon who becomes guilty of a double sin. The aeons appear in *syzygies*, that is, in pairs. However, Sophia wants to generate both *without* her consort and *without* the consent of the Spirit, the supreme authority of the Pleroma. Resulting from her independent way of acting is a miscarriage, her son Yaltabaoth, of whom Sophia is deeply ashamed:

520 Ibid.

521 This is the date of Irenaeus' work *Against Heresies.*

522 See Frederik Wisse, introduction to *The Apocryphon of John (II,1, III,1 IV,1, and BG 8502,2)*, in *The Nag Hammadi Library in English*, trans. and introduced by members of the Coptic Gnostic Library Project of the Institute for Antiquity and Christianity, Claremont, California, ed. James M. Robinson, 3rd, completely rev. ed. (Leiden: Brill, 1988), 104.

523 See ibid.

> And the Sophia of the Epinoia, being an aeon, conceived a thought from herself and the conception of the invisible Spirit and foreknowledge. She wanted to bring forth a likeness out of herself without the consent of the Spirit, – he had not approved – and without her consort, and without his consideration. And though the person of her maleness had not approved, and she had not found her agreement, and she had thought without the consent of the Spirit and the knowledge of her agreement, (yet) she brought forth. And because of the invincible power which is in her, her thought did not remain idle and something came out of her which was imperfect and different from her appearance, because she had created it without her consort. And it was dissimilar to the likeness of its mother for it has another form.
>
> And when she saw (the consequences of) her desire, it changed into a form of a lion-faced serpent. And its eyes were like lightning fires which flash. She cast it away from her, outside that place, that no one of the immortal ones might see it, for she had created it in ignorance. …. And she called his name Yaltabaoth.[524]

Sophia's son Yaltabaoth becomes the creator of the world. He creates angels and aeons[525] who help him to fashion the body of Adam. He, however, is seen as a negative creator. He is "ignorant darkness,"[526] "full of ignorance"[527] and takes a negative attitude towards his creation: "And he (the chief archon) repented for everything which had come into being through him."[528]

However, the one ultimately responsible for the coming into existence of a defective world and a defective humanity is Sophia. She has generated on her own and this is judged negatively. Her "supremacy of the female" in matters of childbirth becomes a "dubious" supremacy. Her wish to generate on her own results in a miscarriage, Yaltabaoth, who creates a defective world. The fact that she had a miscarriage because she had wished to generate on her own is mentioned repeatedly. Sophia is full of distress about the consequences of her transgression of the "Pleromatic laws of generation": "And she became dark because her consort had not agreed with her.

524 *The Apocryphon of John (II,1, III,1 IV,1, and BG 8502,2)*, trans. Frederik Wisse, in *The Nag Hammadi Library in English*, trans. and introduced by members of the Coptic Gnostic Library Project of the Institute for Antiquity and Christianity, Claremont, California, ed. James M. Robinson, 3rd, completely rev. ed. (Leiden: Brill, 1988), 110.

525 See ibid., 110–112.

526 Ibid., 111.

527 Ibid., 24.

528 Ibid., 28, 29.

.... And when the mother recognized that the garment of darkness was imperfect, then she knew that her consort had not agreed with her."[529]

As an attempt to repent Sophia intervenes into the imperfect world and tries to make it better. For example, when Adam's body is created by Yaltabaoth and his angels, Sophia animates it with spirit.[530] However, the figure of Sophia remains tied to the question of gnostic theodicy. She is associated with the deficiency of the world. Thus the supreme God of the Pleroma, the "Mother-Father," dispatches the luminous aeon Epinoia ("Life") who is hiding in Adam "that the archons might not know her, but that the Epinoia might be a correction of the deficiency of the mother."[531]

Sophia's dubious supremacy over the male in matters of childbirth, which has equally dubious consequences, namely, the creation of an imperfect world, is also noted in the *The Sophia of Jesus Christ*. This text is "a revelation discourse given by the risen Christ in response to the questions of his disciples,"[532] most probably written during the latter half of the first century C.E. in Egypt.[533] Sophia's "sinful" wish to generate on her own which then produces defectiveness, reappears as a motif in *The Sophia of Jesus Christ*:

> I want you to know that Sophia, the Mother of the Universe and the consort, desired by herself to bring these to existence without her male (consort). But by the will of the father of the Universe, that his unimaginable goodness might be revealed, he

529 Ibid. 13–14.

530 Ibid., 19: "And when the mother wanted to retrieve the power which she had given to the chief archon, she petitioned the Mother-Father of the All who is most merciful. He sent, by means of the holy decree, the five lights down upon the place of the angels of the chief archon. They advised him that they should bring forth the power of the mother. And they said to Yaltabaoth, 'Blow into his face something of your spirit and his body will arise.' And he blew into his face the spirit which is the power of his mother; he did not know (this), for he exists in ignorance. And the power of the mother went out of Yaltabaoth into the natural body which they had fashioned after the image of the one who exists from the beginning. The body moved and gained strength, and it was luminous."

531 Ibid., 20.

532 Douglas M. Parrott, introduction to *Eugnostos The Blessed (III,3 and V,1)* and *The Sophia of Jesus Christ (III,4 and BG 8502,3)*, in *The Nag Hammadi Library in English*, trans. and introduced by members of the Coptic Gnostic Library Project of the Institute for Antiquity and Christianity, Claremont, California, ed. James M. Robinson, 3rd, completely rev. ed. (Leiden: Brill, 1988), 220.

533 See ibid.

created that curtain between the immortals and those that came afterward, that the consequence might follow ....

every aeon and chaos, that the defect of the female might (appear), and it might come about that Error would contend with her. And these became the curtain of spirit.[534]

However, as in *The Apocryphon of John*, Sophia in *The Sophia of Jesus Christ* is also responsible for the spiritualizing of the lower world. In the case of *The Sophia of Jesus Christ*, she lets a drop of light fall from the divine realm into the visible world.[535]

Again in *The Hypostasis of the Archons*, a Christian work from the third century C.E., containing mainly Jewish elements,[536] Sophia becomes guilty of generating on her own. Again she brings about the distinction between the upper and lower world. Yet, also in *The Hypostasis of the Archons*, it is again the function of Sophia to introduce light into matter:

Sophia, who is called Pistis, wanted to create something, alone without her consort; and her product was a celestial thing.

A veil exists between the world above and the realms that are below; and shadow came into being beneath the veil; and that shadow became matter; and that shadow was projected apart. And what she had created became a product in the matter, like an aborted fetus. And it assumed a plastic form molded out of shadow, and became an arrogant beast resembling a lion. It was androgynous [...] because it was from matter that it derived.

Opening his eyes he saw a vast quantity of matter without limit; and he became arrogant, saying, 'It is I who am god, and there is none other apart from me.'

When he said this, he sinned against the entirety. ....

---

534 *The Sophia of Jesus Christ (III,4 and BG 8502,3)*, trans. Douglas M. Parrott, in *The Nag Hammadi Library in English*, trans. and introduced by members of the Coptic Gnostic Library Project of the Institute for Antiquity and Christianity, Claremont, California, ed. James M. Robinson, 3rd, completely rev. ed. (Leiden: Brill, 1988), 240.

535 Ibid. : "As I have said already, a drop from Light and Spirit came down to the lower regions of Almighty in chaos, that their molded forms might appear from that drop."

536 Roger A. Bullard, introduction to *The Hypostasis of the Archons (II,4)*, in *The Nag Hammadi Library in English*, trans. and introduced by members of the Coptic Gnostic Library Project of the Institute for Antiquity and Christianity, Claremont, California, ed. James M. Robinson, 3rd, completely rev. ed. (Leiden: Brill, 1988), 161.

> And he said, 'If any other thing exists before me, let it become visible to me!' And immediately Sophia stretched forth her finger and introduced light into matter; and she pursued it down to the region of chaos. And she returned up [to] her light.[537]

The Nag Hammadi text, *On the Origin of the World*, has many parallels to the *Hypostasis of the Archons*.[538] However, it is a rather special mix of "various kinds of Jewish views, Manichaean elements, Christian ideas, Greek philosophical conceptions, and figures of Greek or Hellenistic mythology, magic, and astrology, as well as a clear emphasis on Egyptian thought."[539] This points to Alexandria as the probable place of origin for the Greek original of the text.[540]

On the Origin of the World draws the familiar ambivalent picture of Sophia. She is the daughter of the aeon Pistis (faith), and it is said that she assumes an intermediary position between the upper and the lower world: "She [Sophia] functioned as a veil dividing mankind from the things above."[541] Again the motif-complex of matter, miscarriage and the spiritualization of matter appears, closely related to (Pistis) Sophia.[542]

---

537 *The Hypostasis of the Archons (II,4),* trans. Bentley Layton, in *The Nag Hammadi Library in English*, trans. and introduced by members of the Coptic Gnostic Library Project of the Institute for Antiquity and Christianity, Claremont, California, ed. James M. Robinson, 3rd, completely rev. ed. (Leiden: Brill, 1988), 167–168.

538 See Hans-Gebhard Bethge, introduction to *On the Origin of the World (II,5 and XIII,2)*, in *The Nag Hammadi Library in English*, trans. and introduced by members of the Coptic Gnostic Library Project of the Institute for Antiquity and Christianity, Claremont, California, ed. James M. Robinson, 3rd, completely rev. ed. (Leiden: Brill, 1988), 171.

539 Ibid., 170.

540 See ibid.

541 *On the Origin of the World (II,5 and XIII,2)*, trans. Hans-Gebhard Bethge, Bentley Layton, Societas Coptica Hierosolymitana, in *The Nag Hammadi Library in English*, trans. and introduced by members of the Coptic Gnostic Library Project of the Institute for Antiquity and Christianity, Claremont, California, ed. James M. Robinson, 3rd, completely rev. ed. (Leiden: Brill, 1988), 172.

542 Ibid., 173: "And when these things had come to pass, then Pistis came and appeared over the matter of chaos, which had been expelled like an aborted fetus – since there was no spirit in it. For all of it (viz., chaos) was limitless darkness and bottomless water. Now when Pistis saw what had resulted from her defect, she became disturbed. … And when Pistis Sophia desired to cause the thing that had no spirit to be formed into a likeness and to rule over matter and over all her forces, there appeared for the first time a ruler, out of the waters, lion-like in appearance, androgynous, having great authority within him and ignorant of whence he had come into being."

Yet another text that testifies to Sophia bringing about a cosmic disaster by wishing to generate on her own is *The Letter of Peter to Philip*. This Christian Gnostic tractate was most probably written around the end of the second century C.E.[543] *The Letter of Peter to Philip* condemns Sophia's attempt to create by herself: "First of all concerning [the deficiency] of the aeons, this [is] the deficiency, when the disobedience and the foolishness of the mother appeared without the commandment of the majesty of the Father. She wanted to raise up aeons."[544]

Furthermore, *The Letter of Peter to Philip* makes Sophia expressly responsible for human suffering: "My brothers, Jesus is a stranger to this suffering. But we are the ones who have suffered through the transgression of the mother."[545]

As has been shown above, the Nag Hammadi picture of Sophia trying to generate by herself without male participation is highly ambivalent. She is tied to the question of theodicy but also remedies human suffering. The two most important Christian thinkers who wrote about the gnostics, namely Irenaeus and Hippolytus, confirm this picture.

In the first book of his *Against Heresies*, the church father Irenaeus (*between 140 and 160 at Smirna) writes about the understanding of Sophia in the gnostic school of Valentinus. Here Sophia has a consort called Theletós (Desired). However, she acts without him as she tries to reach the "father," who is the highest entity in the Pleroma and remains unknown to all the aeons except *Mind*.[546]

---

543 See Marvin W. Meyer, introduction to *The Letter of Peter to Philip (VIII,2),* in *The Nag Hammadi Library in English*, trans. and introduced by members of the Coptic Gnostic Library Project of the Institute for Antiquity and Christianity, Claremont, California, ed. James M. Robinson, 3rd, completely rev. ed. (Leiden: Brill, 1988), 433.

544 *The Letter of Peter to Philip (VIII,2)*, trans. Frederik Wisse, in *The Nag Hammadi Library in English*, trans. and introduced by members of the Coptic Gnostic Library Project of the Institute for Antiquity and Christianity, Claremont, California, ed. James M. Robinson, 3rd, completely rev. ed. (Leiden: Brill, 1988), 435.

545 Ibid., 436.

546 Irenaeus of Lyon, *Against the Heresies*, trans. Dominic J. Unger, with further revisions by John J. Dillon (New York, N.Y. and Mahwah, N.J.: The Newman Press, 1992), I 2, 2: "But the last and youngest Aeon of the Dodecad [...] namely, Wisdom [Sophia], advanced far ahead of all of them and suffered passion, though without the embrace of Desired, her consort. The passion began in Mind and Truth but spread as by infection to this estranged Aeon [Sophia] under the pretense of love, but in reality out of temerity, because he had no fellowship with perfect Father, as even Mind did.

In Irenaeus' account of Valentinian Gnosticism the *motif* of Sophia's miscarriage comes to the forefront and is linked to several passions, namely, fear, pain, confusion and ignorance. These passions beyond the Pleroma lie at the origin of the material world. Thus Sophia generating dubiously by herself is also the indirect cause for the coming into existence of a dubious world. Sophia herself however, despite her miscarriage, is re-integrated into the Pleroma:

> After she had undertaken the impossible and unattainable affair, she brought forth a formless substance, namely, such a nature as a woman could bring forth. When she looked at it, she was filled first with grief on account of the unfinished nature of her offspring, then with fear lest her very existence should come to an end. After that she was beside herself and perplexed as she sought the cause [of her offspring] and how she might conceal her. While involved in these passions, she changed her mind and tried to return to Father. When she had made the bold attempt for some time and her strength failed, she entreated Father. The other aeons, too, especially Mind, made supplication together with her. Hence, they claim, material substance took its beginning from ignorance and grief, fear and bewilderment.[547]

After her fall Sophia rejoins her *syzygos* and for the sake of the stability of the Pleroma the eternal father emanates another syzygy, namely Christ and the Holy Spirit. Sophia's intention, which remains outside the Pleroma, is called Achamoth. Longing for the Pleroma, but prevented by the aeon Horus-Limes from entering it, Achamoth undergoes a conversion from which the World Soul and the soul of the Demiurge derive[548]. Achamoth is the moving force behind the Demiurge as he creates both the material and the spiritual worlds.[549] As in the Nag Hammadi texts,

---

The passion consisted in seeking after Father; for he wished, so they say, to comprehend his greatness." Ireneo di Lione: Contro le eresie e gli altri scritti: Introduzione, traduzione, note e indici a cura di Enzo Bellini (Milano: Jaca Book, 1979).

547 Ibid., I 2, 3.

548 See ibid., I 4, 1 and I 4,2.

549 Ibid., I 5,1: "First, they say, she gave form out of her ensouled substance to the God, Father and King of all things, also of those who are of the same nature as he, that is, of the ensouled substances – which they also call the right-handed – and of the substances [that came] out of passion and matter – which they also call left-handed. For, they assert, he gave form to all things that exist after him, to which he was secretly urged by his Mother. Hence they also call him Mother-Parent, Fatherless, Demiurge and Father."

Sophia-Achamoth introduces the spiritual element into man when he is created by the Demiurge.[550]

Irenaeus also mentions a doctrine of the Sethians and Ophites regarding the origins of Sophia. Here the coming into existence of Sophia is due to "an accident in the Pleroma,"[551] as Couliano calls it. The enigmatic father generates an immense light with the female entity called *Spirit* ("By illuminating her, [he] generated from her an incorruptible Light"[552]). *Spirit* cannot contain all the light with which she is filled and thus she loses light from her left side. Sophia is born from this loss of Spirit's light.

As in the Nag Hammadi Library, Sophia stands again for an encounter between spirit and matter, full of tension and tragedy. She descends into the material world, although in this version of the myth it is not she but the "pleromatic accident" which is responsible for her "fall." Sophia's creations then, remain in this "dubious" tension, in the *chiaroscuro* where the material and spiritual meet. Through her fall and from her body, both the sky and the first woman's body are formed, before she manages to rise once more to the Pleroma.[553]

---

550 See ibid., I 5, 5–6 and I 30, 6. In Irenaeus, *Against the Heresies*, I 30, 9 Sophia comforts Adam and Eve, suffering from their heavy bodies and the knowledge of their mortality by reanimating in them the consciousness of their spiritual sides. She also helps them to find food after Yaldabaoth has chased them out of paradise.

551 Couliano, *The Tree of Gnosis*, 87.

552 Irenaeus, *Against the Heresies*, I 30, 1.

553 Ibid., I 30, 3: "The Power on the other hand, which overflowed from the Woman, since it was endowed with moisture of light, fell downwards from her Progenitors, they teach, though she of her own will retained the moisture of light, which they call Left-handed, Prounikos, Sophia, and Bisexual. She simply descended into the waters which were in a state of calm and set them in motion by recklessly agitating them to their depths. From them she took a body for herself. They relate that all things ran to meet this moisture of light and clung to it and embraced it. And unless she had possessed that [moisture], she would perhaps have been entirely absorbed by, and submerged in, matter. When, therefore, she was held bound by the body and weighed down very much, she regretted [what had happened] at one time and made an attempt to escape from the waters and ascend to her Mother. She could not accomplish this because of the weight of the body which surrounded her. She felt very bad and schemed to hide the light she had from above, fearing lest it too should suffer from the lower elements as she had. But when she had received power from her moisture of light, she leaped back and was lifted up on high. And having attained the heights, she spread herself out as a covering and thus made out of her body the heaven that is visible. She remained under the heaven that she had made, and still possesses the form of the watery body. But when she was seized by a longing for the higher light

As has already been mentioned, Irenaeus is not the only representative of Christian orthodoxy who wrote against gnosticism thereby transmitting important information on the Sophia myth. Sophia, "the fallen wisdom,"[554] also appears in Hippolytus' *Refutatio Omnium Haeresium*. The way Hippolytus tells the Sophia myth resembles the account of Irenaeus in several aspects. Here Sophia is the youngest aeon of the Pleroma (the twenty-eighth). She manages to ascend towards the enigmatic father of the Pleroma and is impressed with the fact that he has generated aeons without a partner, although all the other aeons have generated as couples.[555] Sophia wants to imitate the father but overestimates her powers to do so. Regarding this point the account of Hippolytus seems to draw upon the Aristotelian theory of generation to explain why Sophia cannot generate on her own. That is to say, while the ungenerated father contains all principles, Sophia, being female, is identified with matter, and therefore lacks the form which is given exclusively by the male principle of generation. Thus Hippolytus finds a "biological" explanation for Sophia's miscarriage: "For in the Unbegotten [...] all things exist together; but among the begotten the female is the projector of substance, but the male gives form to the substance which the female projects. Therefore Sophia projected only that which she could, a substance shapeless and unformed."[556]

Like in the writings of Irenaeus and in the texts of the Nag Hammadi Library, the fact that Sophia generates on her own creates turmoil inside and outside the Pleroma.[557] While Sophia mourns her miscarriage, the aeons are afraid that their generations too would become miscarriages. Finally, the father orders the aeons Nous and Aletheia to generate Christ and the Holy Spirit who separate the product of Sophia's miscarriage from the Pleroma and transform Sophia into a perfect aeon placed outside of it. Furthermore, the aeon Stauros, also called Horos ("border"), keeps Sophia and the outcome of her miscarriage separate from the Pleroma. However, in Hippolytus' *Philosophumena*, suffering and tears continue to

---

and had received power through all things, she put off the body and was freed from it. Now this body which she is said to have put off they style a female from a female." In his Italian translation of this passage Enzo Bellini keeps the word Androginos which Unger translates as Bisexual. See Ireneo di Lione, *Contro le eresie e gli altri scritti*, trans. Enzo Bellini (Milano: Jaca Book, 1979).

554 Couliano, *The Tree of Gnosis*, 85.

555 Hippolytus, *Philosophumena*, VI. 30.

556 Ibid.

557 See for the following ibid., VI. 31.

be attached to the figure of Sophia.[558] Once banned from the Pleroma she is full of fear and longs for Christ and the Holy Spirit. Finally, Christ and all the other aeons take pity on her. Christ – who is sent to Sophia by the aeons – finds her in the grip of four passions, namely Anguish (also translatable as Fear), Pain (also translatable as Grief), Confusion (also translatable as Perplexity) and Supplication.[559] Hippolytus writes:

> Then the Fruit [=Christ] being outside the Pleroma and finding her amid the first four passions (to wit) in fear and grief and perplexity and supplication, corrected her passions, but did not think it seemly in correcting them that they should be destroyed, since they were eternal and special to Sophia, nor yet that Sophia should be among such passions as fear and grief, supplication and perplexity.[560]

Christ changes Sophia's passions into substances: Anguish is transformed into the psychic substance of which the Demiurge consists; Pain becomes material substance; Confusion becomes demonical substance; and Supplication becomes the psychic substance "of the right."[561]

With regard to the change of Sophia's passions into substances it is of the utmost importance that her fall, which occured as a result of her wish to generate on her own, provokes the creation of a "dubious" world. The troubled Sophia provokes the creation of a world perceived to be full of turmoil, and how else could it be, given that the material world is seen as deriving from Sophia's Pain and that the Demiurge, the creator of this world, has its origin in Sophia's Anguish.

How much the Sophia myth actually forms part of the logic of the "dubious" supremacy of the female over the male in matters of childbirth, is clarified, if the versions described so far are compared with the Nag Hammadi text *The Tripartite Tractate*, probably written in the early to mid-third century.[562] In the *The Tripartite Tractate* the masculine aeon

558 See for the following ibid., VI.32.

559 According to Couliano, Supplication is positive and equals Conversion in the version of Irenaeus. See Couliano, *The Tree of Gnosis*, 78.

560 Hippolytus, *Philosophumena*, VI. 32.

561 Ibid.: "He made them fundamental essences. And He made the fear into the essence of the soul, and the grief into that of matter, and the perplexity into (that) of demons, but the conversion and entreaty and supplication He made a path to repentance and (the) power of the soul's essence, which (essence) is called the Right Hand or Demiurge from fear."

562 See Harold W. Attridge and Elaine H. Pagels, introduction to *The Tripartite Tractate (I,5)*, in *The Nag Hammadi Library in English*, trans. and introduced by members

Logos is ultimately responsible for the coming into existence of the first human being and cosmic governance. Harold W. Attridge and Elaine H. Pagels support the view that the Logos in *The Tripartite Tractate* fills the position usually occupied by Sophia. However, the masculine Logos, in contrast to Sophia, is not an ambivalent entity but has exclusively positive connotations:

> In *The Tripartite Tractate* the agent of the rupture in the Pleroma is a masculine aeon, the (Word). His fall, which includes elements of [...] traditional explanations of Sophia's catastrophe, is presented in remarkably positive terms, as a result of his own "abundant love"(76, 19–20). It is also, remarkably enough, in accordance with the father's will (76, 24–77,1). Most importantly, it proceeds from the Logos' free choice (75, 35–76,1), a quality which all entities dependent on him share.[563]

The only time the Logos is depicted with a touch of negativity in *The Tripartite Tractate* is when it splits into two and his better, masculine part returns to the Pleroma to intercede on behalf of his defective, feminine self. Thus the ambivalence of Sophia has to do with her femininity. As a female aeon revealing a supremacy over the male in matters of creation, she becomes "dubious." On the other hand, being in the same position as Sophia, the masculine aeon Logos does not have any "dubious" traits. Significantly, it is his feminine part which is defective. In a similar vein, Couliano interprets Sophia as being comparable to the figure of a female trickster: "The trickstress embodies a number of exaggerated negative traits sometimes attributed to femaleness. ... It seemed in all cases that there was something wrong with the Trickstress's eroticism [...] that she interfered with the male order of the world and sabotaged humankind."[564]

However, maintaning that the problem with Sophia's behaviour in the different versions of the Sophia myth lies with her eroticism can easily lead one astray. Couliano himself identifies Sophia generating without a partner as a constant accusation throughout the texts. Thus it is less the question of erotic behaviour and more the question of how generation takes place that seems to be the core issue of the Sophia story. Sophia presides over childbirth. Like Gaia she generates on her own. However,

---

of the Coptic Gnostic Library Project of the Institute for Antiquity and Christianity, Claremont, California, ed. James M. Robinson, 3rd, completely rev. ed. (Leiden: Brill, 1988), 58.

563 Ibid., 59.

564 Ibid., 86.

in contrast to Gaia, Sophia's behaviour is not connoted positively. Quite the opposite, she is punished and her dubious actions lead to the creation of a dubious world. As Couliano puts it: "By introducing the hypostasis Sophia-Wisdom gnostics try to solve an unfathomable metaphysical problem: How is it possible that impermanence stems from permanence, lack and pain from Fullness and immovibility."[565]

Sophia's independent act of generation becomes a transgression of the Pleroma's and the Father's law, resulting in a miscarriage which produces the world. In contrast to the procosmic creation myth of Gaia involving an independently generating goddess, the creation myth involving Sophia is linked to Gnostic theodicy.

3. Isis and Mary: The Supremacy of the Female and Harmony between Spiritual Birth and Childbirth

As has already been pointed out, the cult of the Graeco-Roman and ancient Egyptian goddess Isis, and the worship of Virgin Mary are two further examples important to the supremacy of the female over the male in matters of childbirth. However, the cults of Isis and Mary are virtually inseparable from the fourth symbolic pattern of childbirth that is concerned with the idea of a harmony between spiritual birth and childbirth. Thus it is preferable to refer to Isis and Mary at a later stage because they stand for an enduring combination of both symbolic patterns of childbirth which can be traced up to current times.[566]

4. Mikhail Epstein: The "Russian-Doll-Principle"

Some passages of Mikhail Epstein's essay *Fatherhood* have already been examined in the context of the first symbolic pattern of childbirth.

565 Couliano, *The Tree of Gnosis*, 73.

566 See section III.4.

However, other passages of the book also testify to the supremacy of the female over the male in matters of childbirth. This is because Epstein metaphorically links the birth of a daughter to parthenogenesis. In Epstein's essay the father experiences the sensation that the mother has generated on her own and reproduced herself without a man:

> The birth of a girl is a bit puzzling. It is like an asexual form of propagation without participation of the opposite sex. The female body reproduces itself just like a cell is reproducing itself by self-division and not by mating like a gamete. It is as if no man had been involved, as if the woman had generated a spitting image of herself while preserving her immaculate virginity. For this reason the father traditionally wants a son of whom he is proud as a proof of his manly force and power over the woman (he has been victorious over her in the love battle, he has implanted himself – his semen and likeness – in her womb). On the contrary, he feels somewhat ashamed of a girl as if he had been weak and the woman had not needed him for such an easy thing because she had simply divided herself into two. This is how this naive unconscious mythology looks like.[567]

Symbolically conceiving of giving birth to a daughter as of a parthenogenetic act distances the father from the child and lets the woman become the primary source of life:

> The fact that a girl had been born made me feel somehow chaste and being pushed aside. This was a light and not a fire. This did not burn but was radiating with a cool, blue, ideal light. I did not feel the triumph of self-assertion and victory but rather gratefulness for having been accepted and regarded worthy, as if not I had done this but this had been done on my behalf.[568]

In *Fatherhood*, the supremacy of the female over the male in matters of childbirth is expressed as a physical supremacy. The mother and child's embrace is pictured as being reminiscent of their fusion during pregnancy. The father, instead, is painfully feeling the comparatively larger physical distance to the child: "She [the mother] is holding the fidgetly child tight to herself because she has born it out of herself – she is pressing its body to her body. But in the fatherly body there is no place of origin for the baby. He is connected to it more by his will than by his flesh."[569]

The strong physical link between mother and child during pregnancy gives the father in Epstein's essay a feeling of inferiority. During pregnancy

567 Epstein, *Tagebuch für Olga*, 37–38.
568 Ibid., 38.
569 Ibid., 220.

he has the sensation that his child is somewhere in an unknown world and that his existence is insignificant for it.[570] This feeling of inferiority, stemming from the greater physical attachment between the mother and her child, persists even after birth:

> Birth is, as it were, an exchange of feelings and rights of possession between the parents, the transition from the father's longing for the invisible child in his wife's womb to the mother's fear for the child she no longer feels in herself. [...] Evidently, compared to my joy over acquiring Olga, even with her fear of loss L. is still infinitely superior to me. The anguish of her body is a sign that the little girl secretly keeps on being inside her, although only in the form of a tormenting absence.[571]

The tension between the supremacy of the female in matters of childbirth and the male's feeling of inferiority resulting from it is creatively resolved in *Fatherhood*. The father indulges in an act of mimesis of the female pregnant body. By embracing his baby he can imitate the fusion of mother and child during pregnancy:

> To carry a baby in one's arms while it is lying in the safe and secure hollow between chin and chest is a blissfulness comparable to nothing else. Suddenly there awakes a new ability in the male body to deepen thus forming a half-closed space and thereby partially emulating the emotions of a mother who gives shelter to her child and looks after it in her flesh.
>
> All other types of touching look cold and distant if compared to the one of a body not cuddling up to another from the outside but enclosing it in itself.[572]

The mimesis of pregnancy gives the father a feeling of happiness. The father's embrace of the child is metaphorically described as an organic fusion like that of a flower and the earth, a cloud and the air:

> She simply exists inside me, in my arms, on my chest, like a flower growing out of the earth or a cloud floating in the air. [...] All my outward appearance immediately gains the qualities of an inner space as soon as it cuddles up to her: it becomes softer and warmer. It has not been my part to carry this fruit to the end but after her birth she started to grow into me.[573]

---

570 Ibid., 65: "Das, was mich während ihrer Schwangerschaft gequält hat, daß Olga irgendwo im Ungekannten ist und ich für sie überflüssig bin."

571 Ibid.

572 Ibid., 66.

573 Ibid., 68.

In summary, the father in Epstein's essay experiences the supremacy of the female in matters of childbirth as something painful to him. The father's mimesis of pregnancy through physical contact with his child heals the suffering imposed by the "physical" supremacy of the female in matters of childbirth. Mimesis bridges the comparatively wider "physical" distance which exists between father and child.

III.4 Harmony between Spiritual/ Theoretical Natality and Childbirth

The following chapter identifies a symbolic pattern of childbirth in which childbirth and birth into the realm of thought/ spirituality are not mutually exclusive[574] but rather are in harmony with each other. The myths, cults, literary and philosophical traditions of the Ancient Egyptian/ Graeco-Roman goddess Isis have been chosen to illustrate such a harmony between spiritual birth and childbirth.

The history of Isis spans from the second millennium before Christ until roughly the fifth century C.E. She became the most important divinity in Egypt during the final stage of Egyptian religious development under the Greek Ptolomeic dynasty.[575] If one takes into consideration the persistent influence of Isiac traditions on Christianity,[576] it could even be argued that the history of Isis has not come to an end yet, because Isis has survived in the figure of Mary.

However, in the following presentation of the goddess as the symbolic carrier of a specific conception of childbirth, it should be taken into consideration that what Karl Jaspers has labelled *Achsenzeit*[577] ("axial age") cuts through the "continuity" between the Isis and Mary worship. Eisenstadt, who elaborates on Jaspers' work, defines the axial age civilizations as civilizations "in which there is an emphasis on the chasm between the transcendental and the mundane order and a conception of a higher moral or metaphysical order."[578] Whereas Isis emerges rather unshaken from axial age culture, the axial age gap becomes visible in the transformation of Isis

574 See section III.2. "Theoretical, Spiritual and Political Natality versus Childbirth" for the contentions between spiritual birth and childbirth.

575 See Wilhelm Heinrich Roscher, *Ausführliches Lexikon der griechischen und römischen Mythologie* (1882–1921; reprint, Hildesheim: Olms, 1993), 360.

576 See for example Samuel Sharpe, *Egyptian Mythology and Egyptian Christianity* (London: Carter and Co, 1896) and Reginald Eldred Witt, *Isis in the Graeco-Roman World* (London: Thames and Hudson, 1971), 269–281.

577 See Karl Jaspers, *Vom Ursprung und Ziel der Geschichte.*

578 Eisenstadt, *The Origins and Diversity of Axial Age Civilisations*, 3.

into Mary. There still is a harmony between spiritual birth and childbirth in the Mary cult, but it differs considerably from the one attached to Isis.

In addition to the examples of Isis and Mary, the forth symbolic pattern of childbirth will be illustrated by some works of the artist Paula Modersohn-Becker and by Mikhail Epstein's "ethics of childbirth."

1. Childbirth, Wisdom and Mystery Religion: The Reign of Queen Isis

The harmonious interplay of childbirth, wisdom and mystery religion in the myths and cults of Isis is as old as the Ancient Egyptian goddess herself. In the following, the way each of these three realms is attached to Isis will be examined. In this manner, a picture will emerge of how the cults and myths of Isis testify to the symbolic pattern of childbirth labeled "Harmony between Spiritual/Theoretical Natality and Childbirth."

Wisdom will be the first concept explored from the Isiac triad, "childbirth, wisdom and mystery." A myth about the unknown name of Ra gives a full account of the earliest reasons which were given for the connection between Isis and wisdom. Here we encounter the goddess setting out to learn the secret name of the chief god Ra.[579] The myth is part of a magical text dated to the nineteenth dynasty (1350–1200 B.C.) which was employed as a conjuration against the bite of a scorpion.[580]

John A. Wilson remarks that in Ancient Egypt, "the name was an element of personality and of power. It might be so charged with divine potency that it could not be pronounced. Or the god might retain a name hidden for himself alone, maintaining this element of power over all other gods and men."[581] The desire of Isis to learn the secret name of Ra expresses her wish to appropriate his power and wisdom to herself. The

579 For Ra creating the world by ejaculation and subsequent mimesis of birthgiving see section III.1.1. of this work.

580 John A. Wilson, "Egyptian Myths, Tales, and Mortuary Texts," in *Ancient Near Eastern Texts: Relating to the Old Testament*, ed. James Bennett Pritchard, 3rd ed. with supplement (1969; reprint, Princeton, New Jersey: Princeton University Press 1992), 12.

581 Ibid.

spell starts with an evocation of the chief god's power. Immediately after this, Isis is juxtaposed with Ra because of her vast knowledge:

> Now Isis was a clever woman. Her heart was craftier than a million men; she was choicer than a million gods; she was more discerning than a million of the noble dead. There was nothing which she did not know in heaven and earth, like Re, who made the content of the earth. The goddess purposed in her heart to learn the name of the august god.[582]

In the following it is told how Isis fashioned a snake from earth mixed with Ra's saliva. The chief god was bitten by the animal and assembled the gods to find a remedy for his pain. On condition that Ra reveals his secret name to her, Isis offers to help. The text narrates, "Isis came with her skill, her speech having the breath of life."[583] At first Ra resists and tries to maintain his secret. He does this by showing himself in all his might as the god of creation but without revealing his secret name:

> I am he who made heaven and earth, who knotted together the mountains, and created what is thereon. I am he who made the waters. [...] I am he who made the bull for the cow, so that sexual pleasures might come into being. I am he who made the heaven and the mysteries of the two horizons, so that the soul of the gods might be placed therein. [...] I am Khepri in the morning, Re at noon, and Atum who is in the evening.[584]

Finally, "the great god divulged his name to Isis, the Great of Magic"[585] in exchange for the antidote to the poisonous snake bite. The transmission of this divine wisdom is nearly a physical act. Ra says, "let thy ears be given to me, my daughter Isis, that my name may come forth from my body into thy body."[586] How powerful and wise Isis has become by the knowledge of Ra's name is revealed by the closing lines of the charm against the scorpion's bite: "The poison is dead through the speech of Isis the Great, the Mistress of the Gods, who knows Re (by) his own name."[587]

---

582 Ibid.
583 Ibid., 13.
584 Ibid.
585 Ibid.
586 Ibid.
587 Ibid., 14.

"Isis's ancient role as Wisdom"[588] accompanied the goddess as she conquered the Graeco-Roman world. Here she became associated with Hermes[589] functioning as her instructor, as can be shown from passages of Diodorus Siculus' *Library*, which was composed in the first century BC. Hermes presided over various types of knowledge and wisdom, including the realms of nature, music, religion, language and philosophy.[590] Diodorus connects Hermes to Isis by quoting an Isiac hymn from a stele in Arabian Nysa. Here it says: "I am Isis, the queen of every land, she who was instructed of Hermes."[591]

The Isiac hymn from Nysa stands in the tradition of Greek and Roman aretology. The term *aretalogia* was used in antiquity "to designate an account of or testimony to the virtues (*aretai*) of Isis as demonstrated to her devotees."[592] An aretology of ancient Maroneia again evokes the connection between Isis and Hermes. Here, with the aid of Hermes, she discovers writing, including the sacred mystical writings.[593] In Greco-Roman times, Hermes was identified with the ibis-headed ancient Egyptian god Thoth, who was a god of scripture and wisdom. In his turn, Thoth had been linked to Isis since the Pyramid Texts.[594] Witt states that in "the

588 Howard Clark Kee, *Miracle in the Early Christian World: A Study in Sociohistorical Method* (New Haven and London: Yale University Press, 1983), 128.

589 For the link between Isis and Hermes see ibid. 115, 123–124, 127, 132.

590 Diodorus of Sicily, *Diodorus of Sicily: In Twelve Volumes*, trans. Charles Henry Oldfather (1933; reprint Cambridge, Mass.: Harvard University Press, 1968), Book I. 16. 1–2:

"It was by Hermes [...] that the common language of mankind was further articulated, and that many objects which were still nameless received an appellation, that the alphabet was invented, and that ordinances regarding the honours and offerings due to the gods were duly established; he was the first also to observe the orderly arrangement of the stars and the harmony of the musical sound and their nature [...] to give thought to the rhythmical movement of the human body and its proper development. He also made a lyre and gave it three strings, imitating the seasons of the year; for he adopted three tones, the high from the summer, the low from the winter, and the medium from the spring. The Greeks were also taught by him how to expound (hermeneia) their thoughts, and it was for this reason that he was given the name Hermes."

591 Ibid., Book I 27.2–4.

592 Kee, *Miracle*, 122.

593 Yves Grandjean, *Une Nouvelle Arétalogie d'Isis à Maronée*, (Leiden: Brill, 1975), 20: "Elle a découvert avec Hermès les écrits, et parmi ceux-ci, les écrits sacrés pour les mystes, et les écrits à caractère public pour tous."

594 See Witt, *Isis in the Graeco-Roman World*, 108.

eclectic religion of the Hellenistic age Isis and Thoth/Hermes grew to be more and more closely associated, and the outcome of all this can be observed in the "Hermetic Books" at the end of the second century A.D."[595] In the Hermetic Literature, Isis talks about "philosophy and magic" as sustaining the soul just as medicine cures the ailments of the body.[596]

With the reference to Hermetic Literature we are already approaching the second concept of the triad "wisdom, mystery and childbirth" to which the goddess is linked. Isis as "Mistress of the mysteries" also presides over a special kind of wisdom, namely, esoteric wisdom. Witt points to the fact that both in Ancient Egypt and in Ancient Greece religious mysteries played an important role and that in both cultures Isis was tied to them.[597]

Having been instructed by Hermes, who is considered to have invented religious rites, Isis starts to preside over these rites herself. In an Isis hymn from Andros it says:

> I have revealed to mankind mystic initiations,
> I have taught reverence for the gods' statues,
> I have established the gods' temples.[598]

The myth which establishes an undissolvable relationship between Isis and the mysteries is the myth of Isis and Osiris. It played an important role both in Ancient Egyptian religion and in the Graeco-Roman cult of Isis. However, there is no complete account of the myth of Isis and Osiris in Ancient Egyptian texts. The most complete version of the divine couple's story can be derived from *De Iside et Osiride* written by Plutarch (*45–125) as part of his *Moralia*. In Plutarch's Greek reception of the myth, the story of Isis and Osiris runs as follows:[599]

Isis and Osiris were the children of Rhea and Cronus. Plutarch depicts them as already enamoured of each other "in the darkness of the womb before their birth."[600] Their brother Typhon conspired against Osiris, by

595 Ibid.

596 See ibid., 189.

597 See ibid., 152–153.

598 Werner Peek, *Der Isishymnus von Andros und verwandte Texte* (Berlin: Weidmann, 1930), 22.

599 See for the following Plutarch, *De Iside et Osiride,* in Plutarch, *Moralia: In Sixteen Volumes*, vol. 5:351C–438E, trans. Frank Cole Babbitt (1936; reprint Cambridge, Mass.: Harvard University Press, 1969), 355 D-358 D.

600 Ibid., 356 A.

secretly measuring the body of Osiris and then making a beautifully ornamented chest which he showed during a festivity. He promised that he would give it to the man whose length would fit it. When Osiris lay down in the chest, Typhon slammed down the lid and fastened it by nails and molten lead. Then he threw the chest into the river, which carried it to the sea.

The news of her brother's death reached Isis who started to mourn and wander around restlessly in search of the chest. Finally, she managed to find it, but again malicious Typhon intervened. He divided the body of Osiris into fourteen parts and scattered them, each in a different place. Again Isis had to look for her brother's body and every time she found a part, she held a funeral for it. Each funeral site became a sacred tomb of Osiris. The only part Isis could not find was the male member because it had been eaten by fish. "But Isis made a replica of the member to take its place, and consecrated the phallus."[601] It was Isis who ordained that the replica of the phallus should be honoured and borne in processions.[602]

The fashioning of tombs for Osiris and the consecration of the image of his phallus turn Isis into the founder of religion and mysteries. In fact, Plutarch writes explicitly that Isis' experiences are at the origin of religious rites:

> But the […] sister and wife of Osiris […] was not indifferent to the contests and struggles which she had endured, nor to her own wanderings nor to her manifold deeds of wisdom and many feats of bravery, nor would she accept oblivion and silence for them, but she intermingled in the most holy rites portrayals and suggestions and representations of her experiences at that time, and sanctified them, both as a lesson in godliness and an encouragement for men and women who find themselves in the clutch of like calamities.[603]

There is one important element in the myth of Isis and Osiris to consider in our context, which is told quite differently by Plutarch as compared to Egyptian sources. This is the conception, procreation and birth of Horus, the son of Isis and Osiris, who is deeply linked to the Isiac mysteries.[604] According to Plutarch, Isis and Osiris had two sons, Hor and

601 Ibid., 358 B.
602 Ibid., 365 C.
603 Ibid., 361 D-E.
604 See for the following Theodor Hopfner, *Plutarch über Isis und Osiris: Text, Übersetzung und Kommentar* (Prag: Orientalisches Institut, 1940), 77–95.

Harpocrates, the latter coming forth from the couple's necrophilous union: "Osiris consorted with Isis after his death, and she became the mother of Harpocrates."[605] However, in the Egyptian sources there is only one son, Horus, who is indeed procreated after the death of Osiris. Another difference between Plutarch and the Egyptian sources is the fact that many Egyptian iconographic and textual representations of Isis depict the goddess (not Osiris) as the active partner in the necrophilous union of which Horus is born. For example, in the temple of Sethi I. in Abydos, and in the temple of Dendera, Isis is represented as a falcon which is reviving the sexual organ of dead Osiris by hovering over it.[606] Likewise, in textual tradition Isis appears as a bird flapping its wings. This is because in both Egyptian and Greek culture the wind was seen as favouring the capacities to procreate.[607] In a hymn to Osiris, flying Isis and her magical powers bringing about the extraordinary conception/procreation and birth of Horus, are depicted as follows:

> Thy sister acted as a protectress to thee. She drove thine enemies away, she averted seasons [of calamity], she recited formulae with the magical power of her mouth, [being] skilled of tongue and never halting for a word, being perfect in command and word. Isis the magician avenged her brother. She went about seeking him untiringly. She flew round and round over the earth uttering wailing cries of grief, and she did not alight on the ground until she had found him. She made light to [appear] from her feathers, she made air to come into being by means of her two wings, and she cried out the death cries for her brother. She made to rise up the helpless members of him whose heart was at rest, she drew from him his essence, and she made therefrom an heir. She suckled the child in solitariness, and none knew where his place was, and he grew in strength.[608]

In the Isis aretology of Maroneia, Isis is again the active partner in her relations with Osiris. Here it says that she took Serapis (Osiris) as her consort.[609] Grandjean comments that this fits the general historical development of the goddess Isis, as she tended to be the more dominant part of

605 Plutarch, *De Iside et Osiride,* 358 E.

606 See Hopfner, *Plutarch über Isis,* 82.

607 See ibid., 81.

608 Ernest Alfred Wallis Budge, *Osiris: The Egyptian Religion of Resurrection* (New York: University Books, 1961), 94.

609 Grandjean, *Une Nouvelle Arétalogie d"Isis*, 55: "Tu as pris Sérapis comme compagnon." The name Serapis is derived from the ideas of Alexandrian Graeco-Egyptian theologians who fused the Greek Zeus, with the Egyptian Apis-bull, identified with Osiris.

the couple from the 2nd century B.C. on.[610] E.A. Wallis Budge also accentuates her prominence, when he writes "in late times, her worship wholly eclipsed that of her male counterpart Osiris."[611]

The necrophilous procreation/ conception of Horus, brought about by the agency of Isis, stands in the mythical tradition W. Brede Kristensen labels "life out of death."[612] In fact, Osiris symbolically continues living because of his son's birth.[613] Moreover, the extraordinary conception/ procreation of Horus is an example for the supremacy of the female over the male in matters of childbirth. Here, in a way, Isis appropriates both female and male procreational activity to herself.[614]

In the conception/procreation myth of Horus, childbirth, mystery and the supremacy of the female in matters of childbirth are closely intertwined with one another. The two main dogmas of Isiac faith, the death of the brother-husband and the birth of the child Horus are mysteriously linked, in that the death of Osiris entailed his rebirth as Horus.[615] Moreover, during the Middle and New Kingdom the life giving forces of Isis were accentuated by the idea that Isis not only revived the procreational faculty of Osiris, but also resurrected him by beating her wings and thus bestowing on him the breath of life.[616]

The ubiquity of *Isis lactans*, that is the representation of the goddess breastfeeding her baby, is another strong indication that Isis stands for a fusion of mystery and childbirth. In the myth of Isis and Osiris, the goddess had to escape from the evil powers of Typhon (in Egyptian, Seth) after she had given birth to Horus. She fled to the marshes where she hid and nourished her child. *Isis lactans* was surely one of the most frequent

---

610 Ibid., 55–56: "Cette prééminence d'Isis n'est pas pour surprendre; dès le IIe siècle avant J.-C., en effet, la déesse tend à prendre une place prépondérante par rapport à Sérapis et cette place ne fera que s'affirmer au cours des siècles."

611 Wallis Budge, *Osiris*, 271.

612 See William Brede Kristensen, *Life out of Death: Studies in the Religions of Egypt and of Ancient Greece*, trans. H. J. Franken and G. R. H. Wright (Louvain: Peeters, 1992).

613 Jan Assmann, *The Search for God in Ancient Egypt*, trans. David Lorton (Ithaca: Cornell University Press, 2001), 130: "Osiris rises in his son, but he himself abides in the netherworld."

614 In fact, Isis "could characterize herself as a woman who turns herself into a male." Witt, *Isis in the Graeco-Roman World*, 44.

615 See Erich Neumann, *The Great Mother*, trans. Ralph Manheim (New York: Pantheon Books, 1955), 64–65.

616 See Witt, *Isis in the Graeco-Roman World*, 36.

representations of the goddess both in Ancient Egypt and in Graeco-Roman times.[617] The milk of Isis had a highly symbolic value. According to Tran Tam Tinh, both milk and breastfeeding were loaded with religious symbolism in the Egyptian belief system.[618] The representations of Isis breastfeeding Horus depict the goddess as a life-giving force. On inscriptions next to *Isis lactans* in the temples of Luxor and Deir el-Bahari, the goddess is compared to Ra, the god of creation. Here it says that the milk, just like Ra, gives life, stability and health.[619] From the depiction of *Isis lactans* on reliefs as part of a shrine, Kee deduces the role of Isis as mistress of the mysteries.[620] Thus Isis appearing as *Isis lactans* is a giver of both life and spiritual life.

The harmony between spiritual birth and childbirth in Isis is further evidenced by a rather special iconographic representation of *Isis lactans*. Tran Tam Tinh analyses several Graeco-Roman representations of the goddess breastfeeding a small Apis Bull, interpreted to be the incarnation of Osiris. In the Osirian mystery religion the *mystes*, that is the initiate, could identify with his god Osiris. Thus Tran Tam Tinh makes the hypothesis that the *mystes* symbolically becoming Apis like Osiris might have been connected to the gods by the milk of Isis.[621]

In everyday life Isis was seen as a goddess presiding over childbirth in Ancient Egypt and in Graeco-Roman times. Witt stresses the fact that, although Isis was *myrionymos*, the one of countless names in Graeco-Roman thought, her identification with Artemis-Eileithyia ("Child-bearing") was of utmost importance.[622] Like Artemis-Eileithyia, Isis could be associated with both maternity and virginity.[623] Both goddesses were represented

617 Ibid.

618 See Vincent Tam Tinh Tran, avec la collaboration de Yvette Labreque, *Isis Lactans: Corpus des monuments greco-romains d'Isis allaitant Harpocrate* (Leiden: E.J. Brill, 1973), 4.

619 Ibid.: "Il [le lait] donne toute vie, toute stabilité, toute santé à toi comme Ra», and: «Celle qui est sur le sommet de la maison de la flamme … donne toute vie, toute santé à toi comme Ra."

620 See Kee, *Miracle*, 132.

621 Tran, *Isis Lactans*, 28 : "Peut-être ce geste symbolique a-t-il encore une signification mystique selon laquelle le myste, devenu apis comme son Dieu Osiris, s'introduit dans le cercle des dieux grâce au lait issu de la déesse."

622 See Witt, *Isis in the Graeco-Roman World*, 151.

623 See ibid., 142. How Isis as Artemis-Eileithyia was transformed into Mary, will be shown in the following section.

with torches, "symbolizing the moon, present to save mother and child in their darkness."[624] In a hymn from Andros, Isis is depicted as the giver of new life, assisting women during childbirth as the heavenly midwife. Here she says:[625] "I have brought forth the new-born babe at the tenth orbit of the moon – fit light for the deed that is consummated."

Another interesting example for the connection between Isis and childbirth is a spell Roscher mentions in his "Encyclopaedia of Greek and Roman Mythology." Here a birthgiving woman, identifying herself with Isis, asks for help from the gods. In the event that they should refuse to help her, she threatens them, and finishes the spell by emphasizing that the threats have been pronounced by Isis and not by herself.[626]

Furthermore, an Egyptian fairy tale tells of Isis helping the mother of three children during birthgiving. The children are destined to become kings. At the birth of each of the boys, Isis speaks some words from which their names derive.[627] Finally, Ovid, in his most famous and moving prayer for his beloved Corinna in *Ars Amatoria*, implores the goddess to take mercy upon Corinna, suffering from the consequences of an abortion. Here also, Isis appears as the one who eases "the labor of women in their pangs, when their bodies are tormented by the hidden burden."[628]

---

624 Ibid., 148.

625 Andros Hymn, 37, quoted in Witt, *Isis in the Graeco-Roman World*, 148.

626 Roscher, *Ausführliches Lexikon*, 502: "Nicht ich sage dies, nicht ich wiederhole es; Isis sagt es, Isis wiederholt es."

627 See ibid., 367. Here again Isis is attached to the knowledge about names. As the one who knows the secret name of Ra, she gives names to the royal children.

628 Ovid, *The Art of Love* (*Ars Amatoria*), trans. Charles D. Young (New York: Horace Liveright Inc., 1931), Book II, XIII.:
"Great Isis, who art fond of Paraetonium and Canopus, of Memphis and Pharos covered with swaying palms, where the great Nile flows swiftly through the seven mouths into the sea, I beseech you by the revered face of Anubis (and may Osiris ever love your rites, the sluggish serpent glide about your altar gifts, and horned Apis be your comrade!) turn towards us your countenance and spare us both: giving life to my lady, she will grant life to me. She was ever zealous in her ministrations to you on the days allotted for your service, where the Gallic squadron rides by your laurel trees.
And you, who ease the labor of women in their pangs, when their bodies are tormented by the hidden burden, do you attend in charity, and harken to my prayers, Ilithyria! She is deserving of your aid, and I beseech you, bid her life! And I accoutered in festive robes, shall offer incense on your smoking altars, and bring you gifts to lay at your feet. My offerings shall bear the legend: "Naso, for Corinna who was saved." Do most graciously give me occasion for both gift and legend."

Up to this point I have used various sources from Ancient Egypt and Greco-Roman times to evidence the harmony between wisdom, mystery religion and childbirth represented by Isis. There are, however, two classical works which show in depth that Isis did in fact unite childbirth and theoretical/spiritual natality, namely *De Iside et Osiride* by Plutarch (*45 C.E.–125 C.E. ca.) and Apuleius' *The Golden Ass* (*Asinus Aureus*). Both works merit longer discussion because they highlight different aspects of the issue. In *De Iside et Osiride*, Isis is primarily depicted as the goddess of wisdom and childbirth, whereas Lucius Apuleius (around 125–180 C.E. ca.) emphasizes her qualities as the mistress of mysteries and the giver of all life in the *Golden Ass*.

1.1 Plutarch's Isis as Idea: The Goddess of Philosophers and the Goddess of Childbirth

In his *De Iside et Osiride* Plutarch attempts to "translate" the goddess Isis into Platonic philosophy. However, quite to the contrary of Plato, who in the *Symposium*, opposes childbirth and philosophy,[629] Plutarch harmonizes philosophy and childbirth with his reception of Isis.

How does Plutarch conceive of reason, philosophy and childbirth then? In a Platonic manner, Plutarch assumes in *De Iside et Osiride* that man's most precious good is reason, and that this becomes a means by which to approach the divine: "The fact is that nothing of man's usual possessions is more divine than reasoning, especially reasoning about the gods; and nothing has a greater influence toward happiness."[630] Plutarch's "reasoning about the gods" in *De Iside et Osiride*, is a rationalization and "demythization" of Egyptian divinities in large part. Plutarch firmly maintains the ascending Greek hierarchy of animal, man and god, and he tries to purify the Egyptian gods from mythical and ritual elements, which seem irrational to him.[631]

629 See section III.2.2. of this work.

630 Plutarch, *De Iside et Osiride*, 378 C-D.

631 A good example for Plutarch's approach is his rather Greek critique of Egyptian animal worship:
"In these matters the Greeks are correct in saying and believing that the dove is the sacred bird of Aphroditê, that the serpent is sacred to Athena, the raven to Apollo, and the dog to Artemis. ....

In accordance with Plutarch's more philosophical approach to the divine, elements of the Isiac myth, such as Isis taking on the shape of a falcon and hovering over dead Osiris to revive his procreational activity, are left out. Instead, the goddess is mainly depicted as the personification of wisdom and truth as is made clear right from the beginning of *De Iside et Osiride*. In the first section of his treatise, Plutarch evokes the Isiac priestess Clea, to whom he dedicates his work. Moreover, he indulges in reflections on the gods whose divine being is identified with their knowledge and intelligence.[632] In the second chapter of *De Iside et Osiride*, Plutarch links Isis to wisdom (*sophia*) and truth. Furthermore, he suggests that the etymological derivation of the word "Isis" is from the Greek "to know":

> Therefore the effort to arrive at the Truth, and especially the truth about the gods, is a longing for the divine. For the search for truth requires for its study and investigation the consideration of sacred subjects, and it is a work more hallowed than any form of holy living or temple service; and, not least of all, it is well-pleasing to that goddess whom you worship, a goddess exceptionally wise and a lover of wisdom [philosophon], to whom, as her name at least seems to indicate, knowledge and understanding are in the highest degree appropriate. For Isis is a Greek word.[633]

Like Diodorus of Sicily, Plutarch establishes a link between Hermes and Isis, and thereby attributes the knowledge of divine mysteries to her.[634] In another instance, Plutarch writes that Isis collected and put together the sacred writings which Typhon had torn to pieces and scattered to the

---

But the great majority of the Egyptians, in doing service to the animals themselves and in treating them as gods, have not only filled their sacred offices with ridicule and derision, but this is the least of the evils connected with their silly practices. ….
The notion that the gods, in fear of Typhon, changed themselves into these animals, concealing themselves, as it were, in the bodies of ibises, dogs and hawks, is a play of fancy surpassing all the wealth of monstruous fable. The further notion that as many of the souls of the dead as continue to exist are reborn into these animals only is likewise incredible" (Ibid., 379 D-F).

632 See ibid. 351D.

633 Ibid. 351 E-F. Also the word Iseion, meaning the Isiac shrine, is linked to knowledge: "The name of her shrine also clearly promises knowledge and comprehension of reality; for it is named Iseion, to indicate that we shall comprehend reality if in a reasonable and devout frame of mind we pass within the portals of her shrines" (Ibid. 352 A).

634 See ibid., 352 B. In the same passage Plutarch speculates about the saying that Isis would be the daughter of Prometheus, "the discoverer of wisdom and forethought." This is still another way to make a connection between the goddess and wisdom.

winds. She then gave these sacred writings "into the keeping of those that are initiated into the holy rites."[635] In this context, Isis is depicted as a founder of religion. However, Plutarch sets up a clear hierarchy between religious rites on the one hand, and the philosophical search for truth on the other. He stresses the importance of the latter for Isiac believers by addressing the priestess Clea with the following words:

> It is a fact, Clea, that having a beard and wearing a coarse cloak does not make philosophers, nor does dressing in linen and shaving the hair make votaries of Isis; but the true votary of Isis is he who, when he has legitimately received what is set forth in the ceremonies connected with these gods, uses reason in investigating and studying the truth contained therein.[636]

Plutarch's basic attitude towards Isis is summarised by Witt who states that "for Plutarch 'wise and wisdom loving' Isis was a 'philosophic' divinity."[637] However, Plutarch's Isis as a "philosophic" divinity goes hand in hand with Isis the goddess presiding over childbirth and generation. Indeed, Plutarch's references to Isis in her relation to childbirth are numerous. When he depicts her as the consort of Osiris, Plutarch develops the link between Isis and childbirth/generation in depth. Here he relies upon the aforementioned Aristotelian and Platonic ideas about generation in regards to the role males and females respectively play, i.e. the male is the active spiritual part and the female the material part in the process of generation.[638] Thus he identifies Isis as the mother and Osiris as the father with their different functions:

> Plato is wont to give to the conceptual the name of idea, example, or father, and to the material the name of mother or nurse, or seat and place of generation, and to that which results from both the name of offspring or generation [...] and so Osiris may be regarded as the origin, Isis as the recipient, and Horus as perfected result.[639]

However, the association Plutarch makes between Isis and receptive female matter does not despiritualize the goddess, given the nature of what she receives. Osiris is essentially imagined as the idea of the good. Osiris is the beginning, "far removed from the earth, uncontaminated and unpolluted

635 Ibid., 352A.

636 Ibid., 352 C.

637 Witt, *Isis in the Graeco-Roman World*, 22–23.

638 See the chapter on Aristotle in section III.1.7.of this work.

639 Plutarch, *De Iside et Osiride*, 373 F–374 A.

and pure from all matter that is subject to destruction and death."[640] He is "that beauty which is for men unutterable and undescribable."[641] As a result of Isis being the consort of Osiris, the "Osirian principles" are now extended to her:

> Some think the seed of Woman is not a power or origin, but only material and nurture of generation. To this thought we should cling fast and conceive that this Goddess also who participates with the first God and is associated with him in the love of the fair and lovely things about him is not opposed to him, but, just as we say that an honourable and just man is in love if his relations are just, and a good woman who has a husband and consorts with him we say yearns for him; thus we may conceive of her as always clinging close to him and being importunate over him and constantly filled with the most dominant and purest principles.[642]

What Plutarch here calls "the most dominant and purest principles" is thoroughly intertwined with generation, both in the metaphorical and in the concrete sense of the word:

> [Isis] inclines always towards the better and offers to it opportunity to create from her and to impregnate her with effluxes and likenesses in which she rejoices and is glad that she is made pregnant and teeming with these creations. For creation is the image of being in matter, and the thing created is a picture of reality.[643]

In Plutarch's reasoning, Isis comes very close to the goddess as creatrix because she not only receives the Osirian principles but "sends them forth from herself": "With this beauty [of Osiris] Isis, as the ancient story declares, is for ever enamoured and pursues it and consorts with it and fills our earth with all things fair and good that partake of generation."[644] Although Plutarch makes explicit references to Plato's *Symposium* when he ascribes yearning for beauty to Isis,[645] which is the essence of Eros in the *Symposium*,[646] the basic logic of Plutarch's *De Iside et Osiride* differs greatly from the *Symposium*. In the latter, childbirth and the birth of ideas are placed in strong opposition, and played out against one another. In *De Iside et Osiride* it becomes impossible to distinguish between creation

640 Ibid., 382 F.
641 Ibid., 383 A.
642 Ibid., 374 F–375 A.
643 Ibid., 372 F.
644 Ibid., 375 B.
645 See ibid., 372 D.
646 See section III.2.2. of this work.

and ideas because childbirth is the expression of the "Osirian principles." Moreover, the process of conception implies that reason is at work in the creative forces of Isis:

> Isis is, in fact, the female principle of Nature, and is receptive of every form of generation, in accord with which she is called by Plato the gentle nurse and the all-receptive, and by most people has been called by countless names, since, because of the force of reason, she turns herself to this thing or that and is receptive of all manner of shapes and forms. She has an innate love for the first and most dominant of all things, which is identical with the good, and this she yearns for and pursues.[647]

Plutarch describes the face of Isis as symbolizing birth.[648] Furthermore, Isis as the principle of generation, has an important spiritual function. It is because of her, the goddess of childbirth, that the evil powers of Typhon can be temporarily overcome. In a passage in which Isis is identified with the moon and Osiris with the sun, Plutarch writes:

> Thus they make the power of Osiris to be fixed in the Moon, and say that Isis, since she is generation, is associated with him. For this reason they also call the Moon the mother of the world, and they think that she has a nature both male and female, as she is receptive and made pregnant by the Sun, but she herself in turn emits and disseminates into the air generative principles. For, as they believe, the destructive activity of Typhon does not always prevail, but oftentimes is overpowered by such generation and put in bonds.[649]

In Plutarch's *De Iside et Osiride*, wisdom, mystery and childbirth – the three regions that form the dominion of Queen Isis – are explored in depth. As the daughter of Hermes, she is the philosophic divinity and founder of the mysteries. As the consort of Osiris, she is filled with the "Osirian principles" which are expressed in generation, and finally, as she sends forth these principles into the world, she becomes the "mother of all" who can limit and temporarily overcome the destructive power of Typhon.

Plutarch calls Isis "the mother of all," or *myrionymos* ("the one of countless names"). The title of *Myrionymos* appears to be rather abstract in *De Iside et Osiride*. Isis is nature and as such can take on every form and shape by the help of reason.[650] However, in a less philosophical sense,

647 Plutarch, *De Iside et Osiride*, 372 E-F.
648 See ibid., 376 E.
649 Ibid., 368 C-D.
650 See ibid., 372 E.

Myrionymos was a most frequent Isiac title in the second century C.E.[651] It is a title that testifies to the fact that Isis was slowly fused with virtually all the pantheon of Graeco-Roman goddesses and thus became many goddesses in one. As Witt puts it beautifully, "Queenly as Hera, mystic and fructifying as Demeter, comely as Aphrodite, victorious as Athena and pure as Artemis, she embraces within her the functions of all."[652] Also in the *The Golden Ass* by Lucius Apuleius the Isiac title of *Myrionymos* figures prominently.

In fact, as will be shown by the following chapter on *The Golden Ass*, Isis became the all-encompassing goddess, giver of life, meaning both physical and spiritual life. Apuleius – just like Plutarch – describes the goddess as presiding over both spiritual birth and childbirth. His approach to Isis, however, is more of a poetic than of a philosophical nature.

1.2 Lucius Apuleius: Isis as "Blessed Queen of Heaven," "Reliever of the Birth Pangs of Women," and "Sovereign of All Things Spiritual"

The last book of the *Metamorphoses* by Lucius Apuleius, commonly known as *The Golden Ass* (*Asinus Aureus*) is another good example of how childbirth and spiritual birth become harmoniously intertwined in the goddess Isis. *The Golden Ass* was most probably written around 170 C.E.[653] It tells the story of a young man called Lucius. Visiting the town Hypata in Thessaly for reasons of business, he notices that his landlord's wife is a witch. Driven by the wish to learn the art of magic from her, he starts a love affair with her slave Fotis. With the help of the slave girl he succeeds in gaining a magic ointment by which he hopes to be transformed into an owl. However, he is not transformed into this, the bird of wisdom, but into an ass which in Apuleius' day typified lust, cruelty and wickedness.[654] Moreover, the ass was

651 Inscriptions addressing Isis as *Myrionymos* were found in a vast area stretching from Nubia, to the Mediterranean up to Northern France and Germany. See Witt, *Isis in the Graeco-Roman World*, 112.

652 Ibid., 110.

653 See John Gwyn Griffiths, introduction to *The Isis-Book: Metamorphoses, Book XI of Apuleius of Madauros*, ed. and trans. John Gwyn Griffiths (Leiden: Brill, 1975), 10.

654 See Robert Graves, introduction to *The Transformations of Lucius otherwise Known as The Golden Ass*, by Lucius Apuleius, trans. Robert Graves (Harmondsworth, Middlesex: Penguin Books, 1951), 13.

sacred to the god Seth/Typhon, the antagonist of Isis and Osiris.[655] The ass Lucius lives through a number of adventures until he is finally rescued by Isis who returns his human shape and initiates him into her mysteries.

Woven into the main plot of *The Golden Ass* are quite a number of autobiographical elements from Apuleius. Like the young man in the story, Apuleius also came from Madaura and was from a noble family.[656] At his death, his father left him a great deal of property, and like the student Thelyrhon (whom the ass meets during his adventures), Apuleius may also have run through his inheritance.[657] The strongest autobiographical element though, seems to be contained in the last book of *The Golden Ass*, which is also called the Isis-Book. Like the Lucius of the story, Lucius Apuleius became an Isiac priest, and in the Isis-Book, he conveys his own experience as an Isiac initiate.[658] In the following it will be shown in which manner the Isis-Book depicts the goddess uniting childbirth and a spiritual rebirth.

The last book of *The Golden Ass* starts with Lucius, the ass, sleeping at the seaside, having found some peace after the many misfortunes of his life. He suddenly wakes up in the middle of the night and sees the full moon rising. He decides to address a prayer to Isis, whose presence he feels to be in the moon. Before praying, Lucius indulges in a rite of purification by bathing in the sea. This ritual bath is a clear foreshadowing of his spiritual purification, that is, his spiritual rebirth, to come. Lucius starts his prayer by evoking the goddess by her countless names:

> O Queen of Heaven [Regina Caeli] – whether thou art Ceres […], or whether thou art heavenly Venus, who didst unite the difference of the sexes in the first beginnings of nature by creating Love, and after bringing forth mankind with its unceasing offspring, art worshipped in the island shrine of Paphos; or the sister of Phoebus, who didst relieve the delivering of young ones by soothing remedies, thus rearing such teeming masses, and art now adored in the celebrated temples of Ephesus; or whether as Proserpine […] thou art propitiated with differing rites – whoever thou art […] help me now in the depth of my trouble.[659]

655 See ibid.
656 See ibid., 15.
657 See ibid.
658 See Griffiths, *Introduction,* 6.
659 Apuleius, *The Isis-Book: Metamorphoses, Book XI of Apuleius of Madauros,* ed. and trans. John Gwin Griffiths (Leiden: Brill, 1975), 267, 4–20.

Isis becomes all things to Lucius in her numerous shapes. He adresses her as Artemis, the sister of Phoebus, presiding over childbirth and links her to the "unceasing offspring" of mankind.

The contents of Lucius' prayer, corrisponds to the way the goddess is describing herself when she mercifully appears to Lucius, the ass, by rising from the middle of the sea. In this context, Isis manifests as a cosmic power presiding over both nature and the spiritual world. Showing herself with all her might, Isis says,

> I am with you, Lucius, moved by your prayers, I am the mother of the universe, the mistress of all the elements, the first off-spring of time, the highest of deities, the queen of the dead, foremost of heavenly beings, the single form that fuses all gods and goddesses; I who order by my will the starry heights of heaven, the health giving breezes of the sea, and the awful silences of those in the underworld: my single godhead is adored by the whole world in varied forms, in differing rites and with many diverse names. ….
>
> Thus the Phrygians […] call me Pessinuntia, Mother of the Gods; thus the Athenians […] call me Cecropeian Minerva; and the sea-tossed Cyprians call me Paphian Venus, the archer Cretans Diana-Dictynna, and the trilingual Sicilians Ortygian Proserpine; to the Eleusinians I am Ceres, the ancient goddess, to others Juno, to others Bellona and Hecate and Phammisia. But the Ethiopians […] together with the Africans and the Egyptians who excel through having the original doctrine, honour me with my distinctive rites and give me my true name of Queen Isis.[660]

In the course of her speech, Isis orders Lucius to eat from a rose garland supposed to be carried by her high priest during a procession in her honour the following day. She promises that by doing so, Lucius will regain his human shape. However, Isis emphasizes to Lucius that his rebirth as a man needs to be linked to his spiritual rebirth (as her devotee). The goddess ordains him: "The eternal laws of religion devote to my worship the day born from this night."[661] With the metaphor of the coming day to be born from the night ("diem, qui dies ex ista nocte nascetur"[662]) both Lucius' physical rebirth and his spiritual birth are alluded to. In the description of the Isiac procession taking place the following day, Apuleius has Isis appear as the mistress of mysteries and as the goddess of childbirth represented by various objects and animals. There is "a golden vessel, rounded in the shape of a woman's

660 Apuleius, *The Isis-Book,* trans. Griffith, 269, 9 – 270, 1.

661 Apuleius, *The Transformations of Lucius*, trans. Graves, 271.

662 Apuleius, *The Isis-Book,* trans. Griffith, 270, 5.

breast, from the nipple of which a thin stream of milk fell to the ground,"[663] and "a cow in upright posture; that cow was the fertile image of the goddess who is the creator of all."[664] During the processional, obeying the goddess, Lucius eats the roses and is transformed into a human being. The followers of the procession praise both his physical and his spiritual birth: "This is the man who has been restored to human shape through the splendid divinity of the all-powerful goddess. …. He is, as it were, born again and has at once pledged himself to service in the sacred rites."[665]

Lucius' initiation into the Isiac mysteries forms part of his spiritual birth. In this initiation process, he is required to die a symbolic death in order to renew his life:

> I approached the very gates of death and set one foot on Proserpine's threshold, yet was permitted to return, rapt through all the elements. At midnight I saw the sun shining as if it were noon; I entered the presence of the gods of the under-world and the gods of the upper-world, stood near and worshipped them.[666]

After his initiation into the Isiac mysteries is completed, a public celebrational ceremony takes place. Referring to the day of this ceremony, Lucius says: "That day was the happiest of my initiation, and I celebrated it as my birthday."[667] Clearly this "birthday" refers to Lucius' spiritual birth which together with his re-birth as a man he owes to Isis.

2. From Isis to Mary

Apuleius' *Golden Ass* and Plutarch's *De Iside et Osiride* are two examples of many documents which testify to Isis' immense significance in the first centuries C.E. In the Roman world during Apuleius' life time the Isis cult was at its height. It is true that before the conquest of Egypt by Alexander the Great, Isis was already being worshiped as *Isis lactans* by the Greek,

663 Apuleius, trans. Graves, 274, 10–12.
664 Apuleius, *The Isis-Book*, trans. Griffith, 274, 18–19.
665 Ibid., 278, 6–9.
666 Apuleius, *The Transformations of Lucius,* trans. Graves, 286.
667 Ibid.

Phoenecians, Carthagians and perhaps also by the Palestinians.[668] However, there was a massive expansion of the Isis cult in the Roman world during the first century C.E.[669]

For several centuries Isiac religion resisted the claims of Christian religious hegemony. Even in the fourth century C.E., when Christianity had become the official religion of the Roman Empire, Isis appeared on Alexandrian coins.[670] The last recorded traces of Isiac cults go back to the sixth century C.E. In 560 Justinian ordered the Isiac temple, on the small Nile island of Philae in Upper Egypt, to be closed. The priests were then imprisoned and the Isis-icons transferred to Constantinople. The temple itself was transformed into a church dedicated to St. Stephanus.[671] However, precisely those centuries that see the end of Isis worship, witness the emergence of Mary from the background to the foreground of Christian scenery.

The ways in which Isis shaped the figure of Mary are manifold. To begin with, a number of Isiac titles were transferred to Mary. Thus just like Isis, Mary too could be called *Theotokos*[672] ("the one giving birth to God"), *Regina* ("Queen"); *Isis Mater* corresponds to the Marian *Mater Domini*, *Isis Furva* to the *Madonna Addolorata* and *Isis Pelagia* to *Maris Stella*. Like *Isis Nike* also Mary could appear as a divinity of victory.[673] Furthermore, there are striking cultic resemblances between Isis worship and the worship of Mary, such as similar types of processions and the rich adornment of both Isis and Mary icons with jewellery and garments.[674] Finally, on an iconographic level, representations of Mary (and Jesus) appear to be highly dependent on representations of Isis (and

668 See Tran, *Isis Lactans*, 9.

669 This can be deduced from the huge production of lamps featuring Isis breastfeeding Horus. It was probably the Greek population of Alexandria who initially created this type of popular art. Another fact which accounts for a real boom of the Isis cult in the Roman Empire during the first centuries C.E., is the appearance of coins picturing the hellenized *Isis lactans*. See ibid., 17.

670 See Roscher, *Ausführliches Lexikon*, 2:424.

671 See ibid., 2:426.

672 Thomas F. Mathews and Norman Muller, "Isis and Mary in Early Icons," in *Images of the Mother of God: Perceptions of the Theotokos in Byzantium*, ed. Maria Vassilaki (Aldershot: Ashgate, 2005), 4.

673 See for this and a longer list of corresponding Isiac and Marian titles Roscher, *Ausführliches Lexikon* 2:428–429.

674 See ibid., 2:429–430.

Horus).[675] In a detailed study comparing the earliest icons of Mary from sixth century Egypt to late Egyptian Isis icons from the second and third centuries, Thomas F. Mathews and Norman Muller come to the conclusion that there are numerous common elements in the iconography of Isis and Mary.[676] Mary has what Mathews and Muller call the "detached 'Isis look.'"[677] Both Isis and Mary have their young son seated on the left thigh; both are pictured on a throne, and they even share a marked double chin.[678]

For the context of symbolic patterns of childbirth, it has to be emphasized that the figure of Mary, the Virgin Mother, essentially derives from the fusion of the two goddesses Isis and Artemis.[679] Both goddesses helped women in labour pain. However, Artemis never took care of a child of her own.[680] According to Witt, Artemis, the goddess presiding over the wild nature of the woodlands "symbolized the belief that for women there was a nobler state than being mated with a husband."[681] Here, virginity can be seen as an expression of independence. It fits perfectly into the picture that Artemis was also "the protecting deity of the Amazons who, like her, were warriors and huntresses and independent of men."[682] Wilamowitz called Artemis "Goddess of the Outside" ("Göttin des Draußen"[683]) because of her love for wild nature. One of her symbols was the cyprus[684] and her cultic places were the woody tops of hills, fountains in the middle of woods, rivers, lakes and brooks.[685]

However, it seems that, to a certain extent, both Mary's motherly and the virginal aspects are "tamed," disembodied versions of how maternity and virginity are expressed in Isis and Artemis. Isis, in contrast to Mary,

675 Occasionally icons of Isis were even mistaken as Mary icons and worshipped as such like in the church of St. Germain des Prez. See ibid., 2:431.

676 See Mathews and Muller, *Isis and Mary*, 3–11.

677 Ibid., 8.

678 See ibid., 8–9.

679 See Witt, *Isis in the Graeco-Roman World*, 146.

680 See ibid.

681 Ibid., 141.

682 Pierre Grimal, *A Concise Dictionary of Classical Mythology*, ed. Stephen Kershaw, trans. A. R. Maxwell-Hyslop (Oxford: Blackwell, 1990), 61.

683 Wilamowitz quoted in Karl Hoenn, *Artemis: Gestaltwandel einer Göttin* (Zürich: Artemis-Verlag, 1946), 20.

684 See ibid., 47.

685 Ibid., 47–48.

conceived her child actively, by expressing her sexual-magical forces. Virginity, in the case of Isis-Artemis, is an expression of female independence, that is, an absence of male power over the woman. The focus is less on sexual behaviour itself than on the power relations it might imply. In contrast to this, the high status of the Virgin Mary and virginity in Christianity are associated with the low status of the sexual body, and then consequently, childbirth. It is therefore precisely the Virgin Birth of Jesus which reconciles spiritual birth and childbirth. As will be shown in the following, this type of a harmony between spiritual birth and childbirth includes various forms of Mary's theological disembodiments which are connected to the Virgin Birth. Giving birth without pain and with a closed uterus, as well as Mary's perpetual virginity even after childbirth represent a disembodiment of childbirth completely alien to the goddess Isis. Thus, though in a rather different way than Isis, Mary – who in the course of the centuries would develop into a goddess like figure herself – continued to preserve both a supremacy of the female over the male in matters of childbirth and a harmony between spiritual birth and childbirth.

3. The Incarnation of the Sacred Through a Woman: Mary as "Spiritual Vessel"

> *Rerum factor fit factura*
> *Virginis in gremio*
> ("The creator of all becomes a creature in a virgin's womb")
> 13th century hymn

> *O womb more spacious than a city! O womb wider than the span of heaven! O womb that contained him whom the seven heavens do not contain. You contained him without pain and held in your bosom him who changed his being into the smallest of things. O womb that bore, concealed in (your) body, the Christ who has been made visible to many. O womb that became more spacious than the whole creation.*
> The Questions of Bartholomew

These quotes from a 13th century hymn[686] and from the apocryphal text *Questions of Bartholomew*[687] testify to the high status Mary acquired in Christianity because she gave birth to Jesus. However, at the beginning of Christianity, the mother of Jesus did not hold such a strong position. In the following, some stages in the historical development of Mary will be sketched. It will be shown how Mary changed from the "handmaid of the Lord" into a goddess-like figure in the course of the centuries.

In the first two centuries of Christianity no evidence can be found of Mary worship (as an independent practice). In fact, Mary played a minor role in the new religion, which was initially centered entirely on Christ.[688] However, in the gospels of Matthew and Luke, God reaches out into the world by means of her, that is by means of a female body[689]: Mary conceives Jesus, the son of God, and gives birth to him.[690]

In the gospel of Matthew, the incarnation of the sacred through a woman manifests itself in a rather surprising way. Seemingly, Jesus' birth relies on the tradition of male, patriarchal generation that we have

686 13th century hymn, quoted in Marina Warner, *Alone of All Her Sex: The Myth and Cult of the Virgin Mary* (1976; reprint, London: Vintage, 2000), 96.

687 *The Questions of Bartholomew*, trans. and ed. Felix Scheidweiler, in *Gospels and Related Writings, revised edition,* vol. 1 of *New Testament Apocrypha*, ed. Wilhelm Schneemelcher, English translation ed. R. McL. Wilson (Cambridge: James Clarke & Co, 1991), 546–547. According to Felix Scheidweiler *The Questions of Bartholomew* belong to an original form of the *Gospel of Bartholomew* presumably from the 3rd century. See Felix Scheidweiler, introduction to *The Questions of Bartholomew*, in *Gospels and Related Writings, revised edition,* vol. 1 of *New Testament Apocrypha*, ed. Wilhelm Schneemelcher, English translation ed. R. McL. Wilson (Cambridge: James Clarke & Co, 1991), 540.

688 See Delius, *Geschichte der Marienverehrung*, 35.

689 Christian theology is sensitive to the issue of which body – male, or female, becomes the *locus* of divine manifestation. In one of his sermons for Christmas (Sermon 184.2.), Augustine writes: "Let men rejoice, let women rejoice. Christ was born Man; He was born of woman. Both sexes have been honored" (Augustine, *Sermons for Christmas and Epiphany*, trans. Thomas Comerford Lawler (New York: Newman Press, 1952), 73). Similarly, in another sermon for Christmas by Augustine (Sermon 190. 2.), it says: "But because He Himself certainly had created both sexes, that is, male and female, even by His being born He wished to honor the sexes which He had come to free. .... Both have been favored by the Lord's Nativity with the hope of salvation. The honor of the male sex comes from the body of Christ; the honor of the female sex is in the mother of Christ." Ibid., 103.

690 The reversal of such a symbolic pattern of childbirth was illustrated by the description of the procreation of Muhammad by Ibn Hisham. See section III.1.11.

encountered before. Matthew gives the genealogical line of men generating one another: "Abraham begot Isaac; and Isaac begot Jacob; and Jacob begot Judas and his brethren; And Judas begot Phares and Zara of Thamar;" etc. down to Joseph.[691] The Italian writer Luigi Santucci has beautifully described the turning-point in the gospel, when he writes: "Matthan begot Jacob; Jacob begot Joseph, the husband of Mary … Go ahead, Matthew! And Joseph? Whom did he beget? But here the chain breaks. Joseph was a virgin."[692]

Joseph, in relation to Jesus, is indeed a "virgin," a patriarch who, according to Matthew, does not procreate his son. Instead it is the birth-giving on behalf of the mother, to which the genealogical line quite unexpectedly shifts: "And Jacob begot Joseph the husband of Mary, of whom was born Jesus, who is called Christ."

This unexpected shift, from Joseph to Mary in Matthew 1:16, has puzzled theologians throughout the centuries. For example, Eusebius of Caesarea comments on the gospel of Matthew, writing that Matthew actually should have given the genealogy of Mary instead of giving Joseph's genealogy, as there was no physical link between Joseph and Jesus.[693] Already the apocryphal *Protevangelium of James* – which has its roots in the second century[694] – puts forth the idea of Mary's Davidic descent so as to support the Davidic descent of Jesus.[695] Moreover, the churchfathers

691 Matthew 1:1–16. Here the translation of the King James Bible is used because the translation of this passage in the King James Bible is more literal than the one of the "New Oxford Annotated Bible." I am grateful to Sonja Ammann for her advice on this matter.

692 Luigi Santucci, *Volete andarvene anche voi? Una vita di Cristo*, 3rd ed. (Torino: Edizioni San Paolo, 2001), 18: "Mathan generò Giacobbe; Giacobbe generò Giuseppe, lo sposo di Maria …
Avanti, Matteo. E Giuseppe chi generò? Ma qui la collana si spezza. Giuseppe fu vergine."

693 See Delius, *Geschichte der Marienverehrung*, 93.

694 See Oscar Cullmann, *The Protevangelium of James*, in *Gospels and Related Writings, revised edition,* vol. 1 of *New Testament Apocrypha*, ed. Wilhelm Schneemelcher, English translation ed. R. McL. Wilson (Cambridge: James Clarke & Co, 1991), 423.

695 See *The Protevangelium of James,* trans. and ed. Oscar Cullmann, in *Gospels and Related Writings, revised edition,* vol. 1 of *New Testament Apocrypha*, ed. Wilhelm Schneemelcher, English translation ed. R. McL. Wilson (Cambridge: James Clarke & Co, 1991), 430.

Justin and Irenaeus also attached Jesus to the house of David, by sustaining that Mary was of Davidic descent.[696]

The gospel of Luke strongly emphasizes Mary's function as the *locus* where the manifestation of the divine takes place. Here the Archangel Gabriel's annunciation to Mary of the conception and birth of Jesus becomes especially important. In Luke 1:28 the angel addresses Mary with the words: "Greetings, favored one! The Lord is with you." The beginning of this verse – which became famous in its Latin translation *Ave Maria, gratia plena* – accentuates the divine blessing that has descended on Mary. From a theological perspective, the annunciation scene correlates with the Gospel of John. Jaroslav Pelikan writes: "What the Gospel of John stated in the language of theology and of Hellenistic Philosophy when it said 'The Word [Logos] was made flesh,' the Gospel of Luke described in the language of drama and dialogue, in the form of an exchange between Mary as the chosen one of God and the angel Gabriel as the emissary of God."[697]

The word descends into a woman's womb. It is Mary giving birth to Jesus and not Joseph "procreating" him. This becomes evident when the angel tells Mary that she will conceive from the Holy Ghost: "The Holy Spirit will come upon you, and the power of the Most High will overshadow you; therefore the child to be born will be holy; he will be called Son of God."[698] The election of Mary, and therefore female fertility, as a transmitter for the incarnation of the divine spirit in Christ, forms part of the logic of a supremacy of the female over the male in matters of childbirth. In Luke 1:46–54 (later known as the *Magnificat*), Mary rejoices God's mercy, as she is certain to become the mother of Jesus:

> And Mary said, "My soul magnifies the Lord,
> and my spirit rejoices in God my Savior,
> for he has looked with favor on the lowliness of his servant.
> Surely, from now on all generations will call me blessed;
> for the Mighty One has done great things for me, and holy is his name.
> His mercy is for those who fear him from generation to generation.
> He has shown strength with his arm; he has scattered the proud in the thoughts of their hearts.
> He has brought down the powerful from their thrones, and lifted up the lowly;
> he has filled the hungry with good things, and sent the rich away empty.
> He has helped his servant Israel, in remembrance of his mercy,

696 See Delius, *Geschichte der Marienverehrung*, 60.

697 Pelikan, *Mary Through the Centuries*, 82.

698 Luke 1:35.

according to the promise he made to our ancestors,
to Abraham and to his descendants forever.[699]

Walter Delius describes the extraordinary function of Mary in the following way: "The breakthrough of the divine world into this world takes place [...] through the pregnancy of Mary."[700] Like Luke, Matthew also accentuates the extraordinary pregnancy of Mary brought about by the Holy Ghost, although his account is more sober. In Matthew 1:18 it says: "Now the birth of Jesus the Messiah took place in this way. When his mother Mary had been engaged to Joseph, but before they lived together, she was found to be with child from the Holy Spirit." In the first few centuries of the Christian era, the status of Mary depends on Christ.[701] The virgin birth helped to underline the extraordinary and divine nature of Christ, which is also recognized by Joseph: He does not touch his wife until Jesus is born.[702] By reporting this Matthew acknowledges the divine conception.[703]

Jesus' conception and birth do not only evidence a supremacy of the female in matters of childbirth, but also represent a harmony between spiritual birth and childbirth. This harmony is attached to the relationship between Jesus and Mary, which was interpreted differently throughout the centuries. The development of this relationship can be best illustrated by closely examining several titles which Mary has acquired through the course of Christian history, namely, *Theotokos,* Blessed Virgin, *Immaculata*, *Mediatrix, Corredemptrix*, *Regina Coeli* and *Sophia*. Furthermore, it will be shown that these titles partially stand for a disembodiment of Mary and the birth of Jesus.

*3.1 Mary-*Theotokos

In 431 C.E., the Council of Ephesus conferred upon Mary the title *Theotokos* ("the one giving birth to God"). Ephesus was the town that had once housed the Artemis temple, one of the miracles of the ancient world. Mary

699 See Delius, *Geschichte der Marienverehrung*, 24 for this interpretation.

700 Ibid., 18: "Der Einbruch der göttlichen Welt in diese Welt geschieht [...] in der Schwangerschaft der Maria."

701 See ibid., 23.

702 Matthew 1: 25.

703 See Delius, *Geschichte der Marienverehrung*, 20.

replaced Artemis-Eileithyia with whom Isis had been so strongly identified.

According to Delius, a first move toward the idea of Mary-*Theotokos* can be seen in the encounter between Elisabeth and Mary[704] as described in Luke 1:43. Here Elisabeth says: "And why has this happened to me, that the mother of my Lord comes to me?" However, this text alone surely could not have led to the proclamation of the *theotokos* title. It has to be kept in mind that the fifth century after Christ is a period of consolidated Christian faith. Therefore, it became possible to re-adopt elements of the ancient goddess cults, namely of Isis and Artemis, without fearing conversions. Additionally, drawing upon the ancient religion could have served as a means to facilitate the spread of Christianity itself.[705] As has been shown in the last section, both Isis and Artemis were goddesses strongly related to childbirth. Isis is actually the paradigm for Mary-*Theotokos* and even the title itself was originally used for Isis.[706]

The question to be pursued here though, is what changed and what remained stable in the Isis to Mary-*Theotokos* transformation? In the following, it will be shown that the unity of childbirth and spiritual birth in Isis continues to be perpetuated in Mary. However, as will be illustrated, this unity, or harmony, comes in a rather different guise.

One of the initial differences between Isis and Mary *Theotokos* lies in the fact that Isis is a goddess representing both childbirth and spiritual birth, whereas Mary is a human being and comes in contact with the divine through the mercy (*gratia*) that God bestows upon her. This means that Mary's status as *Theotokos* depends on the status of her son. To the extent that Jesus is believed to be the divine spirit incarnate, Mary is believed to have birthed a god. In this sense, Elisabeth in Luke 1:42 tells her: "Blessed are you among women, and blessed is the fruit of your womb."

The unity of childbirth and spiritual birth in Mary is on the one hand constituted by her divine election, and on the other, her faith. She chooses to answer the angel in the annunciation scene: "Here am I, the servant of the Lord; let it be with me according to your word."[707] Mary's faith, and therefore her spiritual birth as related to the conception of, pregnancy with, and birthgiving to Jesus, is furthermore expressed in two passages

704 See ibid., 26.

705 See ibid., 33–34.

706 See Mathews and Muller, *Isis and Mary,* 4.

707 Luke 1: 38.

of Luke. After the birth of Jesus, the shepherds to whom the angel of God has appeared visit Mary. Here it says: "But Mary treasured all these words, and pondered them in her heart."[708] In a similar way, Luke 2:51 alludes to the spiritual transformation Mary has undergone because of Jesus. Here it says of Mary, and not of Joseph, that she "treasured all these things in her heart." Augustine alludes to Mary's spiritual birth through the birth of Jesus writing that Mary was conceiving Christ in her mind before she did so in her womb.[709] And even during the Reformation, Mary's spiritual birth in Christ was acknowledged; Calvin writes that Mary was spiritually regenerated through her son with whom she had been pregnant.[710]

The idea of *Theotokos* was not a static concept in the history of Christianity.[711] Two theological tendencies can be identified here. Already at the time of the Council of Ephesus, opponents of the proclamation of the *Theotokos* title pointed out the "danger" that Mary could acquire divine status if this title was conferred upon her. This objection was made by Nestorius, patriarch of Constantinople. According to Jaroslav Pelikan, this line of argument runs as follows: "Mary should be called not Theotokos, which gave the blasphemous impression that she had given birth to the divine nature itself and which therefore sounded like the title of the mother deities of paganism."[712] However, at the Council of Ephesus, this position was anathematized. Indeed, what Nestorius feared actually became symbolic practice in Christian history: by officially bestowing the title of *Theotokos* on Mary, a step was taken towards the divinization of Mary.

However, the controversy over the status of Mary in Christianity was not ended by the Council of Ephesus. Quite the contrary, it continued to occupy the minds of theologians. For example, Thomas Aquinas discusses the *Theotokos* title in the *Summa Theologica*, formulating the question "Whether the Blessed Virgin should be called the Mother of

---

708 Luke 2: 19.

709 Augustine, *Sermons for Christmas*, 130 (Sermon 196.1): "The angel announces; the virgin hears, believes, and conceives. She has faith in her soul, and Christ dwells in her womb."

710 Calvin, quoted in Delius, *Geschichte der Marienverehrung*, 233: "Maria spiritualiter regenita in filio quem utero gestabat."

711 See for the following Pelikan, *Mary Through the Centuries*, 56–60.

712 Ibid., 56.

God?" He recalls the Nestorian position and then dismisses it with Cyril of Alexandria's argumentation.[713]

Contentions about the title *theotokos* also accompanied the rise of Protestantism, dethroning Mary who, in the course of the centuries, had acquired the title and position, "Queen of Heaven" (*Regina Caeli*).[714] Under the influence of Zwingli, the theological war against the *Regina Caeli* – who was supposed to become the simple "Handmaid of the Lord" again – even assumed civic dimensions. In 1529, a law was passed in Bern punishing any citizen carrying a rosary by making them pay ten *gulden*.[715]

However, here the focus will be on the development of the *Theotokos* tradition rather than on its contestation. What is continuous and what has changed in the harmony between spiritual birth and childbirth as expressed first through Isis and then through Mary?

It seems that the divinization of Mary goes hand in hand with a particular construction of her body, that is a disembodiment, totally absent from the myth of Isis (it suffices to remember the conception/procreation of Horus here). The disembodiment of Mary, and one has to add, the millennia-lasting, theological disputes over the degree to which she should be considered to be disembodied, touch upon Mary-*Theotokos* in different ways. In the tradition of the praise and worship of Mary, several aspects of birthgiving undergo a process of disembodiment. Mary gives birth as the perpetual virgin and she does not feel labour pain.

To a certain extent, Mary's disembodiment with regard to childbirth parallels Aristotle's disembodying construction of procreation. As has been shown,[716] Aristotle divided male semen into a physical part and a

---

713 Thomas Aquinas, *Summa Theologica*, Pt. III, Q. 35 Art. 4: *But Cyril, in a letter against Nestorius … answers it thus:* Just as when a man's soul is born with its body, they are considered as one being: and if anyone wish to say that the mother of the flesh is not the mother of the soul, he says too much. Something like this may be perceived in the generation of Christ. For the Word of God was born of the substance of God the Father: but because he took flesh, we must of necessity confess that in the flesh He was born of a woman. *Consequently we must say that the blessed virgin is called the Mother of God, not as though she were the mother of the Godhead, but because she is the mother, according to His human nature, of the Person who has both the divine and the human nature.*

714 However, there also were protestant thinkers such as Feuerbach, P. de Lagarde and Kierkegaard who functioned as advocates for the Mary cult in the protestant church. See Delius, *Geschichte der Marienverehrung*, 202–203.

715 See ibid., 230.

716 See section III.1.7.

part to which the divine *pneuma* was attached. Thus, Aristotle makes male procreation approach the divine by partially disembodying male semen. In Aristotle's *De Generatione Animalium*, male procreation was disembodied to be spiritualized,[717] whereas in the case of Mary and the Virgin Birth without labour pain, giving birth becomes disembodied to approach the divine. May be, in both cases axial age culture – which opens up a chasm between the mundane and the transmundane – is at work. Perhaps it is this chasm which cuts through Aristotle's male procreating body and through Mary's birthgiving body.

The birth of Jesus is an important example for a harmony between spiritual birth and childbirth because it entails the spiritual rebirth of Mary, the spiritual birth of mankind and the connection of childbirth to the divine sphere. Given the fact that Mary's disembodiment is intrinsically linked to the harmony between spiritual birth and childbirth she stands for, in the following chapter special attention will be given to the Virgin Birth without labour pain.

3.2 Mary's Disembodiment and the Painless Virgin Birth

There is a long tradition of the assumption that Mary gave birth to Jesus without pain. Often contrasted to the absence of labour pain during the miraculous birth in Bethlehem, is the Genesis curse inflicting pain upon Eve during childbirth. Thus we get the contrasting pair of Eve the sinner and Mary the redeemer.[718]

One of the earliest texts referring to Mary giving birth without pain is the second part of the apocryphal text *Ascension of Isaiah* (*Ascensio Jesajae*), which describes a heavenly journey of the biblical prophet during which he has a vision of the birth of Jesus.[719] In the *Ascension of Isaiah* the story of the birth of Jesus is told as follows:

---

717 In this sense, Aristotle's *De Generatione Animalium* is not only an example for "The Supremacy of the Male" (see section III.1.7.) but also could have been used as an example for the symbolic pattern "Harmony between Spiritual Birth and Childbirth."

718 For the iconography of Eve and Mary see Ernst Guldan, *Eva und Maria: Eine Antithese als Bildmotiv* (Graz: Böhlau, 1966).

719 C. Detlef G. Müller tentatively dates the origins of this part of *The Ascension of Isaiah* tentatively back to the second century. See C. Detlef G. Müller, introduction to *The Ascension of Isaiah*, in *Writings Relating to the Apostles: Apocalypses and Related Subjects,* revised edition, vol. 2 of *New Testament Apocrypha*, ed. Wilhelm

4. But the angel of the Spirit *appeared* in this world, and after that Joseph did not put Mary away, but kept her; but he did not reveal the matter to anyone. 5. And he did not approach Mary, but kept her as a holy virgin, although she was with child. 6. And he did not [yet] live with her for two months. 7. And after two months, when Joseph was in his house, and his wife Mary, but both alone, 8. it came to pass, while they were alone, that Mary straight away beheld with her eyes and saw a small child, and she was amazed. 9. And when her amazement wore off, her womb was found as it was before she was with child. 10. And when her husband Joseph said to her, "What made thee amazed?" his eyes were opened and he saw the child and praised God, that the Lord had come to his portion. 11. And a voice came to them: "Tell this vision to no one." 12. And the report concerning the child was noised abroad in Bethlehem. 13. Some said, "The virgin Mary has given birth before she was married two months," 14. and many said, "She has not given birth: the midwife has not gone up [to her] and we have heard no cries of pain."[720]

The idea of Mary giving birth without pain has come down through Christian history.[721] Just to give a few examples, Ambrosius refers to the painless birth.[722] In the twelfth century Walter de Mortagne explains the absence of labour pain during the birth of Christ as follows: Labour pain is correlated to lust during conception. As Mary conceived Jesus without lust and without male semen, she gave birth without pain.[723] Thomas Aquinas formulates the question "Whether Christ was born without his mother suffering?" in the *Summa Theologica* and adopts the same reasoning as Mortagne based on Augustine:

The pains of childbirth in the woman follow from the mingling of the sexes. Wherefore (Gen. iii. 16) after the words, in sorrow shalt thou bring forth children, *the following are added:* and thou shalt be under thy husband's power. *But, as Augustine says [...], from this sentence we must exclude the Virgin Mother of God; who,* because she conceived Christ without the defilement of sin, and without the stain of sexual mingling,

Schneemelcher, English translation ed. R. McL. Wilson (Cambridge: James Clarke & Co, 1992), 604.

720 *The Ascension of Isaiah*, ed. and trans. C. Detlef G. Müller, in *Writings Relating to the Apostles: Apocalypses and Related Subjects,* revised edition, vol. 2 of *New Testament Apocrypha*, ed. Wilhelm Schneemelcher, English translation ed. R. McL. Wilson (Cambridge: James Clarke & Co, 1992), 618 (*The Ascension of Isaiah* 11.4–14).

721 See for the following Delius, *Geschichte der Marienverehrung*, 133–179.

722 See Delius, *Geschichte der Marienverehrung*, 133–134.

723 Walter de Mortagne, quoted in Delius, *Geschichte der Marienverehrung*, 179.

> therefore did she bring Him forth without pain, without violation of her virginal identity, without detriment to the purity of her maidenhood.[724]

Aquinas argues further for the absence of pain during the miraculous birth at Bethlehem. He writes:

> The pains of childbirth are caused by the infant opening the passage from the womb. Now it has been said above [...], that Christ came forth from the closed womb of His Mother, and, consequently, without opening the passage. Consequently, there was no pain in that birth, as neither was there any corruption.[725]

Also Luther – despite all the changes he introduced in relation to the figure of Mary – describes the absence of labour pain when Mary gave birth to Jesus.[726] The disembodiment of Mary by depicting her giving birth without pain immediately leads into another dominant configuration around the *Theotokos*: the painless birth cannot be detached from the virgin birth.

The earliest text that refers to Mary's virginity is the annunciation scene in Luke 1:34. Here Mary asks the angel: "How can this be, since I am a virgin?" However, the widespread idea that Mary was not only a virgin before and during conception, but also during and after childbirth,[727] mainly derives from a different source, namely, the apocryphal *Protevangelium of James*, probably dating back to the second century CE.[728] The *Protevangelium of James* belongs to the category of apocryphal infancy gospels, which initiated a theological shift. The infancy gospels changed the focus from the death and resurrection of Jesus that was prevalent in the earliest period of Christianity, to his birth and childhood.[729] The *Protevangelium of James* exercised a lot of influence on future Mariology because it works more as a glorification of Mary and her perpetual virginity than an account of the life of Jesus.[730]

---

724 Thomas Aquinas, *Summa Theologica*, Pt. III, Q. 35 Art. 6 ad 1.

725 Ibid.

726 Luther, quoted in Delius, *Geschichte der Marienverehrung*, 208.

727 *Virginitas ante partum, in partu et post partum.*

728 See Cullmann, *The Protevangelium of James*, 423.

729 See Oscar Cullmann, *Infancy Gospels,* in *Gospels and Related Writings, revised edition,* vol. 1 of *New Testament Apocrypha*, ed. Wilhelm Schneemelcher, English translation ed. R. McL. Wilson (Cambridge: James Clarke & Co, 1991), 414.

730 Cullmann, *The Protevangelium of James*, 423. Cullmann maintains that in antiquity, the Middle Ages and the Renaissance the infancy gospels exercised more influence on literature and art than the Bible itself. See Cullmann, *Infancy Gospels*, 418.

The *Protevangelium of James* starts with the miraculous conception and birth of Mary herself. Her parents, Anna and Joachim, are childless. Joachim fasts for forty days and nights in the wilderness[731] and Anna prays to obtain the divine blessing of a child.[732] Far from being sheer physical acts, conception and childbirth are depicted as moments where the human and the divine meet. Childbirth is seen as both an expression of divine mercy and a human way to please God. In the *Protevangelium of James* this twofold meaning of childbirth is most beautifully put into words in Anna's lament. At the sight of a sparrows' nest in a laurel tree, Anna moans her infertility because it deprives her of close contact with the divine:

> Woe to me, who begot me,
> What womb brought me forth?
> For I was born a curse [before them all and] before the children of Israel,
> And I was reproached, and they mocked me and thrust me out of the Temple of the Lord.
> 2. Woe is me, to what am I likened?
> I am not likened to the birds of the heaven;
> for even the birds of the heaven are fruitful before thee, O Lord.
> Woe is me, to what am I likened?
> I am not likened to the unreasoning animals;
> for even the unreasoning animals are fruitful before thee, O Lord.
> Woe is me, to what am I likened?
> I am not likened to the beasts of the earth;
> for even the beasts of the earth are fruitful before thee, O Lord.
> 3. Woe is me, to what am I likened?
> I am not likened to these waters;
> for even these waters gush forth merrily, and their fish praise thee, O Lord.
> Woe is me, to what am I likened?
> I am not likened to this earth;
> for even this earth brings forth its fruit in its season and praises thee, O Lord.[733]

The lament of Anna links up with biblical approaches to childbirth which harmonize the embodiment of childbirth/procreation and the relationship to the divine: childbirth and procreation do not have to be disembodied in order to be spiritual events.[734] However, the narrative *of the Protevangelium*

731 See *The Protevangelium of James,* 426.

732 Ibid., 427: "O God of our fathers, bless me and hear my prayer, as though didst bless the womb of Sarah [our mother Sarah] and gavest her a son, Isaac."

733 Ibid.

734 See for example Phyllis Trible's study *God and the Rethoric of Sexuality* where she comes to the conclusion that "in the Hebrew scriptures the wombs of women belong

of James starts to move towards a different logic as it comes to the telling of Mary's childhood. Mary, the future mother of Jesus, is symbolically disembodied. When she is six months old, her mother Anna makes "a sanctuary in her bed-chamber, and [...] [does] not permit anything common or unclean to pass through it,"[735] so that she should not touch the ground before she is taken to God's temple where she is supposed to grow up as a virgin. At the age of three she is fed by the hand of an angel in the temple.[736] When she is twelve years old, the high priest marries her to Joseph who is chosen as her husband because of divine signs.[737] However, Joseph respects her virginity. This is elucidated in a scene before the birth of Jesus in a cave in Bethlehem. Referring to Mary's virginity during pregnancy Joseph tells a midwife he wants to bring to the cave: "She is Mary, who was brought up in the temple of the Lord, and I received her by lot as my wife. And (yet) she is not my wife, but she has conceived of the Holy Spirit."[738]

Finally, Mary's virginity after birth is confirmed by the mid-wife's friend Salome who does not want to believe in the virgin birth before she has tested it: "And Salome put (forward) her finger to test her condition. And she cried out, saying: ["Woe for my wickedness and my unbelief; for]" I have tempted the living God; and behold, my hand falls away from me, consumed by fire!"[739]

In the history of Christianity Mary's perpetual virginity became one of her most important characteristics. Her virginity was also expressed by the idea that she gave birth *utero clauso,* that is, with a closed uterus. Already Augustine refers to the perpetual virginity of Mary, when he writes in one of his sermons for Christmas: "A virgin who conceives, a virgin who gives birth; a virgin with Child, a virgin delivered of Child – a virgin ever virgin."[740] To give more of the innumerable examples referring to Mary as the (perpetual) virgin, one could mention Tertullian, seeing Mary as

to God." Trible, *God and the Rethoric*, 36. See also section III.1.9.3. "Reflections on Male Divinities Intervening into Womens' Wombs" of this work.

735 *The Protevangelium of James*, 428 (6.4.).

736 See ibid., 429 (8.1.).

737 See ibid., 429–430 (9.1.).

738 Ibid., 434 (19.1.).

739 Ibid., 434, (20.1.).

740 Augustine, *Sermons for Christmas,* 71 (Sermon 186.1). See for other references to the perpetual virginity in Augustine's Sermons for Christmas ibid. 94 (Sermon 188.4), 103 (Sermon 190.2) and 127 (Sermon 195.2).

having fulfilled the prophecy of Isaiah 7:14 that it will be a divine sign when "a virgin shall conceive and bear a son."[741] Hippolytus writes that the word ["verbum"] "leapt from the sky into the womb of a virgin; it leapt out of the holy belly upon the tree. It leapt from the tree into the underworld, it leapt again from there in this human flesh to the earth."[742] Epiphanius defends the perpetual virginity of Mary[743] as does Ambrosius,[744] Gregory of Nyssa,[745] Walter de Mortagne,[746] Pope Xystus III.,[747] Gregor Strigenicius,[748] Bernard de Clairvaux,[749] Martin Luther,[750] and many others.

As has been shown above, in the Christian tradition Mary is depicted as the virginal *Theotokos*. By way of being disembodied as the perpetual virgin she approaches the divine. This is not dissimilar to the Aristotelian idea of man approaching the divine by way of his semen containing the heavenly *pneuma*. In both cases "disembodiment" of procreational activities is connected to coming close to the divine. In the following, Mary's disembodiment will be explored further with regard to the Immaculate Conception.

3.3 Immaculate Conception

Mary's symbolic disembodiment which links spiritual birth and childbirth, is not only brought about by childbirth being painless and virginal but also by the idea that Mary herself had been conceived without original sin.

Through the thinking of Tertullian and St. Ambrose of Milan early Christian theology established the idea that the propagation of original sin was by sexual intercourse and precisely by male semen as the carrier of

---

741 Tertullian, *De Carne Christi*, 17, quoted in Delius, *Geschichte der Marienverehrung*, 66.

742 Hippolytus, *On the Song of Songs*, 21.2, quoted and trans. in Mark W. Elliott, *The Song of Songs and Christology in the Early Church 381–451* (Tübingen: Mohr Siebeck, 2000), 76.

743 See Delius, *Geschichte der Marienverehrung*, 98.

744 See ibid., 132.

745 See ibid., 95.

746 See ibid., 179.

747 See ibid., 432–440.

748 See ibid., 226.

749 See ibid., 293.

750 See ibid., 208.

original sin–an idea that has been previously explored in the section on the "dubious" supremacy of the male in matters of childbirth.[751] It was probably Ambrose of Milan who linked the sinlessness of Christ to the absence of original sin in Christ and to the virginal conception.[752] In this logic, the virginal conception frees Jesus from sin because he was conceived without male semen which was supposed to transmit original sin.

Going a step further, Augustine considers the possibility that Mary, as the future mother of Jesus, was also granted the mercy to have been conceived without original sin. The following passage from Augustine's *On Nature and Grace* is generally seen as the first text moving in the direction of Mary's Immaculate Conception. Augustine begins by stating that even saints cannot be considered as without sin. In this context he writes:

> I make an exception of the Blessed Virgin Mary, in whose case, out of respect for the Lord, I wish to raise no question at all when the discussion concerns sins-for whence do we know what an abundance of grace for entirely overcoming sin was conferred on her who had the merit to conceive and bear him who undoubtedly was without sin?[753]

From medieval times onward, these lines were often "cited as a proof-text to establish that Augustine taught the doctrine of the immaculate conception of Mary."[754] However, as Gerald Bonner points out, "it is not so much that he [Augustine] declares her personal sinlessness, as that he absolutely refuses to discuss the matter *propter honorem domini*, for the honour of the Lord."[755] In the same vein, Jaroslav Pelikan comments: "But Augustine did not explain this great exception, leaving it to the doctrinal development of the West over the next fourteen centuries to clarify it."[756]

Here it will suffice to outline a few stages in the history of the Immaculate Conception until its dogmatization in 1854. In the ninth century, the *Cogitis me* ("You compel me"), a work attributed to Paschasius Radbertus,

751 See section III.1.10.

752 See Pelikan, *Mary Through the Centuries*, 190.

753 Augustine, *On Nature and Grace*, 41: "Excepta itaque sancta virgine Maria, de qua propter honorem domini nullam prorsus, cum de peccati agitur, haberi volo quaestionem – unde enim scimus quid ei plus gratiae conlatum fuerit ad vincendum omni ex parte peccatum, quae concipere ac parere meruit, quem constat nullum habuisse peccatum?"

754 William J. Collinge, in Augustine, *On Nature and Grace*, note 142.

755 Gerald Bonner, *St. Augustine of Hippo: Life and Controversies* (Philadelphia: Westminster, 1963), 328.

756 Pelikan, *Mary Through the Centuries*, 191.

a Benedictine monk at Corbie, raises the question of whether it would not be appropriate to commemorate the nativity of Mary with a feast. This leads to another question, namely, that of the circumstances of Mary's conception, which the author leaves open.[757] In Lyon, in 1139 the canonics of St. Etienne et St. Jean le Baptiste introduced the feast of the Immaculate Conception.

The scholastics were divided into two parties with regard to the Immaculate Conception. Thomas Aquinas supported Augustine's theory of original sin but made no exceptions for Mary: "Because the Blessed Virgin was conceived in original sin, she was in Abraham as needing to be healed. Therefore she paid tithes in him, as descending from him according to seminal virtue."[758]

In contrast to Aquinas, Duns Scotus held very different views on Mary. Deviating from the Aristotelian idea of the supremacy of the male over the female in matters of childbirth (which Aquinas also adopted),[759] Scotus imagines Mary actively participating in the formation of Christ. He asserts that the mother, drawing from the force pertaining to organic life, may, perhaps, form the child to a higher degree than the father, whose contribution is limited to procreation.[760] Though Duns Scotus accepted the Scholastic creationist idea that the soul is created by God and becomes contaminated by its union with the body, he wondered whether God might have created Mary without sin.[761] For Scotus, Mary "was immaculately conceived because what nature had not given to her, the special grace of God had accomplished in her."[762] These different positions of Scotists and Thomists mark Scholasticism.[763] The contentions about the Immaculate Conception, like the already mentioned contentions about the Marian title *theotokos*, could be interpreted as a disagreement over the degree to which Mary should have been able to approach the divine. In case of the Immaculate Conception the degree to which there was advocacy for her disembodiment may be read as the degree to which she was seen to approach the divine.

757 See ibid., 192.

758 Thomas Aquinas, *Summa Theologica*, Pt. III Q 31, 6 ad 2.

759 See sections III.1.7 and III.1.10 of this work.

760 See Delius, *Geschichte der Marienverehrung*, 184.

761 See ibid., 185.

762 Pelikan, *Mary Through the Centuries*, 197.

763 See Delius, *Geschichte der Marienverehrung*, 240.

At the end of the 14th century the university of Paris adopted Duns Scotus' view on the Immaculate Conception.[764] Nevertheless, the Immaculate Conception has been one of the most widely discussed theological questions since the 14th century.[765] While theologians were debating over the issue, artists started to develop an iconography of the immaculately conceived Mary, thus paving the way for the acceptance of the idea of the Immaculate Conception.[766]

In following the debates on the Immaculately Conceived through the history of the church, the importance of the Council of Basel in 1439 has to be underlined. Here it was declared that the Immaculate Conception was "a pious doctrine, in conformity with the worship of the Church, the catholic faith, right reason, and Holy Scripture." It also prescribed that the doctrine "be approved, held, and professed by all Catholics."[767] However, because of general political conflicts with the Pope, the Council was not entitled to the designation as "ecumenical council."[768] Therefore, the question of the Immaculate Conception still remained open. Nevertheless, "by the end of 15th century [...] the doctrine [of the immaculate conception] had become generally accepted in Western Christendom, believed by the faithful and taught by the doctors of the church."[769]

In the 16th century the contentions about the immaculate conception became part of the theological conflicts during the reformation. The Immaculate Conception was again officially dealt with at the Council of Trent (1545–1563).[770] Here, in the context of pronouncements on the matter of original sin, Mary – as in Augustine's writings – was described as the great exception: she was excluded from the universality of original sin.[771] There are two more important dates in the history of the Immaculate Conception which have to be mentioned here. In the bull of May 24th 1622, public polemics against the Immaculate Conception were prohibited and on December 8th 1661, Pope Alexander VII formulated as a pious

764 See ibid., 180.

765 See ibid., 184.

766 See Mirella Levi D'Ancona: The Iconography of the Immaculate Conception in the Middle Ages and Early Renaissance, New York: College Art Association, 1957, quoted by Pelikan, *Mary Through the Centuries*, 255.

767 Quoted in Pelikan, *Mary Through the Centuries*, 198.

768 See ibid.

769 Ibid.

770 See Delius, *Geschichte der Marienverehrung*, 236.

771 See Pelikan, *Mary Through the Centuries*, 199.

opinion of the church, that Mary's soul had been bestowed upon her during her conception: Mary was freed from original sin thanks to God's special mercy.[772] Finally, with the *Ineffabilis Deus* bull issued by Pope Pius IX on December 8th 1854, the Immaculate Conception became the official doctrine of the Catholic Church. Here it says:

> The doctrine which holds that the Most Blessed Virgin Mary was preserved from all stain of original sin in the first instant of conception, by a singular grace and privilege of Almighty God, in consideration of the merits of Jesus Christ, savior of the human race, has been revealed by God and must, therefore, firmly and constantly be believed by all the faithful.[773]

The doctrine of the Immaculate Conception was opposed both by Eastern Orthodoxy and Western Protestantism holding the position that Mary should be honoured as the mother of the Redeemer,[774] but should not be raised to the status the bull assigns to her.

Linking up with the painless, virginal birth, the Immaculate Conception is one step further in the disembodiment of Mary and thereby in making her approach the divine.

3.4 Mediatrix – Corredemptrix – Regina Caeli

As the disembodied, immaculately conceived, perpetual virgin, giving birth to Christ, Mary sets out to conquer Heaven. Here she becomes the *Mediatrix*, the "mediator" between this world and the divine realm, and the *Corredemptrix*, the "co-redeemer" – a title placing her nearly on the same level as Christ. Here, she becomes the *Regina Caeli*, the Queen of Heaven, a title she shares with Isis but also with the Ancient Oriental goddess Inanna-Ishtar.[775]

From a theological perspective, the three titles *Mediatrix, Corredemptrix* and *Regina Caeli* are linked in the following way: Through her motherhood Mary obtains the status of the Mediator, the Co-Redeemer and the

772 See Delius, *Geschichte der Marienverehrung*, 248.

773 Bull *Ineffabilis Deus*, quoted by Pelikan, *Mary Through the Centuries*, 199.

774 See ibid.

775 See Othmar Keel, *Gott weiblich: Eine verborgene Seite des biblischen Gottes* (Gütersloh: Gütersloher Verlagshaus, 2008), 48.

Queen of Heaven.[776] As the mother of the "king" she becomes the queen. Ultimately then, all of these three titles which are linked to Mary's presence in Heaven, derive from her being the *Theotokos*, the woman giving birth to God. Mary's "admission into Heaven" which is expressed in the titles Mediator, Co-Redeemer and Queen of Heaven mainly depends on two traditions. These are Mary's identification with the biblical "woman clothed with the sun"[777] in the 12th book of Revelation and the apocryphal literature on Mary's assumption. In Revelation 12.1–5 it says:

> Now a great sign appeared in heaven: a woman clothed with the sun, with the moon under her feet, and on her head a garland of twelve stars.
>
> 2. Then being with child, she cried out in labor and in pain to give birth.
>
> 3. And another sign appeared in heaven: behold, a great, fiery red dragon having seven heads and ten horns, and seven diadems on his heads.
>
> 4. His tail drew a third of the stars of heaven and threw them to the earth. And the dragon stood before the woman who was ready to give birth, to devour her Child as soon as it was born.
>
> 5. She bore a male Child who was to rule all nations with a rod of iron. And her Child was caught up to God and His throne.

Throughout the centuries the "woman clothed with the sun" and her child have been identified with Mary and Jesus, notwithstanding the fact that the woman in Revelation 12 suffers labour pain. Epiphanius, Quodvultdeus (a disciple of Augustine) and Oecumenius (d. 550) are the first to apply the apocalyptic vision to Mary. However, as Warner puts it, "patristic testimonies later accumulate, and when Pius XII defined the dogma of the Assumption, he quoted a long tradition in support."[778]

---

776 See Delius, *Geschichte der Marienverehrung*, 297.

777 Revelation 12:1.

778 Warner, *Alone of All*, 94. It is interesting to note that modern theology still clings to the identification of Mary with the woman clothed with the sun. For example, Pierre Prigent sees the woman clothed with the sun as a personification of the people of God. However, he still integrates Mary in his interpretation: "Lorsque Dieu a voulu commencer l'histoire extraordinaire de l'Incarnation, il s'est adressé, par la bouche de son ange, à l'une de ses créatures. Et c'est pour lui demander: voici ce que je veux faire, à travers toi. Est-ce que tu veux bien? Si elle dit non, rien ne se fera. Si elle dit oui… «Qu'il me soit fait selon la volonté de Dieu», répond Marie. Par elle, pour la

The second way of explaining Mary's access to heaven is her assumption. From about the fourth century onwards, apocryphal literature describes Mary's death and ascension into heaven which came to be known under different names: assumption, dormition, falling asleep, passing away, transitus or obsequies.[779] There are many sources in different languages on the assumption. Greek, Latin, Coptic, Syriac, Ethiopic and Arabic manuscripts testify to it.

In the following, the focus will be on a few samples published by J. K. Elliott in his collection of apocryphal Christian literature. Included are the Coptic texts, *The Homily Attributed to Evodius, Archbishop of Rome, The Twentieth Discourse of Cyril of Jerusalem, The Discourse of Theodosius, Archbishop of Alexandria, Sahidic Fragment (Revillout no. 16)*, the Greek text *The Discourse of St John the Divine Concerning the Falling Asleep of the Holy Mother of God*, the Latin texts *The Narrative of Pseudo-Melito* and *The Narrative by Joseph of Arimathaea* and *The Syriac Narratives.*[780] What all these texts have in common is that Mary enters heaven only with Christ's intervention. In several texts,[781] as in the following passage from the *Discourse of Theodosius*, the son comes in all his royal splendour to assist his mother with her transition from life to death and from death to heaven: "There were thunderings and lightnings. Jesus came on a chariot of light with Moses, David, the prophets, and the righteous kings, and adressed Mary […] 'O my beloved Mother, arise, let us go hence.'"[782]

In several transitus-legends the assumption takes place in two steps. After Mary has died she is surrounded by the apostles, who have been miraculously transported to Bethlehem (or Jerusalem) from all over the

première fois dans notre monde, un homme, qui est une femme, fait cette démarche qui fait advenir l'Évangile parmi nous. La femme d'Ap 12 est bien le peuple de Dieu. Mais il faut reconnaître que la première réalité de ce peuple nouveau, c'est Marie qui l'incarne. Rien de plus. Mais rien de moins non plus!" (Pierre Prigent, *L'apocalypse* (Paris: Les Éditions du Cerf, 1998), 129).

779 See J. K. Elliott, *The Apocryphal New Testament: A Collection of Apocryphal Christian Literature in an English Translation Based on M.R. James* (Oxford: Clarendon Press, 1993), 691.

780 See ibid., 691–723.

781 See ibid., *The Homily attributed to Evodius*, *The Sahidic Fragment*, *The Discourse of St John the Divine Concerning the Falling Asleep of the Holy Mother of God*, *The Narrative of Pseudo-Melito*, *The Narrative by Joseph of Arimathaea* and *The Syriac Narratives*.

782 Ibid., 699.

world by clouds, or are even raised from the dead for the occasion.[783] Then Jesus comes to collect his mother's soul. In *The Narrative of Pseudo-Melito* he says: "Come you most precious pearl, enter into the receptacle of eternal life."[784] The apostles see "her soul, and it was of such whiteness that no tongue of mortal men can worthily express it, for it excelled all whiteness of snow and of all metal and silver that shines with great brightness of light."[785]

In several texts on the assumption there is an interval of time between the assumption of Mary's soul and the second part of the ascension of the Blessed Virgin, namely the assumption of her body. The apostles usually bury her after her soul has ascended to heaven and then Jesus returns after some time to take her body as well.[786] *The Discourse of Theodosius, Archbishop of Alexandria* has an impressive description of the reunification of Mary's soul and body:

> He [Jesus] called over the coffin and bade the body arise. …
> The coffin, which had been shut like Noah's ark, opened. The body arose and embraced its own soul, just as two brothers who have come from a strange country, and they were united one with another.[787]

Mary's assumption is firmly rooted in the fact that she has given birth to Jesus. As a result of this she sometimes acquires the traits of the saviour of the world. In *The Discourse of St John the Divine Concerning the Falling Asleep of the Holy Mother of God* the apostles implore Mary on her deathbed: "O mother of the Lord, leave to the world a blessing, for you depart out of it; for you blessed it and raised it up from destruction when you bore the light of the world!"[788]

Mary is the *Theotokos*, the one who has given birth to God. However, in order for this special childbirth to be spiritualized Mary has to be

783 See ibid. 692–723: *The Discourse of St John the Divine Concerning the Falling Asleep of the Holy Mother of God, The Narrative by Joseph of Arimathaea* and the *Syriac Narratives*.

784 Ibid., 711.

785 Ibid.

786 See ibid., 700 (*The Discourse of Theodosius, Archbishop of Alexandria* VIII), 707–708 (*The Discourse of St John the Divine Concerning the Falling Asleep of the Holy Mother of God*, 44, 48), 715 (*The Narrative by Joseph of Arimathaea*, 11, 17).

787 Ibid., 700 (*The Discourse of Theodosius, Archbishop of Alexandria*, VIII–IX).

788 Ibid., 706 (*The Discourse of St John the Divine Concerning the Falling Asleep of the Holy Mother of God,* 41).

disembodied. She becomes the immaculately conceived, perpetual virgin. This is expressed symbolically by the whiteness of her soul or the metaphor of the pearl. Thus the texts unanimously link the assumption and Mary's disembodiment. In this perhaps *The Narrative of Pseudo-Melito* is the most explicit text. Here it says that Jesus tells his mother: "Rise up, my love and my kinswoman: you who did not suffer corruption by union of the flesh shall not suffer dissolution of the body in the sepulchre."[789]

In 591 Emperor Maurice made August 15th the feast of the assumption of Virgin Mary[790] and the feast spread to the Western Church 50 years later.[791] However, it took another 1359 years before the assumption of Mary was dogmatized in the *Constitutio Apostolica Munificentissimus Deus* in 1950. In this dogma, Mary's assumption is closely linked to the fact that she is the Immaculately Conceived Virgin and the mother of God.[792]

---

789 Ibid., 714 (*The Narrative of Pseudo-Melito*, XVII). A poetic expression of the symbolic link between the assumption and the immaculately conceived virgin giving birth can be found in a Georgian liturgical hymn (11th–12th century), where the disembodiment of Mary becomes the condition for being able to give birth to the saviour and thereby to the whole world:

12. Ouvrez joyeusement vos portes, princes du ciel
et recevez la mère et la porteuse
du créateur, l'immaculée
reine de tous.

13. Le Prince du monde ne peut approcher
ton âme. ô immaculée génitrice de Dieu!
et les esprits des air s'écartent
de toi dans la crainte, ô sainte!

14. L'arche d'alliance est portée non plus selon
l'ordre de la Loi mais par la grâce
et les apôtres conduisent avec des cantiques
la mère de Dieu à la tombe.

15. La colombe toute immaculée s'est endormie
dans un repos divin, la bienheureuse
génitrice de Dieu sans mariage,
celle qui a délivré tout le monde.

(Michel van Esbroeck, *Aux origines de la Dormition de la Vierge: Études historiques sur les traditions orientales* (Aldershot: Variorum, 1995), XIV, 11).

790 See ibid., XIV, 4.

791 See Warner, *Alone of All*, 81.

792 See *Constitutio Apostolica Munificentissimus Deus*, 1950, quoted in Delius, *Geschichte der Marienverehrung*, 274–275.

Four years after the proclamation of the assumption dogma, Mary's position was officially further confirmed by the introduction of the feast, Queenship of Mary, which Pope Pius XII announced on the morning of November 1st, 1954. The theological foundations of this feast, which would first be celebrated on May 31, 1956,[793] were laid out in the encyclical "Ad Caeli Reginam" in 1954. Emphasised already in the first passage of the encyclical is that Mary's queenship derives from her motherhood: "Mary, the Virgin Mother of God, reigns with a mother's solicitude over the entire world."[794]

Thus by 1954 Mary was both officially admitted into heaven as the immaculately conceived virgin and celebrated as Queen, the *Regina Caeli* –one of the many titles that she had already unofficially shared with Isis for roughly a millennium and a half.[795] Although the Blessed Virgin Mary officially ascended into heaven as Queen (*Regina*), as late as the twentieth century, beforehand she was already governing from her throne without any dogma. Mary's roles in heaven had mainly been the *Mediatrix* ("the mediator") and the *Corredemptrix* ("the co-redeemer"). As has already been pointed out, from a theological perspective, the three titles *Regina*, *Mediatrix* and *Corredemptrix* are linked and ultimately all of the Marian titles derive from her being the *Theotokos*, the woman who gave birth to God. How did the title of *Mediatrix* develop from that of *Theotokos*?

As early as in the apocryphal literature on Mary's assumption, the Blessed Virgin assumes the role of the mediator for mankind. In *The Discourse of St John the Divine Concerning the Falling Asleep of the Holy Mother of God*, before her assumption, Mary explicitly asks for the privilege of mediating between heaven and earth, and Christ grants it to her:

> 'O Lord, King of the heavens, son of the living God, accept every man who calls upon your name, that your birth may be glorified.' And again she prayed and said, 'O Lord Jesus Christ, who have all power in heaven and on earth, I entreat your holy name

793 See Delius, *Geschichte der Marienverehrung*, 279.

794 *Ad Caeli Reginam: Encyclical of Pope Pius XII*, <www.vatican.va/holy_father/pius_xii/encyclicals/documents/hf_p-xii_enc_11101954_ad-caeli-reginam_en.html> (18 February 2013).

795 See Roscher, *Ausführliches Lexikon*, 428–429 for a longer list of the correspondence between Isiac titles and Marian titles, such as *Regina Caeli*, *Regina Pacis*, *Maris Stella* etc. The title *Regina Caeli* had already been conferred upon Mary by the Ecumenic Council of Nicea in 787 and in the following years was used by countless popes (See Delius, *Geschichte der Marienverehrung*, 297).

> with this supplication: At every time and in every place where there is a memorial of my name, sanctify that place, and glorify those who glorify you through my name, accepting every offering and every supplication and every prayer.' 43. And when she had thus prayed, the Lord said to his own mother, 'Let your heart be glad and rejoice; for every grace and every gift has been given you of my Father who is in heaven and of me and of the Holy Ghost. Every soul who calls upon your name shall not be put to shame, but shall find mercy and consolation and succour and confidence, both in this world and in that which is to come, before my Father who is in heaven.'[796]

Mary's role as mediator is powerfully expressed by her identification with Jacob's ladder in Genesis 28:11–22:

> He [Jacob] came to a certain place and stayed there for the night, because the sun had set. Taking one of the stones of the place, he put it under his head and lay down in that place. And he dreamed that there was a ladder set up on the earth, the top of it reaching to heaven; and the angels of God were ascending and descending on it… . Jacob woke from his sleep and said, 'Surely the Lord is in this place – and I did not know it!' And he was afraid and said, 'How awesome is this place! This is none other than the house of God, and this is the gate of heaven'.[797]

The ladder in Jacob's dream connects heaven and earth, and thus becomes a symbol for Mary in her function as *Mediatrix.* In a Marian hymn by Romanos of Meloden (490–550 ca.) she is seen as the heavenly ladder upon which God descends.[798] Bonaventura explains that Mary is called "ladder" because God came down to earth through her and to go back to God, mankind has to pass through her.[799] Mary is not only identified with Jacob's ladder but also with the expression "gate of heaven" which is again pointing to her function as linking humanity to the divine. In an influential ninth-century hymn, the *Ave, Maris Stella*, it says:

Ave, maris stella,	Hail, star of the sea
Dei mater alma	fostering mother of God
atque semper virgo,	and ever-virgin
felix caeli porta.	happy door to Heaven.[800]

796 Elliott, *The Apocryphal New Testament*, 707 (*The Discourse of St John the Divine Concerning the Falling Asleep of the Holy Mother of God*, 42–43).

797 See Delius, *Geschichte der Marienverehrung*, 115.

798 See Romanos of Meloden, quoted in Delius, *Geschichte der Marienverehrung*, 115.

799 See Bonaventura, quoted ibid., 188.

800 *Ave, Maris Stella*, in *Gotteslob: Katholisches Gebet- und Gesangbuch: Ausgabe für das Erzbistum Köln*, ed. Bischöfe Deutschlands und Österreichs und der Bistümer Bozen-Brixen und Lüttich (Stuttgart: Katholische Bibelanstalt, 1975), 564.

Mary as Jacob's ladder (the means to enter the realm of the divine), also appears in a legend telling the story of a Franciscan monk's dream. Warner summarizes it as the following:

> Leo saw two ladders leading up to heaven, one as red as blood, the other as white as lilies. At the top of the red ladder there appeared Christ, his face full of wrath. St. Francis beckoned to his brothers not to fear and to climb the ladder. They climb, but fall. Francis prays, but Christ displays his wounds and thunders, "Your brothers have done this to me." So St. Francis runs down and leads his brethren to the white ladder, which they scale effortlessly and without mishap, to find Mary at the top, all smiles, to welcome them.[801]

The legend of brother Leo's dream was included in Alphonsus Liguori's, *The Glories of Mary,*[802] a collection of Marian legends which was first published in 1750 and then became one of the most important books on Mary in modern times.[803] The legend of Leo's dream illustrates why Mary's role as *Mediatrix* became so important. During the Middle Ages she was used as a counter-figure to Christ, who was increasingly endowed with the traits of the severe judge at the end of time. Thus, Maria *Mediatrix* "gives Christ the Judge his human face."[804] Michael O'Carroll characterizes the medieval view as working with the idea of two kingdoms, "the kingdom of justice ruled by Jesus and that of mercy by Mary."[805] In innumerable representations of Mary and John the Baptist, they lift their hands in supplication before Christ's celestial throne.[806] Mary's kingdom of mercy, the kingdom of the *Mediatrix*, is perhaps best expressed in the eleventh-century prayer *Salve Regina*. In this it says:

> Hail holy queen, mother of mercy,
> Hail our life, our sweetness and our hope.
> To you do we cry poor banished children of Eve,
> To you do we send up our sighs mourning and weeping in the valley of tears
> Turn then, most gracious advocate
> your eyes of mercy toward us.

801 Warner, *Alone of All*, 326.
802 See Delius, *Geschichte der Marienverehrung*, 251.
803 Michael O'Carroll, *Theotokos: A Theological Encyclopedia of the Blessed Virgin Mary* (Wilmington, Delaware: Michael Glazier, 1983), 14.
804 Warner, *Alone of All*, 316.
805 O'Carroll, *Theotokos,* 14.
806 See ibid., 319.

And after this, our exile,
Show us the fruit of your womb, Jesus.
O clement, O loving, O sweet Virgin Mary.[807]

It was in the eleventh century that Mary who already was considered to be the helper of the sinner (*adiutrix*) also became the advocate of the sinner (*advocata nostra*). This title paved the way for her function as *Mediatrix* which was further enhanced when the *Ave Maria* – originally a prayer of the Eastern Church – was introduced into the Western Church in the thirteenth century.[808] In 1568, Pope Pius V officially recognized the Ave Maria's closing formula "Pray for us sinners, now and at the hour of our death."[809]

Mary *Mediatrix*, on the threshold between heaven and earth, also figures prominently in world literature. This will be shown in the following by the two examples of Dante's *Divine Comedy* and Goethe's *Faust II.* In both cases Mary intervenes to save people from the devil.

In Dante's *Divine Comedy*, on his journey through hell, purgatory and paradise, the poet praises Mary's intercession. She intervenes on behalf of Buonconte da Montefeltro, saving him from hell,[810] and the princes in purgatory's valley of neglectful rulers ask for her pity. Finally, it is Mary's position in heaven that points to her role as *Mediatrix*. In the *Divine Comedy*, Mary is placed just below Christ and is evoked as the mystical rose which worked the miracle of a special childbirth, namely, the miracle of incarnation. "*Regina Coeli*" is sung in heaven[811] and Beatrice – guiding Dante in paradise – tells him to contemplate Mary: "Why does my face so enamour thee that thou turnest not to the fair garden which blossoms beneath the rays of Christ? Here is the Rose, in which the Divine Word became flesh: here are the lilies by whose odor the good way was taken."[812] In the *Divine*

807 *Salve Regina*, in *Gotteslob*, 546–547: "Salve, Regina, mater misericordiae; vita, dulcedo et spes nostra, salve. Ad te clamamus, exsules filii Evae. Ad te suspiramus, gementes et flentes in hac lacrimarum valle. Eia ergo, advocata nostra, illos tuos misericordes oculos ad nos converte. Et Jesum, benedictum fructum ventris tui, nobis post hoc exsilium ostende. O clemens, o pia, o dulcis Virgo Maria."

808 See Delius, *Geschichte der Marienverehrung*, 167.

809 See Warner, *Alone of All*, 306.

810 Dante Alighieri, *La Divina Commedia*, ed. Natalino Sapegno (Firenze: La Nuova Italia, 1977), Purgatorio V, verses 94–108.

811 Ibid., paradiso XXIII, verse 128.

812 *The Divine Comedy of Dante Alighieri*, trans. Charles Eliot Norton (Chicago: William Benton Publisher, 1978), paradise XXIII, verses 70–75; Dante Alighieri, *La Divina Commedia*, paradiso XXIII, verses 70–75: "Perché la faccia mia sí t'innamora,/ che

Comedy Mary herself accentuates the fact that she was pregnant with and gave birth to the Redeemer ("I am Angelic Love, and I circle round the lofty joy which breathes from out the womb which was the hostelry of our Desire"[813]). This *motif* returns in the context of the supreme mediation that Mary works in the *Divine Comedy.* St. Bernard, in C*anto* XXXIII of Paradise, prays to Mary asking her to intervene on Dante's behalf so that he may contemplate the divine. Imploring for her intercession, St. Bernard praises Mary as the *Theotokos*: "Thou art she who didst so ennoble human nature that its own Maker disdained not to become its creature. Within thy womb was rekindled the Love through whose warmth this flower has thus blossomed in the eternal peace."[814]

Mary as *Mediatrix* not only intercedes for medieval Dante – with the result that he has a vision of the divine – but she is also capable of saving Goethe's Faust, who sold his soul to the devil. In *Faust II*, Mephistopheles, the devil, wants to take Faust's soul to hell after his death. However, the angels come with roses – Mary's flowers[815] – and the devil has to surrender.[816] Dr. Faustus, ascending to heaven, becomes *Doctor Marianus*, worshipping Mary:

> O contrite hearts, seek with your eyes
> The visage of salvation;
> Blissful in that gaze, arise,
> Through glad regeneration.
> Now may every pulse of good
> Seek to serve before thy face,

---

tu non ti rivolgi al bel giardino/ che sotto i raggi di Cristo s'infiora?/ Quivi è la rosa in che il verbo divino/ carne si fece; quivi son li gigli/ al cui odor si prese il buon cammino."

813 Ibid., XXIII, 103–105: "Io sono amore angelico, che giro/l'alta letizia che spira del ventre/che fu albergo del nostro disiro."

814 Ibid., XXXIII, 4–9: "Tu se' colei che l'umana natura/ nobilitasti sí, che 'l suo fattore/ non disdegnò di farsi sua fattura./ Nel ventre tuo si raccese l'amore/ per lo cui caldo nell'eterna pace/ cosí è germinato questo fiore."

815 As has been shown in section III.4.1.1.2 of this work, roses were also the flowers of Isis.

816 See Johann Wolfgang von Goethe, *Faust: Der Tragödie erster und zweiter Teil: Urfaust*, ed. Erich Trunz (München: Beck), 2010, verses 11735–11825 of *Faust II*.

Virgin, Queen of Motherhood [literally: Virgin, Mother, Queen[817]]
Keep us, Goddess, in thy grace.[818]

In the last verse quoted above, it is interesting to note that Goethe explicitly recognizes Mary as a goddess in the *crescendo* of "Virgin, Mother, Queen, Goddess." Goethe shows through the succession of the Marian titles how the fact that Mary conceived and gave birth to Jesus, results in her becoming Queen. The word "goddess" exalts Mary even further. Here protestant Goethe celebrates the glory of the divine, he conceives of as feminine,[819] an idea that he also expresses at the very end of *Faust II* in the famous *Chorus Mysticus*:

---

817 My remark.

818 Johann Wolfgang von Goethe, *Faust: Parts One and Two*, trans. Philip Wayne (Chicago: Encyclopaedia Britannica, 2003), 162; Goethe, *Faust: Der Tragödie zweiter Teil*, verses 11735–11825: "Blicket auf zum Retterblick,/ Alle reuig Zarten,/ Euch zu seligem Geschick/ Dankend umzuarten./ Werde jeder beßre Sinn/ Dir zum Dienst erbötig;/ Jungfrau, Mutter, Königin,/ Göttin, bleibe gnädig!"

819 The opinion that Goethe here imagines the ultimate transcendental instance as feminine was held by Prof. Erwin Koppen in his seminar on Faust II in 1988/89 at the University of Bonn. However, Mary is not the only figure by which Goethe allows the feminine life-giving force to emerge as the crucial transcendental power. In fact, Mary is paralleled by the myth of "the mothers" ("die Mütter") in Act One of *Faust II*. Here, Faust wishes to see Helena and Paris; Mephistopheles tells him to descend to "the mothers," who are depicted as the only powers able to fulfil this wish. (Erwin Koppen held the view that with the figures of "the mothers" Goethe was actually inventing a myth). However, being confronted with the idea of having to descend to the mothers, Faust is grasped by a sudden terror:
"Mephistopheles. Loth am I now high mystery to unfold:
Goddesses dwell, in solitude, sublime,
Enthroned beyond the world of place or time;
Even to speak of them dismays the bold.
These are The Mothers.
Faust. Mothers?
Mephistopheles. Stand you daunted?
Faust. The Mothers! Mothers – sound with wonder haunted.
Mephistopheles. True, goddesses unknown to mortal mind,
And named indeed with dread among our kind.
To reach them, delve below earth's deepest floors;
And that we need them, all the blame is yours.
Faust. Where lies the way?
Mephistopheles. There is none. Way to the Unreachable,
Never besought! Is your soul then ready?"

All things corruptible
Are but a parable;
Earth's insufficiency
Here finds fulfillment;
Here the ineffable
Wins life through love;
Eternal Womanhood
Leads us above.[820]

With these verses Goethe touches upon Mary's role as the Coredemptress which – like her other titles – has its own history that will be sketched in the following.

From a theological perspective, redemption seen in relation to Mary is one aspect of Mediation.[821] The idea of Mary as Coredemptress may

---

(Goethe, *Faust: Parts One and Two*, 82). Mephistopheles here describes the mothers as chontic, primordial goddesses, beyond time and space. In fact, Goethe's myth of the mothers actually fits the symbolic pattern of childbirth labeled "The Supremacy of the Female." The powers of "the mothers" are illustrated as follows:
And by that glow shall you behold The Mothers.
Some of them seated, some erect, while others
May chance to roam: Formation, Transformation,
Eternal Mind's eternal recreation.
Around them float all forms of entity.
(Goethe, *Faust: Parts One and Two*, 83). The mothers represent the mystic origin of life. Therefore Faust feels a sacred terror every time Mephistopheles evokes them, i.e. he feels *Ungeheure* ("the shock of fear"):
"Mephistopheles.
It's hidden powers you soon may understand.
This key will scent the true trail from all others;
Follow it down, 'twill giude you to The Mothers.
Faust (shuddering).
The Mothers – still I feel the shock of fear.
What is this Word, that I must dread to hear?"
(Goethe, *Faust: Parts One and Two*, 83). Mary and "The Mothers" in Faust II are two sides of the same coin. Both represent life-giving, feminine, transcendental forces. However, while the mothers underline the terrifying aspect of the mystery of life, Mary's role is to gently soothe: sacred terror becomes mystical maternal mercy, linked to the idea of redemption.

820 Goethe, *Faust: Parts One and Two*, 162; Goethe, *Faust: Der Tragödie zweiter Teil*, verses 12104–12111: "Alles Vergängliche/ Ist nur ein Gleichnis;/ Das Unzulängliche,/ Hier wird's Ereignis;/ Das Unbeschreibliche,/ Hier ist's getan;/ Das Ewig-Weibliche/ Zieht uns hinan."

821 See O'Carroll, *Theotokos*, 305.

have had its early origins in the work of Irenaeus who argued that "Mary was a cause of salvation to herself and all mankind."[822] Also St. Ambrose made an important step towards Mary's role as Coredemptress, creating a link between incarnation and redemption: "Alone Mary has worked the salvation of the world and conceived the redemption of all ... Mary, who gave birth to the victor, has defeated the devil."[823] Together with Mary's role in the incarnation (conception and birth of Christ), her sufferings at the death of her son were contemplated (Milo of St. Amand, St. Peter Damian and St. Anselm) and related to redemption (Arnold of Bonneval, disciple of St. Bernard).[824] Finally, thirteenth-century theology developed the idea of a partnership between Jesus and Mary (Richard of St. Laurent, Pseudo-Bonaventure and Pseudo-Albert).[825] In the following centuries the title Coredemptress is in use[826] and becomes a major focus of theological debate between the end of World War II and Vatican Council II.[827]

To a certain extent one could argue that in the 20th century Mary was not only perceived as the *Corredemptrix* but also as the "Redemptrix," i.e. that she was not only considered to be "assisting" with redemption, but to be a divine redeemer herself. It seems that in the course of history, Mary moved from her position of the mother of Jesus to the position of the Mother of All. Indeed, in the encyclical on the Queenship of Mary (*Ad Caeli Reginam*, 1954) Mary's position is officially sanctioned as "the most Blessed Virgin, the Queen of all creatures, the Queen of the world, and the Ruler of all."[828]

822 Ibid.

823 Ambrose, quoted in O'Carroll, *Theotokos*, 305.

824 See ibid.

825 See ibid., 306. O'Carroll sees the origin of this idea in 12th century thinking, namely Ekbert of Schönau's conception of Mary as the associate of Christ, deriving from her collaboration in the work of incarnation and Hermann of Tournai's ideas giving "*a new dimension to the new Eve concept by the use of Gen:18, 'a helper like himself.'*"

826 See ibid.

827 The question of corredemption was the theme of the French Marian Congress in 1947 and then again at the International Mariological Congress in Rome in 1950. See ibid.

828 Encyclical *Ad Caeli Reginam* of Pope Pius XII, 22.

3.5 *Mary-Sophia*

Among the Marian titles testifying to a harmony between spiritual birth and childbirth there is also that of *Sophia*, which Mary shares with Isis. The identification of Mary with Wisdom relies on a transposition of the biblical conception of God's Wisdom to Mary. From the tenth century onwards the text from Proverbs VIII, "The Lord created me at the beginning of his work", referring to God's Wisdom, was chosen to commemorate Mary's Nativity.[829] The notion of a special relationship between Wisdom and Mary grows through medieval times.[830] Like Isis, Mary also became associated with philosophy. Odo of Canterbury (d. c. 1200), Benedictine Abbot of Battle Abbey, links Mary as the seat of wisdom with her role as *Mediatrix*. She gave birth to Christ and thus to obtain the wisdom of Christ one has to pass through her:

> Philosophy is called the pursuit or love of wisdom. Mary is, therefore, the philosophy of Christians for whoever desire to find true wisdom must direct all their love and endeavour towards Mary. But Christ who is called the power and the wisdom of God, is the true Wisdom. He is strictly the true Wisdom of Christians for to another beyond him the Christian cannot go. Whoever desires to have this wisdom must direct his study towards the Mother for in Mary must he study who is to find Christ. For through Mary we come to Christ as through a mother to a son, through the Mother of mercy to Mercy himself.[831]

The theme of Mary and Wisdom is taken up and developed throughout Christian history up to modern times.[832] Pius XII repeatedly called Mary by her title "Seat of Wisdom,"[833] an invocation which was already part of the eleventh century *Litany of Loreto*, a long list of Marian titles also including other invocations of Mary pointing to a harmony between spiritual birth and childbirth such as "spiritual vessel" (*vas spirituale*).[834]

829 See O'Carroll, *Theotokos*, 368.
830 Ibid.
831 Odo of Canterbury, quoted ibid.
832 See ibid.
833 See ibid.
834 *The Litany of Loreto*, in *Gotteslob*, 1063–1067.

3.6 *Two Examples for Different Conceptions of Mary: Augustine and Friedrich Schleiermacher*

So far the way in which Mary has stood for a harmony between spiritual birth and childbirth has been illustrated by exploring some of the titles conferred upon her throughout the course of Christian history: *Theotokos*, *Blessed Virgin*, *Immaculate*, *Mediatrix*, *Corredemptrix*, *Regina Coeli* and *Sophia*. It has been shown that with regards to Mary childbirth was spiritualized by disembodiment, that is, by the ideas of the painless, *utero clauso* virgin birth and the Immaculate Conception. As will be shown in the following, Augustine's *Nativity Sermons* lay some foundations for this tradition, which also has consequences for the understanding of birth when it comes to ordinary women and children. This is because Augustine places the birth of Jesus in opposition to birth in general.

Contrastingly, an investigation into Friedrich Schleiermacher's text *Christmas Eve*, will evidence that Mary has the potential to spiritualize childbirth in general. Thus Mother Mary can be put up against all other mothers as does Augustine, or every mother may become a Mary as in Schleiermacher's text.

3.6.1 *Augustine's* Nativity Sermons: *Mother Mary against the Mothers*

In Augustine's *Nativity Sermons*, Mary holds the privileged position of being able to unite spiritual birth and childbirth. The special birth of Jesus is spiritualized. This is achieved by claiming that Mary was a virgin in the conception and birthgiving process. Virginity and the miracle of the Virgin Birth are seen as a divine gift:

> True it is, fertility in marriage is good; but virginity in a life of piety is better. For this reason Christ as man who as God – for He was both God and man – was able to give both, could never have given His Mother the gift which the married cherish, and thus deprive her of that better gift for the sake of which virgins pass over the opportunity of being mothers.[835]

However, the harmony of childbirth and spiritual birth Mary represents is seen as exceptional in the *Nativity Sermons*. Augustine emphasizes that

835 Augustine, *Sermons for Christmas,* 94 (Sermon 188.4).

only Mary could achieve it, whereas any other virgin would have to choose between spiritual birth in Christ and having children:

> She, then, whose footsteps you follow, not only did not cohabit with a man that she might conceive, but in giving birth remained a virgin. Imitate her to the best of your ability-not in her fecundity, for this you cannot do and still preserve your virginity. She alone was privileged to have both, and of these it is your wish to have only one; because if you wished to have both, you would lose the one. She alone could have both, for she gave birth to the Omnipotent, through whom this was made possible for her. [...] And you must not think of yourselves as sterile merely because you remain virgins. For it is precisely this holy purity of the flesh that also leads to fruitfulness of the spirit. [...] Since you are not considering *the things of the world, how you may please your husbands*, consider *the things that belong to God, how you may please Him* in all things. And do this so that you may have, not a womb fruitful with offspring, but a spirit fruitful with virtues.[836]

With this passage, Augustine conceives of a religious life devoted to Christ and childbirth as mutually exclusive options for earthly virgins. Thus, when it comes to the birth of ordinary children, Augustine plainly shares the attitudes towards childbirth as illustrated in the section "Theoretical, Spiritual and Political Natality versus Childbirth" of this work. The hierarchies between spiritual birth and childbirth are made clear when Augustine compares the virgin, the widow and the mother to each other, putting the latter on the lowest rung of the ladder leading to a spiritual life in Christ:

> Rejoice, you virgins of Christ! The mother of Christ is one of you. You have not been privileged to give birth to Christ; but because of Christ you have not wished to bear children. He who was not born of you, but He was born for you. [...] Rejoice, you widows of Christ! To Him who has made virginity fruitful, you have vowed holy continence. Rejoice also, all you who live in nuptial chastity, living faithfully with your spouses! What you have lost in your bodies preserve in your hearts. Where the flesh can no more be inviolate because of the use of marriage, let your good conscience in matters of the faith be a virgin, in the same sense that the universal Church is a virgin. [...] Conceive Him by faith, give birth to Him through your works, so that your heart may be doing in the law of Christ what the womb of Mary did in the flesh of Christ.[837]

In Augustine's logic only one special woman, namely the Blessed Virgin, can enjoy the divine privilege of uniting spiritual birth and childbirth, whereas for all other women these are separate options. Thus the disembodiment of Mary, which may be read as the axial age gap cutting

836 Ibid., 110 (Sermon 191.4).

837 Ibid., 113–114 (Sermon 192.2).

right through her body, separates Mary from all other women. This gap between Mary and ordinary women is closed in Schleiermacher's text *Christmas Eve*.

3.6.2 Friedrich Schleiermacher: Every Mother a Mary

In 1806 Friedrich Schleiermacher first published his short book entitled *Christmas Eve: Dialogue on the Incarnation* ["Die Weihnachtsfeier: Ein Gespräch"]. The German protestant philosopher and theologian, models *Christmas Eve* on typical Platonic style, characterized by conversations among several people occupying different standpoints with regard to a specific question. The focus of the book, as the title already indicates, is on Christmas. In *Christmas Eve* several families are celebrating Christmas together and during the festivities, the adults Frederike, Ernestine, Agnes, Leonhardt, Ernst and Eduard start talking about the meaning of the feast. Little Sofie provides the impetus for discussion by saying that she could imagine her mother as the happy mother of the divine child: "Oh, Mother, you might just as well be the happy mother of the divine babe."[838] Sofie's mother confirms that there is some truth to the analogy drawn by her daughter. She sees the revelation of the divine in every child. Thus she can identify with Mary worshipping divine revelation in her son:

> In a way I feel she [Sofie] did not say too much when she thought that I might as well be the mother of the blessed child. For I can in all humility honor the pure revelation of the divine in my daughter, as Mary did in her son, without in the least disturbing the proper relation of mother and child.[839]

838 Friedrich D. E. Schleiermacher, *Christmas Eve: Dialogue on the Incarnation*, trans. with introduction and notes Terrence N. Tice (Lewiston, New York: The Edwin Mellen Press, 1990), 33. Friedrich D. E. Schleiermacher, *Die Weihnachtsfeier: Ein Gespräch* in Friedrich D. E. Schleiermacher, *Werke: Auswahl in vier Bänden*, ed. Otto Braun and Johannes Bauer (Leipzig: Fritz Eckhardt Verlag, 1911), 4:473–532; 19 (of the original impagination which is also reported by Braun and Bauer and will be used in the following): "O Mutter! Du könntest ebensogut die glückliche Mutter des göttlichen Kindleins sein."

839 Schleiermacher, *Christmas Eve*, 36. Schleiermacher, *Die Weihnachtsfeier*, 25: "Wahrlich ich fühle es, daß sie [Sofie] in einer Hinsicht nicht zu viel gesagt hat, als sie sagte, ich könnte wohl auch die Mutter des angebeteten Kindes sein, weil ich in der Tochter, wie Maria in dem Sohne, die reine Offenbarung des Göttlichen recht demütig verehren kann."

In *Christmas Eve*, Schleiermacher endows each mother-child relationship with the aura of the divine emanating from Mary and Jesus. At the same time he humanizes Mary and her son. This mother-Mary analogy is most directly expressed in a scene in which Ernestine recalls a childhood memory. She remembers the Christmas Eve on which she attended midnight mass for the first time in her life. The priest and the church environment turned out to be more annoying than inspiring for the little girl until she suddenly became aware of a mother and her young child sitting apart from the crowd. Ernestine identifies the mother and her child with Mary and Jesus, after which the whole atmosphere of the church immediately appears permeated with holiness. The scene culminates in Ernestine's sensation that the place where the mother and her child are sitting looks like a chapel inside the church:

> My eye caught something. It was a lady sitting in an open pew just under a lovely old monument, holding a small child to her bosom. Apparently giving little heed to the preacher, the singing, or anything else about her, she seemed to be sunk deep in her own thoughts, and her eyes were fixed upon the child. Irresistibly was I drawn toward them, and my companion was obliged to follow as I moved closer. There, at that moment, I had suddenly come upon the sanctuary, the holy place, I had been seeking so long in vain.
>
> I stood before the noblest scene I had ever witnessed. The woman was simply dressed. Her grand and gentil bearing made of the open bench an enclosed chapel. […] Her countenance seemed to display gladness one moment, then dejection; her breath now trembling with joy, now holding the sighs of contentment back. Yet what was communicated through it all was a sense of affable serenity, of loving devotion – radiating gloriously from her dark, downcast eyes, which would have been completely hidden from me had I been any taller. The child also seemed to me uncommonly lovely. It stirred energetically and yet quietly, and seemed absorbed in a half-unconscious dialogue of love and yearning with its mother.
>
> It was as if I were viewing an artist's picture of Mary and child in living exemplar. I was […] deeply entranced.[840]

Schleiermacher's *Christmas Eve* does not only postulate a harmony between spiritual birth and childbirth but also includes the symbolic pattern of childbirth here referred to as "The Supremacy of the Female." Women are depicted as being closer both to childbirth and to spiritual birth than men. Childbirth becomes the "sacred fire"[841] to which women

840 Schleiermacher, *Christmas Eve*, 58.

841 Ibid., 37.

have the privilege to tend to whereby men indulge in finding compensations for their lack of an immediate access to childbirth and the spiritual birth that comes with it:

> Women who devote themselves to this holy service fittingly dwell within the temple, vestals watching over the sacred fire. But we must venture forth into the world in strict array, practicing discipline and preaching penance, or as pilgrims cleaving fast to the cross and girding ourselves with swords in order to seek out some holy object or sanctuary and to recover it.[842]

A gender difference with regards to attitudes towards childbirth is also constructed in other passages of *Christmas Eve*. Thus in a dialogue between Leonhardt and Agnes, Leonhardt emphasizes the joy of educating, and "forming" the child according to one's ideals. Agnes, instead, sharply opposes Leonhardt's focus on education. She argues that prior to any education, the love for a child comes from the beautiful and the divine within him/her. Ernestine agrees with her, by again referring to the mother-Mary analogy: Mothers have divine, eternal children, when children are understood as the expression of a higher spirit:

> "And so you are indifferent, then," queried Leonhardt, "as to whether you can cultivate what you would like for your child or whether it may be torn from you in the first helpless stage of life?"
>
> "Indifferent? Who would say that?" she retorted. "But the inner life, the status of one's soul, is not destroyed thereby. Do you believe, then, that love is directed to what a child can be formed into? What can we form, actually? No, love is directed to what we believe to be lovely and divine in him already, what every mother looks for in every movement of her child, as soon as its soul begins to find expression."
>
> "You see," said Ernestine, "in this sense every mother is another Mary. Every mother has a child divine and eternal, and devoutly looks out for stirrings of the higher spirit in it.[843]

Although the milieu is Protestant, Mary is declared the patroness of the women present at Schleiermacher's Christmas Eve, and Christmas as their feast.[844] The women – despite the shocked Leonhardt – quote a Novalis

842 Ibid., 37.
843 Ibid., 48.
844 See ibid., 56.

poem about Mary that depicts the divine mother as the *mediatrix* through whom the poet feels Heaven in his soul:

> I see thee in a thousand forms,
> O Mary, lovingly expressed;
> Yet none can show thy deeper charms
> That move the soul within my breast.
> I only know the world's uproar
> Appears now as a vanished dream;
> And joys of Heaven, unknown before,
> Through all my heart for ever stream.[845]

In Schleiermacher's *Christmas Eve*, several elements characterizing Mary in Catholicism have been transformed. The gaps that separate the virginal mother from the mother, and the immaculately conceived/conceiving from the woman conceived/conceiving in sin are closed. Mary's virginity and the question of original sin disappear from the stage of philosophical-theological inquiry. Virginity is no longer seen as an ideal state preferred to motherhood.[846] The human does not have to be disembodied in order to approach the divine. Hand in hand with this view, Schleiermacher enables Mary to maintain her holy features without necessiting a special emphasis on the virgin birth. On the contrary, Mary's holiness, manifested in her giving birth to Christ, spreads to every woman giving birth.

4. Paula Modersohn-Becker: The Pregnant Mystic

Paula Modersohn-Becker's paintings provide good examples of childbirth as being in harmony with spiritual birth. Her perception of childbirth is linked to personal beliefs that deviate from official religion. In a way Paula

---

845 Schleiermacher, *Christmas Eve*, 59; Schleiermacher, *Die Weihnachtsfeier*, 76: "Ich sehe dich in tausend Bildern,/ Maria lieblich ausgedrückt;/ Doch keins von allen kann dich schildern/ Wie meine Seele dich erblickt./ Ich weiß nur, daß der Welt Getümmel/ Seitdem mir wie ein Traum verweht,/ Und ein unnennbar süßer Himmel/ Mir ewig im Gemüte steht."

846 On the contrary, the nun is seen as missing out on the happiness that comes with childbirth. Leonhardt says on the nun: "However you look at it, the finest way of life destined for women and their richest happiness is foresworn" (Ibid., 37).

Modersohn-Becker arrives at Schleiermacher's conclusion that every mother can be "a Mary" without there being the need for Mary, Christ or God.

Paula Modersohn-Becker was a member of the Worpswede colony of artists, near Bremen. She died in 1907, a fortnight after she had given birth to her daughter Mathilde. She left behind a huge amount of paintings, in which female nudes, mother and child groups, adolescent girls and portraits of women (including a considerable number of self-portraits) form recurring themes. In the art of Paula Modersohn-Becker, the births of children form an integral part of her religious and artistic experience. Especially her self-portraits made during and just before pregnancy are interesting for a symbolic pattern of childbirth that reconciles spiritual natality and birth. In the analysis of two of Modersohn-Becker's paintings from 1907 made during her pregnancy, namely the *Self-Portrait with Camellia Branch* [*Selbstbildnis mit Kamelienzweig*] and the *Self-Portrait, Two Flowers in the Raised Hand* [*Selbstbildnis mit Doppelblüte*], as well as the *Self-Portrait on the Sixth Wedding Anniversary* [*Selbstbildnis am 6. Hochzeitstag*] from 1906, it will be shown how she integrated childbirth into her identity as an artist[847] and into religious experience.[848] Moreover, some of her letters and sections of her journals will prove useful in revealing how pregnancy and childbirth acquire a spiritual dimension.

4.1 Self-Portrait on the Sixth Wedding Anniversary

The *Self-Portrait on the Sixth Wedding Anniversary* expresses both an attitude toward pregnancy in general and the attitude Paula Modersohn-Becker took towards pregnancy in relation to herself (as an artist). The painting is a half nude and critics have mostly agreed that Modersohn-Becker represents herself here as being pregnant,[849] although her daughter was not conceived until spring of the following year. In this sense the picture expresses

847 Self-Portrait on the Sixth Wedding Anniversary.

848 Self-Portrait with Camellia Branch and Self-Portrait, Two Flowers in the Raised Hand.

849 See Renate Berger, *Malerinnen auf dem Weg ins 20. Jahrhundert* (Köln: DuMont, 1982), 276; Carl Georg Heise, *Paula Modersohn-Becker – Mutter und Kind* (Stuttgart: Reclam, 1961), 13; Christa Murken-Altrogge, *Paula Modersohn-Becker: Leben und Werk* (Köln: DuMont, 1980), 71; Perry, *Paula Modersohn-Becker*, 54.

a wish, a fantasy and a projection. For this, as for all of her female nudes, it can be said that Modersohn-Becker discovered a new dimension in the representation of the naked human being.[850]

Her approach to the female body is not one of erotic tension, as it often was in the paintings of her male colleagues.[851] She instead emphasizes what Busch calls the *Kreatürliche.*[852] As will be shown in the analysis of the painting, her attitude toward pregnancy does not connect female fertility with immanence, but rather with a spiritual dimension. Her belly is thrust out and she is holding it "as if to denote the sacred nature of this part of her body."[853] The colours of the cloth just below her belly and the gesture of the left hand are most important in this context. It has often been stated that there is a certain puzzling paradox in this gesture.[854] Actually the hand does not really "hold" the cloth covering the artist below. Thus the impression conveyed is that the cloth sticks to the body by invisible forces. Such a physical paradox may be interpreted symbolically. The light blue-and-white cloth evokes the sky and is the most immaterial point of the whole painting.[855]

---

850 See Günter Busch, *Paula Modersohn-Becker: Malerin, Zeichnerin* (Frankfurt/M: Fischer, 1981), 54.

851 In this sense, the fact of not seeing the woman exclusively in connection to a male counterpart, but in other contexts as well, Paula Modersohn-Becker did the big advance in art that Virginia Woolf was only hoping for to come in literature, when she wrote the following in *A Room of One's Own*:
"It was strange to think that all great women of fiction were, until Jane Austen's day, not only seen by the other sex, but seen only in relation to the other sex. And how small a part of a woman's life is that; and how little can a man know even of that when he observes it through the black or rosy spectacles which sex puts upon his nose. Hence, perhaps the peculiar nature of women in fiction; the astonishing extremes of her beauty and horror; her altenations between heavenly goodness and hellish depravity – for so a lover would see her as his love rose or sank, was prosperous or unhappy. .... Suppose, for instance, that men were only represented in literature as the lovers of women, and were never the friends of men, soldiers, thinkers, dreamers. [...] How literature would suffer! We might perhaps have most of Othello; and a good deal of Antony; but no Caesar, no Brutus, no Hamlet, no Lear, no Jacques – literature would be incredibly impoverished, as indeed literature is impoverished beyond our counting by the doors that have been shut upon women." (Virginia Woolf, *A Room of One's Own* (1929; reprint, London: Grafton, 1989), 79–80).

852 See Busch, *Paula Modersohn-Becker*, 54.

853 Perry, *Paula Modersohn-Becker,* 54.

854 See Berger, *Malerinnen auf dem Weg ins 20. Jahrhundert*, 276.

855 See for this and the following Brigitte Uhde-Stahl, *Paula Modersohn-Becker: Frau, Künstlerin, Mensch* (Stuttgart and Zürich: Belser, 1989), 102.

Thus the dimension hinted at is one which is not supposed to be ruled by the laws of physics, but to function according to other principles. Other symbols emphasizing wholeness and transcendance also pervade the picture. Paula Modersohn-Becker wears a round Bernstein-necklace, hinting at the symbol of the circle, and following, at eternity. Her eyes gaze self-consciously and with a quiet smile at the spectator. These are eyes full of confidence, which seem to "know." She stands in front of a luminous background where light green spots could stand for the colour of freshly grown leaves in spring. Thus the whole scene gives the impression of a new beginning.

Modersohn-Becker signed this self-portrait with the words: "This I painted, 30 years old, on my 6th wedding anniversary P.B." ["Dies malte ich mit 30 Jahren an meinem 6. Hochzeitstag P.B."]. This sentence reads somehow like a programme.[856] The painter signs with her maiden name and it would seem that she wanted to be considered as a single entity and independent from her family ties. Such an interpretation is supported by some remarks from her journal dating from 1906, following a crisis in her marriage: "I am no longer Paula Modersohn, but neither am I any longer Paula Becker. I am myself and intend always to become myself." ["Ich bin nicht mehr Paula Modersohn, aber ich bin auch nicht mehr Paula Becker. Ich bin ich und gedenke es immer zu werden"]. From this perspective one could interpret the self-portrait as the utmost expression of individuality through – or at least including – the potentiality of female fertility in pregnancy. Such an interpretation is supported by the fact that – in contrast to many of her other self-portraits – in this painting, Paula Modersohn-Becker tries to represent herself according to her real outer appearance.[857] Thus she actually seems to say, "that's me" and includes a potential pregnancy as part of her (artistic) self. In this sense it is not death that becomes the carrier of individuality as in Rilkean or Heideggerian thought, but pregnancy and birthgiving. Furthermore, pregnancy not only becomes the carrier of individuality but also places individuality in a larger spiritual context. The pregnant body is simultaneously represented as hers, as something belonging intrinsically to her identity and as sacred.[858]

856 See Berger, *Malerinnen auf dem Weg ins 20. Jahrhundert*, 276.

857 See Uhde-Stahl, *Paula Modersohn-Becker*, 102

858 I will come to this point further down by linking the Weltanschauung of Paula Modersohn-Becker to her self-portraits.

4.2 *Self-Portrait, Two Flowers in the Raised Hand*

This portrait was painted during the last months of Modersohn-Becker's pregnancy and was the last one she did of herself. As in many of her paintings, here she works with the symbolism of the flower, which in general stands for a link between human beings and nature.[859] In her raised left hand she holds two blossoms, springing forth from the same plant, an obvious allusion to the union of mother and child during pregnancy. There is something triumphant in this gesture.[860] Her right hand is placed on her belly, which is thrust out. Framed by the round face of pregnancy, her eyes look calmly and intensely at the spectator. She seems to be filled with something that is the child and at the same time goes beyond. It was stated that in Modersohn-Becker's art, female fertility is presented both mystically and as full of human warmth.[861] This expresses very much the atmosphere of the painting. Modersohn-Becker emphasizes both the circularity of life and death, and the renewal of life through pregnancy. In the *Self-Portrait, Two Flowers in the Raised Hand*, she celebrates life renewing itself by using many colours in the picture, particularly with the many shades of red (in her face and the two blossoms). Nevertheless, such a celebration does not forget about death, as it integrates and understands the "finiteness of flower and fruit."[862] Pregnancy to Modersohn-Becker is a mystical event, but she also sees the woman as an individual as the active protagonist of this event. This becomes even clearer in the *Self-Portrait with Camellia Branch*.

4.3 *Self- Portrait with Camellia Branch*

If it is true that in general the distinctive characteristic of Paula Modersohn-Becker's self-portraits is a deep sense of mystery in her eyes,[863] this characteristic probably reaches its purest expression in the *Self*

859 See Murken-Altrogge, *Paula Modersohn-Becker*, 57.

860 See Uhde-Stahl, *Paula Modersohn-Becker*, 114.

861 See Murken-Altrogge, *Paula Modersohn-Becker*, 20.

862 Heise, *Paula Modersohn-Becker*, 16. Probably one should place in this context, what Paula Modersohn-Becker told her mother in her last summer, namely that she should paint more flowers (See Uhde-Stahl, *Paula Modersohn-Becker*, 114). Actually when the painter died, it was the *Blumenstilleben mit Sonnenblumen und Malven* to be the last picture on her easel.

863 See Murken-Altrogge, *Paula Modersohn-Becker*, 52.

Portrait with Camellia Branch. Once again, this portrait seems to convey much of the artist's personality. Karl Ernst Osthaus, to whom it belonged, has stated that it is the only one of her self-portraits that corresponds to his memories of the living artist.[864] In this painting, Modersohn-Becker's look has the hint of an antique mask meant to connect its wearer to the gods and to the dead.[865] The portrait was greatly influenced by a collection of Egyptian mummy portraits of Fayum – reproductions of which she received as a gift from her husband on her 31st birthday. In Hellenistic Egypt, such portraits were painted during a person's lifetime and were placed on the face of the mummy after his or her death. This custom was supposed to guarantee that the facial traits of a person would be preserved, so that he or she would be able to live on in his or her original shape after death.[866]

In contrast to the Fayum portraits Modersohn-Becker integrates her bust into the painting.[867] This is most probably to connect the symbolism of the Fayum portraits to her perception of pregnancy. From the lower part of her body grows a green camellia branch, an allusion to the growing child. The highest leaf of the branch touches the necklace she is wearing. Thus, the new growing life is linked to the woman who lets it grow out of her womb and to eternity symbolized by the circular necklace. In this way Modersohn-Becker dissolves traditional oppositions such as body versus soul, matter versus spirit. She links pregnancy to the eternal renewal of life and thus turns it into a means of transcending one's own existence. This is shown even more clearly by a closer analysis of the position that the fingers are in while holding the camellia branch. The round space formed by the extremely vague contours of the thumb and the middle finger reminds one of a bud or a seed,[868] or one might think directly of the vagina. From this space an ascending line passes through the camellia branch, skirting the necklace, the mouth, the nose and the parting of her hair. There is an intense luminosity in the background – especially around her head and neck – deriving from a blue, which is turquoise, *the* colour of spirituality *par excellence*, referring to the process of "letting go" while dying.[869]

---

864 See Liselotte v. Reineken, *Paula Modersohn-Becker* (1983; reprint, Reinbek bei Hamburg: Rowohlt, 1993), 134.

865 See ibid., 105.

866 See Uhde-Stahl, *Paula Modersohn-Becker*, 111.

867 See ibid., 112.

868 Boda Hülsmann, *Paula Modersohn-Becker: In Freiheit zu sich selbst* (Stuttgart: Urachhaus, 1988), 72.

869 See Uhde-Stahl, *Paula Modersohn-Becker*, 112.

It seems that the link between the Fayum portraits and the Camellia Branch Portrait lies in the reference to eternity and immortality, although Modersohn-Becker's reception of Ancient Egyptian art is very special. More than a way of integrating death into life,[870] Modersohn-Becker transcends death in life by linking corporeality and a "mortal immortality" through pregnancy. The Egyptian understanding of an afterlife integrating the body is reinterpreted as the immortality of the body being achieved by generation. The accent is laid on the eternal renewal of life, just like in the Platonic dialogue between Socrates and Diotima in the *Symposium*, where the Mantinean woman states: "It is a divine affair, this engendering and bringing to birth, an immortal element in the creature that is mortal."[871]

All of the mummy portraits were subjected to a canon of representation, which –although conserving individual traits – characterized the person as not existing any more.[872] Although Modersohn-Becker integrates various elements of this canon in her painting (the motionless position of the head and the upper parts of the body, the fixed gaze of the face[873]), she at the same time goes beyond the mummy portraits. By incorporating parts of the canon she places herself in the context of universal humanity. The act of pregnancy is linked both to eternity and to death. This is what she articulates with colour in the self-portrait and what she articulates with words in this way: "Motherhood and death, these remain the greatest things on this earth" ["Muttertum und Tod, das sind doch die größten Dinge dieser Erde"].[874] The hint of the smile gives her face warmth. This makes the self-portrait differ considerably from the mummy portraits. Modersohn-Becker's hidden smile alludes to her child, which is growing in spite of death.

The extent to which Modersohn-Becker's paintings, *Two Flowers in the Raised Hand* and *Self-Portrait with Camellia Branch* are actually linked to the religious attitudes of the painter, can be deduced from a conversation she once had with the poet Rainer Maria Rilke. Modersohn-Becker

870 For this interpretation see Günter Busch, "Über Gegenwart und Tod – Edvard Munch und Paula Modersohn-Becker," in *Edvard Munch. Probleme, Forschung, Thesen*, eds. Henning Bock and Günter Busch (München: Prestel, 1973), 164.

871 Plato, *Symposium*, 206c.

872 See Berger, *Malerinnen auf dem Weg ins 20. Jahrhundert*, 287.

873 Murken-Altrogge, *Paula Modersohn-Becker*, 56.

874 Paula Modersohn-Becker, quoted in Heinrich Wigand-Petzet, *Das Bildnis des Dichters: Paula Modersohn-Becker und Rainer Maria Rilke: Eine Begegnung* (Frankfurt/M: Insel, 1976), 129.

expressed her astonishment about the fact that Rilke mentioned God so frequently, and she told him: "To me God means >she<, the one who brings, who has life and who gives life"[875] ["Mir ist Gott überhaupt >sie<, die Natur, die Bringende, die das Leben hat und schenkt"]. This statement was interpreted as coming close to the Greek conception of *physis,*[876] or to the Greek goddess Demeter, although the latter should not be misunderstood as a simple belief in nature.[877] The fact that Modersohn-Becker opposes a Demeter-like understanding of religion to the Rilkean god, summarizes and explains her attitudes towards birthgiving. Demeter does not stand for creation, but for a continuous process of re-creation – the "necessity of and the will to death where something new wants to be born."[878] In the latent metaphor of the goddess, the artist expresses her view of life as mysteriously renewing itself by generation. For Modersohn-Becker, birthgiving and pregnancy transcend the limits of her own life.

By symbolically linking pregnancy to the divine mystery of the eternal renewal of life, she gives it a mystical meaning. In this sense, her serene smile of *Self-Portrait with Camellia Branch* is the smile of a mystic – a pregnant mystic.

5. Mikhail Epstein: Towards an Ethics of Childbirth

> *This day, all people are children to me,*
> *and just for that reason they are dear.*
> Friedrich Schleiermacher

Mikhail Epstein's work *Fatherhood* has already been discussed from the perspective of the symbolic patterns of childbirth labelled "The Supremacy of the Male" and "The Supremacy of the Female." Here I will discuss *Fatherhood* for a last time as the pattern of a harmony between spiritual/theoretical natality and childbirth is also woven into the essay. This is done through the elaboration of three ideas, namely, the identification of the

875 Paula Modersohn-Becker, quoted in Wigand-Petzet, *Das Bildnis des Dichters*, 32.
876 See ibid.
877 See Hülsmann, *Paula Modersohn-Becker*, 69.
878 Ibid., 70.

child with an access to a beginning, the identification of the newborn with a transcendental sphere, and the development of an ethics of childbirth.

As to the first idea, Epstein sees the father as being carried away by a wave of spiritual renewal thanks to the birth of his child. The newborn guarantees the father access to a beginning and thereby makes him come closer to the divine creator:

> I wish a motto of the apostle Paul to precede this diary of a father:
>
> "Ye have put off the old man with his deeds; And have put on the new man, which is renewed in knowledge after the image of him that created him."[879] The father who procreates the new-born and understands it in all its striking novelty, is renewed himself in the liking of the eternal father. [...] The most important thing I wanted to transmit in this book is this feeling of the incessant, shattering novelty which so powerfully breaks into the life of the father, [...] who resembles the Creator more than in the former "pre-paternal" life.[880]

Epstein is very much in agreement with Hannah Arendt's idea that with the birth of a human being, the utterly new comes into the world. According to Epstein, the parent has privileged access to this "beginning of the beginnings" which can help him/her to undergo a spiritual renewal. This spiritual experience exceeds any other experience, even that of love. Epstein compares Dante's work *Vita Nova*, in which the poet is spiritually reborn due to his encounter with his beloved Beatrice, to the experience of birth. He argues that the experience of renewal through the birth of a child exceeds the experience of renewal through love, as here actual birth and spiritual birth coincide with one another:

> Dante called his novel on Beatrice "Vita Nova" – "New Life" because by this encounter he was born anew. But how much more striking and powerful is this novelty if it coincides with a real birth – if it does not only reveal itself to the gaze of one human being but to the whole cosmos! ....
>
> How new a human being is who has just been born. With the love for the daughter, all of Dante's symbols for a spiritual renewal gain an extremely real embodiment in life. Here love is rooted in the birth, in the source of all being, and on earth it cannot go further. What is love at first sight compared to love at first breath?[881]

879 Colossians 3:9–10.

880 Epstein, *Tagebuch für Olga*, 8–9.

881 Epstein, *Tagebuch für Olga*, 84.

The fusion of spiritual birth and childbirth is furthermore beautifully expressed by Epstein's interpretation of some verses by Goethe from the *West-Eastern Divan*. Goethe writes about the necessity of continuous spiritual renewal, which is metaphorically expressed by the cycle of death and "becoming" ("Werden"). For Epstein, the moment of spiritual birth coincides with the birth of his daughter:

> Goethe writes
> "And till you can meet this test:
> Die, renew your being! [Literally: Die and become!"[882]]
> You are just a dismal guest
> In earth's dark unseeing."[883]
>
> In this way I also was a dismal guest until new life came to me and transformed me into a host. To understand Goethe's "becoming" as the birth of a child and not as one's own resurrection, seems easier to me for the time being though it basically means the same: the overcoming of death, the way out of the non-being. Not to leave this earth to set out for other realms but to receive the newcomers from far away on earth: this is what turns you into a host and into the lord of the house. You are a guest as long as you have not received a guest yourself.[884]

Epstein's idea of the utterly new coming into the world with the birth of a child leads him to reflect on Camus' way of philosophizing about suicide. Epstein confronts Camus' attitude of seeing suicide as the most radical act of individualization, of mastering one's existence from the "philosophy of birth" perspective. Suicide and the creation of new life are two ways of transcending one's own life. However, Epstein argues that in an existentialist view, the decision to create new life is more radical than the decision to take one's own life:

> The birth of a child is the only real alternative to suicide if one is done with one's own life and has to transcend it either by moving on to death or to a new life. [...] If I commit suicide I only change the timetable, but I accept the given conditions. I agree with the course of existence and its law leading up to death. The more radical and riskier question is: Shall I continue to live my existent life which I have already received or shall I myself create new life?

882 My remark.

883 Johann Wolfgang von Goethe, *Poems of the West and East: West-Eastern Divan – West-Östlicher Divan*, bi-lingual edition of the complete poems, trans. John Whaley (Bern: Peter Lang, 1998), 47: "Denn solang du das nicht hast:/ Dieses stirb und werde –/ Bist du nur ein trüber Gast/Auf der dunklen Erde."

884 Ibid.

> This is the only question standing above Hamlet's one: "To be or not to be?" – because here it is decided whether somebody else shall be or shall not be. Here I do not accept the conditions which have been imposed on me from my birth onwards – the inevitability of death – but I create them myself as a free being. Only by creating another life I completely overcome my own createdness. [...] Birth is more innovative and liberating than death. [...] Death is preconditioned by birth, but birth is not preconditioned, it is a matter of free choice. By creating new life a human being shows his own volition and freedom more completely and profoundly than by killing himself.[885]

The contrast between Epstein's "philosophy of birth" and Camus' "philosophy of suicide" parallels the contrast between Arendt and Heidegger which has been illustrated in section II of this work. A "philosophy of birth" may link up with the idea of "being-towards-birth" whereby Camus' "philosophy of suicide" builds upon the Heideggerian "being-towards-death." In the logic of the conception of childbirth which has been outlined in this work[886] it can be argued that Epstein transposes the situation of the birthgiving woman characterized by a "Being-towards-another-*Dasein*"[887] into a general theory of existence defined more from a perspective of birth than from the perspective of death. In Epstein's reasoning, the creation of new life can become an expression of individual will and an introduction of a divine element into human existence:

> If one wants to claim a Mangodhood, that is if one wants to compete with God, one should choose, as a conscious action, giving birth to somebody else rather than taking one's own life. A whole life resembling yours, comprising immeasurable contents, world encompassing thoughts, pleasure, suffering, and death – all this can be or not be and is rooted in your will.[888]

In Epstein's essay, the *motif* of the transcendence of one's own life by means of childbirth, is linked to the idea of the "mortal immortality" that comes with children. All the parental care of and dedication to the child cannot outweigh the gift of eternity the child gives to the parent.[889]

In a striking transposition of Dante's Beatrice to the figure of the daughter, it is the child who leads the father's soul on the path to immortality, just as Beatrice leads the soul of the poet in paradise:

---

885 Ibid., 104–105.

886 See section II. of this work.

887 See ibid.

888 Epstein, *Tagebuch für Olga*, 106.

889 Ibid., 116: "Are all the efforts the parents make for their children – caring, education, self-sacrifice – just a small compensation for such a gain like eternity?"

> Through Olja I can look further into my future than through anybody else. The paths of all the people I know and love may end earlier and part from my path. But my daughter is always waiting ahead of me. As much as I am the only trustworthy memory of her beginning she is the only trustworthy prediction of my end, that is of what will become of me in this and perhaps in another life. Actually now my future is walking by my side. I can touch it and follow its development like a soul which runs ahead of its body, looking over the rim of its existence and following the track of immortality which has been predestined for it. Like Dante, it follows a path at the end of which it is awaited by the one who already had become his soul on earth: Beatrice.[890]

The fact that the child is granting the parent both access to a beginning and a "mortal immortality" is not the only way in which childbirth is spiritualized in Epstein's work. Both the unborn and the newborn are depicted as coming from "another world," which (still) affects them to such a high degree that they can actually function as a bridge between the parent and the spiritual sphere from which they have originated. The child is not only connected to immortality because s/he bestows a "mortal immortality" on the parent but also because s/he has reached this world from eternity: "I know that in the eternity from which you have come there is no separation of the souls."[891] To Epstein the child's origin is a mystery, symbolically expressed by the navel.[892] The mystery of the child's origin connects the parent to eternity and leads to the fact that the young child – being still in touch with the mystery of life – is perceived much more as a spiritual than a physical entity. Children – as opposed to adults – have a stronger spiritual force which tends to spread, even over their material environment:

> It is unpleasant to see the rumpled bedclothes of an adult, the wrinkled linen sheets, the scattered clothes no matter how beautiful and attractive the person himself/ herself may be: The impression on the cloth has something of cast offs and lifelessness to it revealing a certain lack of freshness of the body itself which has stayed behind its soul and has acquired a certain lifelessness during the years it has lived through. [...] Quite the contrary with the child there is so much soul in the body that it wants to get out into the open, leaving its impression on the wrinkled linen sheets, the scattered toys and the whole mess of the children's room. And if the author of this all is absent you even feel more how each thing in a moving way is filled with something, how

890 Epstein, *Tagebuch für Olga*, 197–198. See also ibid. 116 and 164 for other references to the "mortal immortality" that comes with children.

891 Ibid., 160.

892 Ibid., 185: "The navel is, as it were, a dead end street overgrown with thicket, leading to a barred gate and evoking the feeling of a strange, unknown life."

> every single object by having been displaced or by a seemingly coincidental location is radiating with certain spiritual waves. It looks as if the soul which has just entered this world has not decided yet clearly where and as what it should become embodied. And while with determination it is busy building up the body it also spreads over all the things close to it with unrestrained eruptions into this world, drawing them into the same creative whirling as the particles which it still has not rejected in their unfamiliarity and out of which with haste and ecstatic delight jointly with cells, blood and muscles it forms a new wonderful creature.[893]

In summary, *Fatherhood* endows the child with spiritual significance in various ways. The child comes from eternity and grants both access to a supreme beginning and a mortal immortality. Thus it is not surprising that childbirth, towards the end of Epstein's book, also becomes the catalyst for the development of a special ethics. Epstein takes the parent-child relationship as a model for human interaction in general. As God the Father loves humanity, and as the father loves his child, the neighbour should love his/her neighbour. Thus Epstein transforms the "You shall love your neighbor as yourself" of Matthew 22:39 into "You shall love your neighbor as your child":

> And only when within myself I had changed this rule and had told myself: "Thou shalt love thy neighbour as thy child" those who seemed to be far away and not dear to me felt immediately closer and my being started to envelop them with warmth as if they had really ended up in my body. It is sufficient to imagine that childlike nature in an unfamiliar face, or to realize that it has once been in it and immediately that face becomes less strange and unfamiliar. This is because inside me the father's nature awakens which has once enveloped this child. And occasionally with many people around me in the streets this child like nature finds its expression. Though I am by myself among them I start to understand the creator better and I also understand why He loves them all.[894]

It is interesting to note that to Epstein, the love between parent and child is the paradigm for the love of the neighbour precisely because it comes from a depth beyond rationally decided love: "Neither with socio-rational love nor with an enthusiastic-humanist love, with no other love am I able to grow fond of strangers than the one which penetrates them at this protected entrance where they are like my children and will remain children until their deaths."[895] To see the childish fragility and neediness of the

893 Ibid., 148–149.
894 Ibid., 205–206.
895 Ibid., 204.

adult, to lead him/her back to his/her mysterious origin is the means by which to unite humanity:

> Beforehand I was confused because I thought that people needed something else than what I needed. Now actually I have the idea that they need the same as children: tenderness, warmth, all encompassing compassion. And this need is so simple and obvious that one can and has to fulfil it immediately. [...] It is sufficient to imagine the other as a child to feel for him what oneself needs: love, compassion, the desire to embrace from all sides, to include, to protect. It is this one thing where all human beings come from that later on makes it most easy to feel united with them.[896]

Finally – and with this thought I will conclude the analysis of Epstein's "ethics of childbirth" – the essay *Fatherhood* proposes an awareness of the mystery of birth upon which every human being should be able to identify with either the parent or the child. The miracle of birth is thus continuously activated by a process of taking care or being taken care of, in which people switch between the role of the parent and the role of the child:

> Suddenly I saw in all people whom I know by their reliable familiar side a secret breach which is probably only visible to their parents as they have learnt how to hide it in good time. None of us comes into this world by himself. With everybody there remains an opening which is not overgrown and through which the soul enters at birth and leaves at death. We can only form a whole when we unite by means of our child-like incompleteness. Anybody is at the same time a child, a father or a mother to anybody else.[897]

896 Ibid., 206.
897 Ibid., 205.

IV. Final Remarks: A Baby Has Been Born – So What?

"And what shall we do now?", this was my daughter's question at the age of three after she had seen a dead kitten on a carpet. In the preface to this work I wrote about Yasmin's question to make the cultural constructions of birth and death tangible. In the course of this book I have examined four ways of giving meaning to the birth of children, that is four ways of answering the question, "What shall we do now?" in relation to birth.

One way of giving meaning to childbirth is to see the mother as the supreme life-giving force. This symbolic pattern was called "The Supremacy of the Female" and most probably derives from the deep physical involvement of the woman with childbirth. Man's contribution to the coming into existence of a child is less tangible than woman's. Thus, on a symbolic level, the child is more related to her than to him.

To describe the symbolic construction of the supremacy of the female over the male with regard to childbirth, I used myths of goddesses from antiquity who were depicted as mothers of the gods and the origin of the world; the gnostic myth of the creation of the world by Sophia; texts and representations related to the cults of the goddess Isis, who creates life out of death; and the birth of Jesus by Mary whose cult reaches up to our time. I closed this section with a passage from the essay by the contemporary writer Mikhail Epstein, where he describes his impression that a daughter – in opposition to a son – seems to derive from the mother only, as if the mother had split in two miraculously.

The long lasting Isis and Mary worship also testifies to another symbolic pattern of childbirth labelled "Harmony between Spiritual/Theoretical Natality and Childbirth." This is because Isis and Mary are not only supreme givers of life ("The Supremacy of the Female"), but also the path to religious mysteries and wisdom. Further examples for a harmony between spiritual birth and childbirth are some paintings of the artist Paula Modersohn-Becker and again a passage from Mikhail Epstein's *Fatherhood.*

A child has been born. So what? The greater physical distance of man from childbirth, compared with the intense involvement of woman in the process of generation, may be bridged symbolically by ways of constructing and accentuating "procreation." This happens in the symbolic pattern labelled "The Supremacy of the Male." Thus in Ancient Egyptian cosmogony the world comes into existence by ejaculation; in Genesis Eve is born from Adam and Hesiod describes the birth of Anadyomène from the genitals of Ouranos. Furthermore, in the genealogical lines of the Old Testament and of Prophet Muhammad, men procreate sons seemingly without women; in the twelfth tablet of the Gilgamesh Epic men have sons, who are viewed as a means of approaching the divine, whereas nothing is written about the fertility of women. Further examples illustrating the supremacy of the male over the female in matters of childbirth are the births of Dionysos and Athena: Zeus gives birth to them through a mimetic act of female fertility.

A most influential tradition of "The Supremacy of the Male" parts from Aristotelian philosophy. Aristotle assigns more importance to male semen than to female "matter" with regard to the coming into existence of a child. Tertullian, Augustine and Thomas Aquinas share the Aristotelian patrimony of man's superior role with regard to childbirth. Thomas Aquinas describes how God himself takes on the role of the man as the Holy Ghost intervenes into Mary's body to "procreate" Jesus. Finally, Ibn Hisham suggests in his *sirat* that God intervened into the body of Prophet Muhammad's father to grant the special procreation of his Prophet.

"The Supremacy of the Male" is by no means a symbolic pattern from the distant past. This was shown by a short story of Hemingway and by a passage from Mikhail Epstein's *Fatherhood.* In Hemingway's short-story, *Indian Camp*, a male doctor mimetically performs all stages of birthgiving. Mikhail Epstein draws a parallel between male procreation and divine creation.

A baby has been born. So what? To be able to conceive of childbirth from the viewpoint of philosophy this work explored the situation of the birthgiving woman by making use of Heidegger's conception of death. It was shown that many of the outstanding features Heidegger assigns exclusively to death equally apply to the woman giving birth. A second philosophical approach to childbirth was based on the elaboration of Hannah Arendt's philosophy of natality by Patricia Bowen-Moore. The birth of a child ("primary natality"), birth into the timelessness of thought ("theoretical natality") and birth into the realm of action ("political natality") can be understood as three different ways of accessing a beginning and a "mortal immortality." To these three categories I added the category of "spiritual natality," meaning the birth into the realm of religion. Spiritual natality equally brings with it an access to a beginning and a "mortal immortality."

Such a philosophical conception of birth helped to explain the symbolic pattern of childbirth called "Theoretical, Spiritual and Political Natality versus Childbirth". This symbolic register is characterized by the effort to gain access to a theoretical, political or spiritual natality and its specific "mortal immortality," by opposing it to primary natality. Thus the Babylonian myth of creation affirms the supremacy of the power of words over female fertility. In the *Symposium*, Plato prefers virtues as the deathless children of philosophers to children of flesh and blood. In the Justinian myth of Edem and Elohim, the latter abandons, for the idea of the good, the world he created. Abraham chooses faith, when he is confronted with the dilemma of deciding between his faith and the life of his son. Agamemnon sacrifices Iphigeneia for Hellas, the fatherland. In the gospel of Luke, Jesus subordinates the status of women giving birth to children and breastfeeding them to the status of those "who hear the word of God and obey it."[898] Gregory of Nyssa and Macrina devalue childbirth as being part of the realm of the body that is the realm of death as opposed to spirit and eternal life. The martyrs Perpetua and Felicitas value faith above their children. Medieval Héloise refuses to live with Abélard and argues that a baby and a philosopher mutually exclude each other in the same household. Rilke sees an opposition between life (which also includes childbirth) and art: a true woman artist is not supposed to have children. Simone de Beauvoir views giving birth and procreation as a subordination of the individual to the species. For her, childbirth results in a tragic loss of individuality, which she links with transcendance. Finally, in his *Ethics of Genetic Control* Joseph Fletcher values children who owe their existence to "rational procreation" controlled by science over children resulting from the "blind chance of sexual roulette."[899]

The symbolic pattern of childbirth constructing the inferiority of children to various spiritual/theoretical goods may have had a peculiar variant in the twentieth century. Rather than being born, or being

898 Luke 11:28.

899 Fletcher, *Ethics*, XIV–XV.

"procreated," children may also become mere products of the mind. In his novel *Headbirths*, Günter Grass describes the endless debates of the couple Dörte and Harm Peters about whether, or whether not, to have a child. The child remains an idea. Similarly in *Who is Afraid of Virginia Woolf?* Edward Albee describes a couple inventing a child growing up with them as the years go by.

In summary, the question "A child has been born – so what?" was answered by pointing to "The Supremacy of the Male," "The Supremacy of the Female," "Harmony between Spiritual/ Theoretical Natality and Childbirth," and "Theoretical, Spiritual and Political Natality versus Childbirth" as different ways of attributing meaning to generation.

The investigation of the four symbolic patterns of childbirth described above aimed at making visible a tiny part of that "dark side of the moon"[900] in society and culture that is usually taken for granted. Recognizing unconscious mental habits in symbolic registers may also re-introduce a dynamic element into a cultural construction. The multiplicity of meaning related to childbirth highlights the multiple possibilities of intervention in social life. People may choose, adopt, perpetuate, or undo one symbolic pattern rather than another. In this regard what first seemed to be a given fact may appear as one out of many possibilities which can be experimented with as structures of meaning, and, in this sense, also as patterns for social relations:

> It is not only that historical tradition and the natural order of life constitute the unity of the world in which we live as men;[901] the way that we experience one another, the way that we experience historical traditions, the way that we experience the natural givenness of our existence and of our world, constitutes a truly hermeneutic universe, in which we are not imprisoned, as if behind insurmountable barriers, but to which we are opened.[902]

---

900 Monica Greco has applied this expression to describe the work of Foucault as examining those socio-cultural structures usually taken for granted.

901 Here the translator William Glen-Doepel chooses the word "men" to translate "Menschen." However, "human beings" to me seems a more adequate translation of Gadamer's "Menschen."

902 Hans-Georg Gadamer, *Truth and Method*, trans. William Glen-Doepel, 2nd ed. (London: Sheed and Ward, 1979), XiV. Hans-Georg Gadamer, *Hermeneutik I: Wahrheit und Methode: Grundzüge einer philosophischen Hermeneutik*, vol. 5 of *Gesammelte Werke* (Tübingen: Mohr, 1986), 4: "Nicht nur daß geschichtliche Überlieferung und natürliche Lebensordnung die Einheit der Welt bilden, in der wir als Menschen leben – wie wir einander, wie wir geschichtliche Überlieferungen, wie wir

However, the four symbolic patterns of childbirth which have been investigated cannot be placed next to each other, as if it was a matter of indifference. “The Supremacy of the Male” and “The Supremacy of the Female” constitute gender in relation to childbirth rather differently and thereby also potentially bring with them different types of power relations in society. Furthermore, the three symbolic patterns “The Supremacy of the Male,” “The Supremacy of the Female” and “Harmony between Spiritual/Theoretical Natality and Childbirth,” generally are characterized by a strong identification with life. Although I maintain that spiritual, theoretical, and political natality can be accessed on their own without having to be connected to the natality which comes with the birth of children, a strong opposition between primary natality and other types of natality may be highly problematic. This specific configuration of a body-mind dichotomy transposed into a dichotomy of different natalities ultimately puts life itself into question. Perhaps, to borrow an image from Valentinian Gnostic thinking, in whatever form, a “syzygy of Logos and Life” is needed.

die natürlichen Gegebenheiten unserer Existenz und unserer Welt erfahren, bildet ein wahrhaft hermeneutisches Universum, in das wir nicht wie in unübersteigbare Schranken eingeschlossen, sondern zu dem wir geöffnet sind.” Though Gadamer here to a certain extent still assumes the factual givenness of the natural which has to be problematized (see section II.2. Childbirth, Sex and Gender) this quote beautifully describes the potential openness of cultural constructions.

Bibliography

Ackerman, Susan. *Under Every Green Tree: Popular Religion in Sixth-Century Juda*. Atlanta, Georgia: Scholars Press, 1992.

The Acts of the Christian Martyrs. Introduction, Texts and Translations by Herbert Musurillo. Oxford: Clarendon Press, 1972.

Atti dei Martiri. Introduzione, traduzione e note di Giuliana Caldarelli. Milano: Edizioni Paoline, 1985.

Ad Caeli Reginam: Encyclical of Pope Pius XII, 1954. <http://www.vatican.va/holy_father/pius_xii/encyclicals/documents/hf_p-xii_enc_11101954_ad-caeli-reginam_en.html> (18 February 2013).

Aeschylus. *Agamemnon*. In *Aeschylus in Two Volumes*. Translated by Herbert Weir Smyth. 1926. Reprint, Cambridge, Mass.: Harvard University Press, 1971.

—. *Eumenides*. In *Aeschylus in Two Volumes*. Translated by Herbert Weir Smyth. 1926. Reprint, Cambridge, Mass.: Harvard University Press, 1971.

—. *The Libation-Bearers*. In *Aeschylus in Two Volumes*. Translated by Herbert Weir Smyth. 1926. Reprint, Cambridge, Mass.: Harvard University Press, 1971.

Albee, Edward. *Who's Afraid of Virginia Woolf? : A Play*. New York: Atheneum, 1962.

The Apocryphon of John (II,1, III,1 IV,1, and BG 8502,2). Introduced and translated by Frederik Wisse. In *The Nag Hammadi Library in English*. Translated and introduced by members of the Coptic Gnostic Library Project of the Institute for Antiquity and Christianity, Claremont, California. Edited by James M. Robinson. 3rd, completely rev. ed., 105–123. Leiden: Brill, 1988.

Apollodorus. *The Library*. Translated by Sir James George Frazer. 1921. Reprint, Cambridge, Mass.: Harvard University Press and London: William Heinemann LTD, 1939.

The Ascension of Isaiah. Edited and translated by C. Detlef G. Müller. In *Writings Relating to the Apostles: Apocalypses and Related Subjects*. Revised Edition. Vol. 2 of *New Testament Apocrypha*. Edited by Wilhelm Schneemelcher. English translation edited by R. McL. Wilson. 605–620. Cambridge: James Clarke & Co, 1992.

Apuleius. *The Isis-Book: Metamorphoses, Book XI*. Edited and translated by John Gwyn Griffiths. Leiden: Brill, 1975.

—. *The Transformations of Lucius otherwise Known as The Golden Ass*. Translated by Robert Graves. Harmondsworth, Middlesex: Penguin Books, 1951.

Arendt, Hannah. *The Human Condition*. 1958. Reprint, Chicago and London: The University of Chicago Press, 1974.

—. *The Origins of Totalitarianism*. 1951. Reprint, New York: Harcourt Brace Jovanovich, 1978.

—. *Thinking*. Vol. 1 of *The Life of the Mind*. London: Secker and Warburg, 1978.

Aristotle. *Generation of Animals*. Translated by A. L. Peck. 1942. Reprint, Cambridge, Mass.: Harvard University Press, 1979.

—. *On the Heavens*. Translated by W. K. C. Guthrie. 1939. Reprint, Cambridge, Mass.: Harvard University Press, 1971.

—. *On the Soul*. Translated by W. S. Hett. 1936. Reprint, Cambridge, Mass.: Harvard University Press, 1975.

—. *The Metaphysics*. Translated by Hugh Tredennick. Cambridge, Mass.: Harvard University Press, 1962.

Armour, Robert A. *Gods and Myths of Ancient Egypt*. 1986. Reprint, Cairo: The American University In Cairo Press, 1987.

Assmann, Jan. *The Search for God in Ancient Egypt*. Translated by David Lorton. Ithaca: Cornell University Press, 2001.

Aster, Ernst von. *Geschichte der Philosophie*. 1932. Reprint, Stuttgart: Kröner, 1980.

Attridge, Harold W. and Elaine H. Pagels. Introduction to *The Tripartite Tractate (I,5)*. In *The Nag Hammadi Library in English*. Translated and introduced by members of the Coptic Gnostic Library Project of the Institute for Antiquity and Christianity, Claremont, California. 3rd, completely revised edition, edited by James M. Robinson, 58–60. Leiden: Brill, 1988.

Augustine. *Four Anti-Pelagian Writings: On Nature and Grace, On the Proceedings of Pelagius, On the Predestination of the Saints, On the Gift of Perseverance*. Translated by John A. Mourant and William

J. Collinge. Washington, D. C.: The Catholic University of America Press, 1992.
— (Augustin). *La crise Pélagienne II: De Gratia Christi et de peccato originali libri II, De natura et origine animae libri IV.* Vol. 22 of *Œuvres*. Introduction, traduction et notes par J. Plagnieux et F.-J. Thonnard. Paris: Desclée de Brouwer, 1975.
—. *Sermons for Christmas and Epiphany*. Translated by Thomas Comerford Lawler. New York: Newman Press, 1952.
Bahador, Syed Ahmed Khan. *Essays on the Life of Mohammed and Subjects Subsidiary Thereto*. 1870. Reprint, Delhi, India: Idarah-i Adabiyat-i Delli, 1991.
Baumgarth, William I. and Richard J. Regan, S. J. *On Law, Morality and Politics: Saint Thomas Aquinas*. Indianapolis/Cambridge: Hackett, 1988.
Beauvoir, Simone de. *Le deuxième sexe*. 2 vols. 1949. Renouvelé en 1976. Reprint, Paris: Gallimard, 1989.
—. *The Second Sex*. Translated and edited by H. M. Parshley, London: Vintage, 1997.
Berger, Renate. *Malerinnen auf dem Weg ins 20. Jahrhundert*. Köln: DuMont, 1982.
Bethge, Hans-Gebhard. Introduction to *On the Origin of the World (II,5 and XIII,2)*. In *The Nag Hammadi Library in English*. Translated and introduced by members of the Coptic Gnostic Library Project of the Institute for Antiquity and Christianity, Claremont, California. 3rd, completely revised edition, edited by James M. Robinson, 170–171. Leiden: Brill, 1988.
Bhikhu, Parekh. *Hannah Arendt and the Search for a New Political Philosophy*. London: Macmillan, 1981.
The Bible. The New Oxford Annotated Bible. New Revised Standard Version. Edited by Michael D. Coogan, 3rd ed. Oxford: Oxford University Press, 2007.
The Bible. King James Version with the Apocrypha. Edited. by David Norton. London: Penguin, 2006.
Bolman, Elizabeth S. "The Enigmatic Coptic Galaktotrophousa and the Cult of the Virgin Mary in Egypt." In *Images of the Mother of God: Perceptions of the Theotokos in Byzantium,* edited by Maria Vassilaki, 13–22. Aldershot: Ashgate, 2005.

Bonner, Gerald. *St. Augustine of Hippo: Life and Controversies.* Philadelphia: Westminster, 1963.

Bowen-Moore, Patricia. *Hannah Arendt's Philosophy of Natality*. London: MacMillan, 1989.

Brede Kristensen, William. *Life out of Death: Studies in the Religions of Egypt and of Ancient Greece*. Translated by H. J. Franken and G. R. H. Wright. Louvain: Peeters, 1992.

Brown, Peter. *The Body and Society: Men, Women and Sexual Renunciation in Early Christianity*. London: faber and faber, 1988.

Bullard, Roger A. Introduction to *The Hypostasis of the Archons (II,4)*. In *The Nag Hammadi Library in English*. Translated and introduced by members of the Coptic Gnostic Library Project of the Institute for Antiquity and Christianity, Claremont, California. 3rd, completely revised edition, edited by James M. Robinson, 161–162. Leiden: Brill, 1988.

Burkert, Walter. *Greek Religion*. Translated by John Raffan, Cambridge, Mass.: Harvard University Press, 1985.

Busch, Günter. *Paula Modersohn-Becker: Malerin, Zeichnerin.* Frankfurt/M: Fischer, 1981.

—. "Über Gegenwart und Tod – Edvard Munch und Paula Modersohn-Becker." In *Edvard Munch. Probleme, Forschung, Thesen*, edited by Henning Bock and Günter Busch, 161–176. München: Prestel, 1973.

Butler, Judith. *Bodies That Matter: On the Discursive Limits of Sex*. 1993. Reprint, New York: Routledge, 2011.

—. *Gender Trouble: Feminism and the Subversion of Identity*. 1990. Reprint, New York: Routledge, 2008.

Caldarelli, Giuliana. Introduction to *Atti dei Martiri*. Translated by Giuliana Caldarelli, 7–47. Milano: Edizioni Paoline, 1985.

—."La passione delle sante Perpetua e Felicita e dei loro compagni." In *Atti dei Martiri*, translated by Giuliana Caldarelli, 185–188. Milano: Edizioni Paoline 1985.

Carpinello, Mariella. *Libere donne di Dio: Figure femminili nei primi secoli cristiani*. Milano: Mondadori, 1997.

Cavarero, Adriana. *Nonostante Platone: Figure femminili nella filosofia antica*. Roma: Editori Riuniti, 1992.

Cerný, Jaroslav: Ancient Egyptian Religion, London: Hutchinson's University Library, 1952.
Clark, Robert Thomas Rundle. *Myth and Symbol in Ancient Egypt.* London: Thames and Hudson, 1959.
Clement of Alexandria. *The Instructor (Paedagogus)*, in *Fathers of the Second Century: Hermas, Tatian, Athenagoras, Theophilus, and Clement of Alexandria.* Vol. 2 of *The Ante-Nicene Fathers: Translations of the Writings of the Fathers Down to A.D. 325.* Translated by Alexander Roberts and James Donaldson. 1867–97. Reprint, Grand Rapids, Mich: Eerdmans, 1979.
Collinge, William J. Introduction to *On Nature and Grace*, by St. Augustine. In St. Augustine. *Four Anti-Pelagian Writings: On Nature and Grace, On the Proceedings of Pelagius, On the Predestination of the Saints, On the Gift of Perseverance.* Translated by John A. Mourant and William J. Collinge. Washington, D. C.: The Catholic University of America Press, 1992, 3–21.
Couliano, Ioan Peter. *The Tree of Gnosis: Gnostic Mythology from Early Christianity to Modern Nihilism.* Translated by H.S. Wiesner. San Francisco: Harper, 1992.
Cullmann, Oscar. *Infancy Gospels.* In *Gospels and Related Writings: Revised Edition.* Vol. 1 of *New Testament Apocrypha.* Edited by Wilhelm Schneemelcher. English translation edited by R. McL. Wilson. 414–420. Cambridge: James Clarke & Co, 1991.
—. *The Protevangelium of James.* In *Gospels and Related Writings: Revised Edition.* Vol. 1 of *New Testament Apocrypha.* Edited by Wilhelm Schneemelcher. English translation edited by R. McL. Wilson. 421–425. Cambridge: James Clarke & Co, 1991.
Curtius, Ernst Robert. *Europäische Literatur und lateinisches Mittelalter.* 1948. Reprint, Tübingen and Basel: Francke Verlag, 1993.
Dante Alighieri. *La Divina Commedia.* Edited by Natalino Sapegno. Firenze: La Nuova Italia, 1977.
—. *The Divine Comedy of Dante Alighieri.* Translated by Charles Eliot Norton. Chicago: William Benton Publisher, 1978.
Delius, Walter. *Geschichte der Marienverehrung.* München and Basel: Ernst Reinhardt Verlag, 1963.

Diodorus of Sicily. *Diodorus of Sicily: In Twelve Volumes*. Translated by Charles Henry Oldfather. 1933. Reprint, Cambridge, Mass.: Harvard University Press, 1968.

Duden, Barbara. *A Doctor's Patients in Eighteenth-Century Germany*. Translated by Thomas Dunlap. 1987. Reprint, Cambridge, MA: Harvard University Press, 1991.

Eisenstadt, Shmuel Noah, ed. *The Origins and Diversity of Axial Age Civilisations*. New York: SUNY Press, 1986.

Eliade, Mircea. *Rites and Symbols of Initiation: The Mysteries of Birth and Rebirth*. Translated by Willard R. Trask. 1958. Reprint, New York: Harper & Row, 1975.

Elliott, J. K. *The Apocryphal New Testament: A Collection of Apocryphal Christian Literature in an English Translation Based on M. R. James*. Oxford: Clarendon Press, 1993.

Elliott, Mark W. *The Song of Songs and Christology in the Early Church 381–451*. Tübingen: Mohr Siebeck, 2000.

Eom, Seon-Ae. *Todesvertrautheit: Deutungen der Orpheus-Gestalt in Rilkes Dichtung*. Frankfurt/M: Lang, 1988.

Epstein, Mikhail. *Tagebuch für Olga: Chronik einer Vaterschaft (Fatherhood)*. Translated by Otto Markus. München: Roitman Verlag, 1990.

Esbroeck, Michel van. *Aux origines de la Dormition de la Vierge: Études historiques sur les traditions orientales*. Aldershot: Variorum, 1995.

Euripides. *Iphigeneia at Aulis*. In *Euripides. In Four Volumes*. Edited by G. P. Goold. Translated by Arthur S. Way. 1912. Reprint, Cambridge, Mass.: Harvard University Press, 1978.

Feyerabend, Paul. *Killing Time*. Chicago and London: The University of Chicago Press, 1995.

Fletcher, Joseph. *The Ethics of Genetic Control: Ending Reproductive Roulette*. New York: Prometheus Books, 1988.

Foster, Benjamin R., trans. *Enuma Elish*. In *Before the Muses: An Anthology of Akkadian Literature*, translated and edited by Benjamin Foster, 452–473. 3rd. ed. Bethesda, Maryland: CDL Press, 2005.

Foucault, Michel. *L'usage des plaisirs*. Vol. 2 of *Histoire de la sexualité*. 1984. Reprint, Paris: Éditions Gallimard, 1997.

Frenzel, Elisabeth. *Stoffe der Weltliteratur*. Stuttgart: Kröner, 1983.

Fromm, Erich. *The Forgotten Language: An Introduction to the Understanding of Dreams, Fairy Tales and Myths*. 1951. Reprint, New York: Grove Press, 1957.
Gadamer, Hans-Georg. *Hermeneutik I: Wahrheit und Methode: Grundzüge einer philosophischen Hermeneutik*. Vol. 5 of *Gesammelte Werke*. Tübingen: Mohr, 1986.
—. *Truth and Method*. Translated by William Glen-Doepel. 2nd ed. London: Sheed and Ward, 1979.
Gies, Frances and Joseph Gies. *Women in the Middle Ages*. New York: Crowell, 1978.
The Babylonian Gilgamesh Epic. Introduction, Critical Edition and Cuneiform Texts. Translated and edited by A.R. George. Oxford: Oxford University Press, 2003.
The Gilgamesh Epic and Old Testament Parallels. Translated by Alexander Heidel. 2nd ed. Chicago: Chicago University Press, 1963.
The Epic of Gilgamesh. Translated and edited by Benjamin R. Foster. New York and London: Noton & Company, 2001.
Gilmore, David D. *Manhood in the Making: Cultural Concepts of Masculinity*. New Haven and London: Yale University Press, 1990.
Goethe, Johann Wolfgang von. *Faust: Der Tragödie erster und zweiter Teil: Urfaust*. Edited by Erich Trunz. München: Beck, 2010.
—. Faust: Parts One and Two. Translated by Philip Wayne. Chicago: Encyclopaedia Britannica, 2003.
—. *Poems of the West and East: West-Eastern Divan – West-Östlicher Divan*. Bi-Lingual Edition of the Complete Poems. Verse Translation by John Whaley. Bern: Peter Lang, 1998.
Gotteslob: Katholisches Gebet- und Gesangbuch: Ausgabe für das Erzbistum Köln. Edited by Bischöfe Deutschlands und Österreichs und der Bistümer Bozen-Brixen und Lüttich. Stuttgart: Katholische Bibelanstalt, 1975.
Grandjean, Yves. *Une Nouvelle Arétalogie d'Isis à Maronée*. Leiden: Brill, 1975.
Grass, Günter. *Headbirths or The Germans Are Dying Out*. Translated by Ralph Manheim. San Diego: Harvest, 1990.
—. *Kopfgeburten*. 1980. Reprint, Frankfurt/M: Luchterhand, 1982.

Graves, Robert. Introduction to *The Transformations of Lucius otherwise Known as The Golden Ass*, by Lucius Apuleius. Translated by Robert Graves. 8–16. Harmondsworth, Middlesex: Penguin Books, 1951.

—. *The Greek Myths*. London: Penguin Books, 1992.

Gregory of Nyssa. *On the Soul and the Resurrection*. Translated by William Moore and Henry Austin Wilson. Vol. 5 of A Select Library of Nicene and post-Nicene Fathers of the Christian Church: Gregory of Nyssa, edited by Philip Schaff and Henry Wace, 428–468. 1892. Reprint, Grand Rapids, Michigan: Eerdmans 1988.

—. *On Virginity*. Translated by William Moore and Henry Austin Wilson. Vol. 5 of A Select Library of Nicene and post-Nicene Fathers of the Christian Church: Gregory of Nyssa, edited by Philip Schaff and Henry Wace, 343–371. 1892. Reprint, Grand Rapids, Michigan: Eerdmans 1988.

Griffiths, John Gwyn. Introduction to *The Isis-Book: Metamorphoses, Book XI*, by Apuleius of Madauros, Edited and translated by John Gwyn Griffiths. 6–14. Leiden: Brill, 1975.

Grimal, Pierre. *A Concise Dictionary of Classical Mythology*. Edited by Stephen Kershaw. Translated by A. R. Maxwell-Hyslop. Oxford: Blackwell, 1990.

Guldan, Ernst. *Eva und Maria: Eine Antithese als Bildmotiv*. Graz: Böhlau, 1966.

Hänsch, Anja. "Barbara Duden, Judith Butler, and Birth: Contentions about Body Theory Revisited." In *Birth and Death in British Culture: Liminality, Power, and Performance*, edited by Anette Pankratz, Claus-Ulrich Viol, and Ariane de Waal, 15–32. Newcastle upon Tyne, UK: Cambridge Scholars Publishing, 2012.

—."The Body of the Woman Artist: Rainer-Maria Rilke and Paula Modersohn-Becker on Giving Birth and Art." *European Journal of Women's Studies*, no. 4 (November 1997): 435–449.

Hanson, Paul D. "Masculine Metaphors for God and Sex-Discrimination in the Old Testament." *The Ecumenical Review* 27 (1975): 316–24.

Haraway, Donna. *Simians, Cyborgs, and Women: The Reinvention of Nature*. London: Free Association Books, 1991.

Heidegger, Martin. *Being and Time*. Translated by John Macquarrie and Edward Robinson. Oxford: Blackwell, 1978.

—. *Sein und Zeit*. 17th ed. Tübingen: Max Niemeyer Verlag, 1993.

Heidel, Alexander. Introduction to *The Babylonian Genesis*. Translated by Alexander Heidel. 1942. Reprint, Chicago: The Chicago University Press, 1963, 1–15.

—, trans. *The Babylonian Genesis*.1942. Reprint, Chicago: The Chicago University Press, 1963.

Hein, Hilde. "Liberating Philosophy: An End to the Dichotomy of Spirit and Matter." In *Beyond Domination: New Perspectives on Women and Philosophy*, edited by Carol Gould, 123–141. Totowa, NJ: Rowman & Allanheld, 1984.

Heise, Carl Georg. *Paula Modersohn-Becker – Mutter und Kind*. Stuttgart: Reclam, 1961.

Hemingway, Ernest. *In Our Time*. 1925. Reprint, New York: Charles Scribner's Sons, 1958.

Hesiod. *Theogony*. Edited and translated by Glenn W. Most. Cambridge, Mass.: Harvard University Press, 2006.

—. *The Works and Days, Theogony, The Shield of Herakles*. Translated by Richmond Lattimore. 1959. Reprint, Ann Arbor, MI: The University of Michigan Press, 1991.

Hippolytus. *Philosophumena or the Refutation of All Heresies*. Translated by F. Legge. New York: The Macmillan Company, 1921.

Hoenn, Karl. *Artemis: Gestaltwandel einer Göttin*. Zürich: Artemis-Verlag, 1946.

Hopfner, Theodor. *Plutarch über Isis und Osiris: Text, Übersetzung und Kommentar*. Prag: Orientalisches Institut, 1940.

Hülsmann, Boda. *Paula Modersohn-Becker: In Freiheit zu sich selbst*. Stuttgart: Urachhaus, 1988.

The Hypostasis of the Archons (II,4). Translated by Bentley Layton. In *The Nag Hammadi Library in English*. Translated and introduced by members of the Coptic Gnostic Library Project of the Institute for Antiquity and Christianity, Claremont, California. 3rd, completely revised edition, edited by James M. Robinson, 162–169. Leiden: Brill, 1988.

Ibn Ishaq. *Das Leben Muhammeds*. Translated and edited by Ferdinand Wüstenfeld. Göttingen: Dieterichsche Universitäts-Buchhandlung, 1860.

—. *The Life of Muhammad*. Translated and edited by A. Guillaume.1955. Reprint, Lahore: Oxford University Press, Pakistan Branch, 1970.

Irenaeus of Lyon. *Against the Heresies*. Translated by Dominic J. Unger. With further revisions by John J. Dillon. New York, N.Y. and Mahwah, N.J.: The Newman Press, 1992.

—. *Contro le eresie e gli altri scritti*. Translated by Enzo Bellini. Milano: Jaca Book, 1979.

Irigaray, Luce. *L'éthique de la différence sexuelle*. Paris: Les Éditions de Minuit, 1985.

Jaspers, Karl. *The Origin and Goal of History*. Translated by Michael Bullock. London: Routledge, 1953.

—. *Vom Ursprung und Ziel der Geschichte*. München: Piper, 1949.

Jonsen, Albert R. *Reproduction and Rationality*. Paper presented at the International Bioethics Institute Conference on Designs on Life, San Francisco, CA, April 15, 1994.

Katsh, Abraham I. *Judaism in Islam*. New York: New York University Press, 1954.

Kee, Howard Clark. *Miracle in the Early Christian World: A Study in Sociohistorical Method*. New Haven and London: Yale University Press, 1983.

Keel, Othmar. *Gott weiblich: Eine verborgene Seite des biblischen Gottes*. Gütersloh: Gütersloher Verlagshaus, 2008.

—, and Silvia Schroer. *Eva – Mutter alles Lebendigen: Frauen- und Göttinnenidole aus dem Alten Orient*. 2nd ed. Fribourg, Switzerland: Academic Press Fribourg Schweiz, 2006.

Kierkegaard, Søren. *Fear and Trembling: Repetition*. Translated and edited by Howard V. Hong and Edna H. Hong. Princeton, New Jersey: Princeton University Press, 1983.

The Glorious Koran. Translated, edited, introduction and notes by Muhammad Marmaduke Pickthall. 1930. Reprint, Albany: State University of New York Press, 1976.

Kramer, Samuel Noah. *From the Poetry of Sumer: Creation, Glorification, Adoration*. Berkeley: University of California Press, 1979.

Larrington, Carolyne. *Women and Writing in Medieval Europe*. London and New York: Routledge, 1995.

The Letters of Abélard and Héloise. Translated by B. Radice. Harmondsworth: Penguin, 1974.

The Letter of Peter to Philip. Translated by Frederik Wisse. In *The Nag Hammadi Library in English*. Translated and introduced by members

of the Coptic Gnostic Library Project of the Institute for Antiquity and Christianity, Claremont, California. 3rd, completely revised edition, edited by James M. Robinson, 434–437. Leiden: Brill, 1988.
Loraux, Nicole. *Les enfants d'Athéna*. Paris: La Découverte, 1984.
Maihofer, Andrea. *Geschlecht als Existenzweise*. Frankfurt: Helmer, 1995.
Mathews, Thomas F. and Norman Muller. "Isis and Mary in Early Icons." In *Images of the Mother of God: Perceptions of the Theotokos in Byzantium*, edited by Maria Vassilaki, 3–11. Aldershot: Ashgate, 2005.
Meyer, Marvin W. Introduction to *The Letter of Peter to Philip*. In *The Nag Hammadi Library in English*. Translated and introduced by members of the Coptic Gnostic Library Project of the Institute for Antiquity and Christianity, Claremont, California. 3rd, completely revised edition, edited by James M. Robinson, 431–433. Leiden: Brill, 1988.
Müller, C. Detlef G. Introduction to *The Ascension of Isaiah*. In *Writings Relating to the Apostles: Apocalypses and Related Subjects*. Revised Edition. Vol. 2 of *New Testament Apocrypha*. Edited by Wilhelm Schneemelcher. English translation edited by R. McL. Wilson. 603–605. Cambridge: James Clarke & Co, 1992.
Murken-Altrogge, Christa. *Paula Modersohn-Becker: Leben und Werk*. Köln: DuMont, 1980.
Musurillo, Herbert: The Acts of the Christian Martyrs. Introduction, Texts and Translations, Oxford: Clarendon Press, 1972.
Neumann, Erich. *The Great Mother*. Translated by Ralph Manheim. New York: Pantheon Books, 1955.
O'Carroll, Michael. *Theotokos: A Theological Encyclopedia of the Blessed Virgin Mary*. Wilmington, Delaware: Michael Glazier, 1983.
On the Origin of the World (II,5 and XIII,2). Translated by Hans-Gebhard Bethge, Bentley Layton, Societas Coptica Hierosolymitana. In *The Nag Hammadi Library in English*. Translated and introduced by members of the Coptic Gnostic Library Project of the Institute for Antiquity and Christianity, Claremont, California. 3rd, completely revised edition, edited by James M. Robinson, 171–189. Leiden: Brill, 1988.
Ovid. *Metamorphoses*. Translated by A. D. Melville. With an Introduction and Notes by E. J. Kenney. Oxford and New York: Oxford University Press, 1986.

—. *The Art of Love* (*Ars Amatoria*). Translated by Charles D. Young. New York: Horace Liveright Inc., 1931.

Parrott, Douglas M. Introduction to *Eugnostos The Blessed (III,3 and V,1)* and *The Sophia of Jesus Christ (III,4 and BG 8502,3)*. In *The Nag Hammadi Library in English*. Translated and introduced by members of the Coptic Gnostic Library Project of the Institute for Antiquity and Christianity, Claremont, California. Edited by James M. Robinson. 3rd, completely rev. ed., 220–221. Leiden: Brill, 1988.

Passmore, Nancy F. W. "A Consciousness Manifesto." In *The Politics of Women's Spirituality*, edited by Charlene Spretnak, 163–171. New York: Anchor Press, 1982.

Peck, Arthur Leslie. Introduction to *Generation of Animals*, by Aristotle, vii–lix. 1942. Reprint, Cambridge, Mass.: Harvard University Press, 1979.

Peek, Werner. *Der Isishymnus von Andros und verwandte Texte*. Berlin: Weidmann, 1930.

Pegis, Anton C. Introduction to *Summa Contra Gentiles*, by Thomas Aquinas. Vol. 1, *God*. Translated by Anton C. Pegis, 9–25. 1955. Reprint, Notre Dame, Ind.: University of Notre Dame Press, 1975.

Pelikan, Jaroslav. *Mary Through the Centuries: Her Place in the History of Culture*. New Haven and London: Yale University Press, 1996.

Perry, Gillian. *Paula Modersohn-Becker: Her Life and Work*. London: Women's Press, 1981.

Piankoff, Alexandre and Natacha Rambova. *The Shrines of Tut-ankh-amon,* 24. New York: Pantheon Books, 1955. Quoted in Mircea Eliade, *Gods, Goddesses and Myths of Creation: A Thematic Source Book of the History of Religions* (New York: Harper & Row, 1974), 96–97.

Pindar. *The Odes of Pindar*. Translated by Sir John Sandys. 1915. Reprint, 2nd ed. Cambridge, Mass.: Harvard University Press, 1968.

Plato. *Lysis, Symposium, Gorgias*, Translated by W.R.M. Lamb. 1925. Reprint, Cambridge, Mass.: Harvard University Press, 1975.

Plutarch. *De Iside et Osiride*. In Plutarch, *Moralia: In Sixteen Volumes*. Vol. 5:351C-438E. Translated by Frank Cole Babbitt.1936. Reprint, Cambridge, Mass.: Harvard University Press, 1969.

Prigent, Pierre. *L'apocalypse*. Paris: Les Éditions du Cerf, 1998.

The Protevangelium of James. Translated and edited by Oscar Cullmann. In *Gospels and Related Writings: Revised Edition.* Vol. 1 of *New Testament Apocrypha*. Edited by Wilhelm Schneemelcher. English translation edited by R. McL. Wilson. 426–439. Cambridge: James Clarke & Co, 1991.

The Questions of Bartholomew. Translated and edited by Felix Scheidweiler. In *Gospels and Related Writings: Revised Edition.* Vol. 1 of *New Testament Apocrypha*. Edited by Wilhelm Schneemelcher. English translation edited by R. McL. Wilson. 540–553. Cambridge: James Clarke & Co, 1991.

Reiger, Kerreen and Rhea Dempsey. "Performing Birth in a Culture of Fear: An Embodied Crisis of Late Modernity." *Health Sociology Review* 15, no. 4 (2006): 364–373.

Reineken, Liselotte von. *Paula Modersohn-Becker*. 1983. Reprint, Reinbek bei Hamburg: Rowohlt, 1993.

Rilke, Rainer Maria. *Das Florenzer Tagebuch*. Edited by Ruth Sieber-Rilke and Carl Sieber. Frankfurt/M and Leipzig: Insel, 1994.

—. *Die Aufzeichnungen des Malte Laurids Brigge*. Frankfurt/M: Insel, 1982.

—. "Requiem for a Friend." In Rainer Maria Rilke. *Sämtliche Werke*. Edited by Rilke-Archiv in Collaboration with Ruth Sieber-Rilke, 1:645–656. Frankfurt/M: Insel, 1987.

—. "Requiem für eine Freundin." Rainer Maria Rilke, "Requiem for a Friend." In Rainer Maria Rilke. *Requiem and Other Poems*. Translated with an Introduction and Notes by J.B. Leishman, 129–136. London: Hogarth Press, 1949.

Roscher, Wilhelm Heinrich. *Ausführliches Lexikon der griechischen und römischen Mythologie*. 1890–1894. Reprint, Hildesheim: Olms, 1993.

Santucci, Luigi. *Volete andarvene anche voi? Una vita di Cristo*. 3rd ed. Torino: Edizioni San Paolo, 2001.

Schami, Rafik. *Die Sehnsucht fährt schwarz. Geschichten aus der Fremde.* München: Deutscher Taschenbuch Verlag, 1988.

Scheidweiler, Felix. Introduction to *The Questions of Bartholomew*. In *Gospels and Related Writings: Revised Edition.* Vol. 1 of *New Testament Apocrypha*. Edited by Wilhelm Schneemelcher. English translation edited by R. McL. Wilson. 539–540. Cambridge: James Clarke & Co, 1991.

Schleiermacher, Friedrich D. E. *Christmas Eve: Dialogue on the Incarnation.* Translated by Terrence N. Tice. Lewiston. New York: The Edwin Mellen Press, 1990.

—. *Die Weihnachtsfeier: Ein Gespräch* in Friedrich D. E. Schleiermacher. *Werke: Auswahl in vier Bänden*, edited by Otto Braun and Johannes Bauer, 4:473–532. Leipzig: Fritz Eckhardt Verlag, 1911.

Schwenger, Peter. *Phallic Critiques: Masculinity and Twentieth-Century Literature.* London: Routledge and Kegan Paul, 1984.

Seaman, Gerald. "Signs of a New Literary Paradigm: The 'Christian' Figures of Chrétien de Troyes," in *Nominalism and Literary Discourse: New Perspectives.* Edited by Hugo Keiper, Christoph Bod, and Richard J. Utz, 87–110. Amsterdam, Atlanta, GA: Editions Rodopi B.V., 1997.

Seters, John van. *Abraham in History and Tradition.* New Haven and London: Yale University Press, 1975.

Sharpe, Samuel. *Egyptian Mythology and Egyptian Christianity.* London: Carter and Co, 1896.

Sherif, Faruq. *A Guide to the Contents of the Qur'an.* Reading: Ithaca Press, 1995.

The Sophia of Jesus Christ (III,4 and BG 8502,3). Translated by Douglas M. Parrott. In *The Nag Hammadi Library in English.* Translated and introduced by members of the Coptic Gnostic Library Project of the Institute for Antiquity and Christianity, Claremont, California. Edited by James M. Robinson. 3rd, completely revised edition. 222–243. Leiden: Brill, 1988.

Szakolczai, Arpád. *Max Weber and Michel Foucault: Parallel Life-Works.* London: Routledge, 1998.

Tertullian. *De Anima.* Edited by J. H. Waszink. Amsterdam: North-Holland Publishing Company, 1947.

—. *L'anima.* Translated and edited by Martino Menghi. Venezia: Marsilio Editori, 1988.

—. *On the Soul.* Vol. 2 of *The Writings of Quintus Sept. Flor. Tertullianus.* Translated by Peter Holmes. Edinburgh: T. & T. Clark, 1870.

Thomas Aquinas. *Summa Theologica.* Translated by the Fathers of the English Dominican Province. 1948. Reprint, Westminster, MD.: Christian Classics, 1981.

Tran, Vincent Tam Tinh. Avec la collaboration de Yvette Labreque. *Isis Lactans: Corpus des monuments greco-romains d'Isis allaitant Harpocrate*. Leiden: Brill, 1973.

Trible, Phyllis. *God and the Rhetoric of Sexuality*. Philadelphia: Fortress Press, 1978.

Turner, Victor. *Blazing the Trail: Way Marks in the Exploration of Symbols*. Edited by Edith Turner. Tucson, Arizona and London: The University of Arizona Press, 1992.

— and Edith Turner. *On the Edge of the Bush: Anthropology as Experience*. Tucson, Arizona: The University of Arizona Press, 1985.

Uhde-Stahl, Brigitte. *Paula Modersohn-Becker: Frau, Künstlerin, Mensch*. Stuttgart and Zürich: Belser, 1989.

Valverde, I. de. *Historia de la composicion del cuerpo humano*. Rome 1556. Quoted in Julia O'Faolain and Lauro Martines, *Not in God's Image: Women in History from Greeks to Victorians* (London: Virago, 1973), 121–122.

Veith, Ilza. *Hysteria: The History of a Disease*. Northvale, NJ: Aronson, 1993.

Voß, Heinz-Jürgen. *Making Sex Revisited. Dekonstruktion des Geschlechts aus biologisch-medizinischer Perspektive*. Bielefeld: transcript Verlag, 2010.

Waithe, Mary Ellen. "Diotima of Mantinea." In *A History of Women Philosophers*, edited by Mary Ellen Waithe, 1:22–31. Dordrecht: Martinus Nijhoff Publishers, 1987.

Wallis Budge, Ernest Alfred. *Osiris: The Egyptian Religion of Resurrection*. New York: University Books, 1961.

Warner, Marina. *Alone of All Her Sex: The Myth and Cult of the Virgin Mary*. 1976. Reprint, London: Vintage, 2000.

Wirsching, Michael. *Paar- und Familientherapie: Grundlagen, Methoden, Ziele*. München: Beck, 2005.

Wigand-Petzet, Heinrich. *Das Bildnis des Dichters: Paula Modersohn-Becker und Rainer Maria Rilke: Eine Begegnung*. Frankfurt/M: Insel, 1976.

Wikan, Unni. *Culture, Identity and Emotion: Lessons from Research on New Immigrants into Europe*. Lecture given at the European University Institute/Florence, March 11, 1996.

Wilson, John A. "Egyptian Myths, Tales, and Mortuary Texts." In *Ancient Near Eastern Texts: Relating to the Old Testament*, edited by James Bennett Pritchard, 3rd ed. with supplement, 3–36.1969. Reprint, Princeton, New Jersey: Princeton University Press, 1992.

Wisse, Frederik. Introduction to *The Apocryphon of John (II,1, III,1 IV,1, and BG 8502,2)*. In *The Nag Hammadi Library in English*. Translated and introduced by members of the Coptic Gnostic Library Project of the Institute for Antiquity and Christianity, Claremont, California. 3rd, completely revised edition, edited by James M. Robinson, 104–105. Leiden: Brill, 1988.

Witt, Reginald Eldred. *Isis in the Graeco-Roman World*. London: Thames and Hudson, 1971.

Woolf, Virginia. *A Room of One's Own*. 1929. Reprint, London: Grafton, 1989.

Wüstenfeld, Ferdinand. Introduction to *Das Leben Muhammeds*, by Ibn Ishaq. Translated and edited by Ferdinand Wüstenfeld, 2:xi–xxxviii. Göttingen: Dieterichsche Universitäts-Buchhandlung, 1860.

www.ingramcontent.com/pod-product-compliance
Ingram Content Group UK Ltd.
Pitfield, Milton Keynes, MK11 3LW, UK
UKHW020200290926
15471UKWH00005B/988

9 783039 104321